Clinical Manual of Supportive Psychotherapy

Second Edition

Clinical Manual of Supportive Psychotherapy

Second Edition

Peter N. Novalis, M.D., Ph.D.

Virginia Singer, D.N.P., PMHNP-BC, CARN-AP

Roger Peele, M.D., DLFAPA

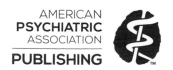

AMERICAN
PSYCHIATRIC
ASSOCIATION
PUBLISHING

If you wish to buy 50 or more copies of the same title, please go to www.appi.org/specialdiscounts for more information.

Copyright © 2020 American Psychiatric Association Publishing

ALL RIGHTS RESERVED

Second Edition

Manufactured in the United States of America on acid-free paper
23 22 21 20 19   5 4 3 2 1

American Psychiatric Association Publishing
800 Maine Avenue SW
Suite 900
Washington, DC 20024-2812
www.appi.org

Library of Congress Cataloging-in-Publication Data
Names: Novalis, Peter N., author. | Singer, Virginia, author. | Peele, Roger, author. | American Psychiatric Association Publishing, issuing body.
Title: Clinical manual of supportive psychotherapy / Peter N. Novalis, Virginia Singer, Roger Peele.
Description: Second edition. | Washington, D.C. : American Psychiatric Association Publishing, [2020] | Includes bibliographical references and index.
Identifiers: LCCN 2019020721 (print) | ISBN 9781615371655 (paperback ; alk. paper) | ISBN 9781615372737 (ebook)
Subjects: MESH: Psychotherapy—methods | Professional-Patient Relations | Psychotherapeutic Processes
Classification: LCC RC489.S86 (print) | LCC RC489.S86 (ebook) | NLM WM 420 | DDC 616.89/14—dc23
LC record available at https://lccn.loc.gov/2019020721
LC ebook record available at https://lccn.loc.gov/2019981117

British Library Cataloguing in Publication Data
A CIP record is available from the British Library.

Contents

PART I
Principles

PART II

Diagnostic Applications

PART III
Interactions and Special Settings

List of Tables

Introduction to the Second Edition

It has been a generation since the *Clinical Manual of Supportive Psychotherapy* saw the light of day. Since then, we have had the privilege of training psychiatry residents and student therapists using this manual, with the knowledge that it has remained effective and accurate even with the background that was available 25 years ago.

One of our original authors, Dr. Rojcewicz, did not participate in the writing of this edition, but his wise and incisive contributions to the first edition can still be found in many spots, especially covering historical issues and schizophrenia. However, we have been much pleased that we now have an advanced practice nurse, Virginia Singer, D.N.P, PMHNP BC, CARN-AP, as a major contributor, and a special chapter on anxiety disorders from our clinical psychologist colleague, Victor Chavira, Ph.D. Therefore, much of the material you see is new or revised, including many new clinical vignettes, but we have also kept many of the "good old parts," as valid now as in the past.

No longer do therapists treat supportive psychotherapy like a stepchild of psychoanalysis or reserve its use for severely impaired psychiatric inpatients who supposedly cannot achieve insight into their unconscious mental processes. Supportive therapy has been recognized as one of the principal psychotherapies required in training for psychiatry residents. Supportive techniques also underlie most other psychotherapies, so that support is found not only in the eponymous therapy but in the other enumerated "psychotherapies" that continue to proliferate (although some of the 400 have become moribund or "proscribed" rather than "prescribed").

To be sure, through the years much has changed and much remains the same. What remains the same is the basic organization of the book, which starts with describing the techniques and then applies the therapy to specific mental disorders and, in the last two parts, special adaptations and interactions and special settings. The academic literature on supportive psychotherapy has mushroomed, and we found hundreds of articles covering both specific populations and technical issues. As was true in the past, we are all practicing clinicians and not academic researchers, but we have tried to reference the relevant literature for those inclined to read further.

Surprisingly, and one of the reasons you are seeing a new edition of our book, there is an absence of any recent textbook on the subject other than the well-known primer *Learning Supportive Psychotherapy,* also from American Psychiatric Association Publishing. Although the authors of that text use extended case presentations and discussions of technique, we have tried to maintain our goal of using both a technique- and a disease-oriented presentation, and have continued to use brief vignettes to illustrate important points. We have streamlined the section on technique to make room for new chapters on co-occurring disorders; special considerations for therapy with residential populations, including detention and corrections, and with intellectually disabled patients; and guidance regarding use of supportive psychotherapy in community settings (which incorporates our previous chapters on working with families and case management). Finally, as in 1993, we end with a discussion of ethics, broadened to reference organizational ethics in psychology and counseling, and augmented with guidance on cultural and religious sensitivity. So in our opinion, that last chapter is a "must read," but you can pick and choose your diagnoses and settings in the middle of the book.

We are pleased to bring you this new edition.

Peter N. Novalis, M.D., Ph.D.
Virginia Singer, D.N.P., PMHNP-BC, CARN-AP
Roger Peele, M.D., DLFAPA

Introduction to the First Edition

This book, the *Clinical Manual of Supportive Psychotherapy*, has been written to fill what we believe is a significant gap in the otherwise plentiful literature on psychotherapy. It is addressed to a wide audience, including residents in psychiatry and nonpsychiatric physicians, as well as more experienced psychiatrists and psychotherapists who would like a comprehensive guide to the specific modality of supportive psychotherapy. This is the type of therapy most often prescribed for persons in crisis or with chronic mental or physical illness, but we believe in, and have tried to document, its wider applicability. We have tried to produce a text that would also be appropriate for novice psychotherapists who are beginning to apply their theoretical knowledge of psychiatric diagnosis to real patients.

While offering a comprehensive and self-contained manual, we have taken pains to refer readers to other resources and current research when needed. For convenience, references have been attached to chapters, but the project was always conceived as a unitary one.

The *principles* of Part I progressively develop the background and techniques of supportive psychotherapy, dividing the latter into explanatory and directive interventions. The *applications* of Part II represent various modifications and adaptations of supportive psychotherapy to major psychiatric and patient populations. In this part we have presented a consistent approach to supportive psychotherapy but have also given attention to identifying guidelines for distinguishing patients who will benefit most appropriately from supportive work. The *interactions* of Part III cover significant issues that arise in supportive work: the interplay between medication, therapy, and compliance; the relationships between therapist, patient, family, and other members of the treatment team; and the interactions between technique and values that generate ethical problems.

As in all finite projects, many topics (especially those germane to psychotherapy as a whole) have been passed over lightly or excluded to conserve both space and the supportive focus of the enterprise. Individual treatment is the overriding emphasis. The chapter on family issues covers the most vital issues for an individual therapist but does not presume to offer a complete guide to the diverse field of family therapy. Group treatments could be applied to most of the problems encountered here, but they are mentioned only when it is especially important not to neglect them. Cultural, racial, sexual, and socioeconomic issues in therapy, as well as the multiple problems of public sector psychotherapy, have also not been given their due. Despite these necessary omissions, we believe we have offered the reader the most comprehensive text yet available on the application of supportive psychotherapy to specific patient populations and diagnostic groups, showing in each case how basic principles must be modified to meet individual needs.

Each of us practices psychiatry in the public sector. We have had extensive experience with both public clinic and private practice patients, and both groups are represented in the cases given here. Both the clinical and theoretical materials were also field-tested by each of us in different courses that over the last few years were presented to first- and second-year psychiatry residents; master's- or doctoral-level therapists in psychology, nursing, social work, education, and art therapy; and pastoral counselors. Lastly, the material developed for this book was presented in a course primarily for psychiatrists at the annual meeting of the American Psychiatric Association in 1992. We are most grateful for the comments we received. And, of course, we are indebted to our patients, who taught us much about how to teach *them*; and our significant others, who have helped to bring this project to fruition, even though our original estimate of the work required was off by a factor of 10.

Peter N. Novalis, M.D., Ph.D.
Stephen J. Rojcewicz Jr., M.D.
Roger Peele, M.D.

Notes on Usage

In the first edition, we used mostly third-person sentences like "The therapist should do this" rather than "You should do this." We also used the somewhat epicene construction "he or she" to avoid sexism, but in retrospect we think that these stylistic decisions impaired readability and made the materials somewhat formal and distant from the reader, that is, YOU. Since this is indeed a clinical manual of instructions, it does seem more appropriate now to address the reader more often in the second person, and we have alternated the "he" and "she" examples to achieve balance without "conjunction dysfunction."

There are also some folks who remind us that there is a difference between "supportive psychotherapy" and "supportive therapy," the latter being a rubric that covers many nonpsychological treatments such as pet therapy or nutrition being supportive therapies for cancer treatment. We understand the difference, but we shall lapse into "supportive therapy" for stylistic reasons, and in the context of this book, it is simply a shortened form of "supportive psychotherapy." Many other writers in the field use "supportive therapy" in the same manner. Our prequel article title "What Supports Supportive Therapy?" had a much better ring to it than the longer version of the term. It is available online, so we apologize if it attracts an occasional pet therapist or dietitian.

Acknowledgments

Dr. Novalis acknowledges the help of and dedicates this book to Carol Novalis, who is a family educator and teacher in her own right. She reviewed and edited the entire manuscript several times and wrote substantial portions of the chapters on family and community involvement and intellectually disabled populations, and sections on active listening and ethics. She was offered a co-authorship, and even a portion of the royalties, but she graciously declined. But she will not be allowed to decline this appreciation for a lifetime of friendship, love, and marriage.

Dr. Singer acknowledges the help of and dedicates this book to Donald Singer, for his love, encouragement, and support, which kept her motivated; and for his endless trips to the office supply store for paper and ink. And for taking Blinky to the dog park while she worked.

PART I

Principles

The Basis for Supportive Psychotherapy

What Is Supportive Psychotherapy?

Supportive therapy is a type or mode of psychotherapy. A *psychotherapy*, in turn, is a collection of rules or techniques used to conduct mental health treatment, having a relevant set of goals, between a professionally trained person known as a *therapist* and a recipient or subject of the therapy known as the *client* or *patient*. Of course, there are therapies involving couples or groups. Supportive group psychotherapy is indeed an important modality of treatment, and we shall make some mention of it—but coverage of group therapy is not the focus of this book.

Rule Books and Clinical Manuals

You might compare a psychotherapy to a serious game or any organized activity of which you may think. To learn the game, you might ask, "Who are the players?" and "Where is it played (on a board, etc.)? How long does a game last? What are the rules? Where is the rule book? Who starts the game and what are they allowed to do? What goals do the players seek to reach? What does it take to win the game? Is there a prize for winning a game? What skills do serious players have that help them to win games? What are the penalties for people who don't play by the rules?" And of course, in the field of psychotherapy, there are many books that set out the rules of the relevant "game" one is learning.

In fact, you are reading a rule book for psychotherapy. Many therapies have been codified into manuals that give fairly detailed instructions on how to perform the therapy and how to develop a therapeutic relationship (or working alliance) with the patient, respond to the patient's questions or behaviors, develop goals and a treatment plan, manage difficult issues and emotions, periodically measure the effectiveness of the therapy, move the therapy through phases of treatment, and eventually terminate the therapy.

This *clinical manual* does do all those things but in a laissez-faire manner, which gives the therapist a considerable amount of leeway in performing the therapy. Therapy manuals that are more directive and present highly structured advice do abound in the psychotherapy field and do exist for supportive psychotherapy. A much referenced one by Luborsky (1984) is a free-standing book as well but also contains instruments to create goals of the therapy, monitor its effectiveness, and so on. The book is still readily available, and at least two manualized versions are posted online for treatment of marijuana and cocaine use disorders. That manual is still used by researchers, and an update of such studies may be found (Leichsenring and Leibing 2007). The authors of the learning series mentioned in our introduction (Winston et al. 2012) also used a manualized treatment. (A brief but complete treatment manual for time-limited, short-term supportive individual therapy can be found in Piper et al. 2002.) However, our conceptualization of supportive psychotherapy is somewhat different from these manualized versions, for reasons we make clear in the next few chapters.

So-called manualized therapies have an important role to play in training and research, because they enable head-to-head comparisons of the effectiveness of different therapies in differing populations, and so on. However, it is still debatable whether one should conduct one's therapy with patients using a strict treatment protocol or manual. It could certainly be boring to do so and would not allow for the eclecticism that we figure is central to supportive therapy. Once more, there is considerable research and debate on the place of highly manualized treatments versus looser and unstructured treatment protocols.

Until recently, the very mention of psychotherapy suggested a particular mode of psychotherapy known as *psychodynamic psychotherapy*, itself being an outgrowth of Sigmund Freud's (and others') psychoanalytic therapy and theory. However, supportive psychotherapy historically was conducted to an extent thousands of years ago by the ancient Greeks and was simply overshadowed by the Freudian-era focus of treatment on making the unconscious conscious.

It is helpful to define supportive therapy both by its collection of techniques and by its goals of treatment. For example, we have already suggested that supportive therapy does *not* have the goal of making unconscious processes conscious. Although some researchers prefer to define the therapy with its techniques, you cannot do only that. For example, Freud might have encouraged ventilation of emotions to assist someone in interpreting her dream. A supportive psychotherapist might also encourage ventilation to reduce a patient's anger, a very different goal. Perhaps the best way to clarify this is to define not the supportive therapy but the supportive therapist, as a therapist who uses the techniques of supportive therapy in a supportive therapeutic alliance with the patient to meet the aims of supportive therapy.

To explain and elucidate what supportive psychotherapy is, we will be discussing the goals, techniques, and patient-therapist relationship that characterize supportive psychotherapy: the goals of supportive therapy (see Table 1–2 later in this chapter), the techniques of supportive therapy (see Tables 3–1, 3–2, and 4–1), and the components of a supportive patient-therapist relationship (see Tables 2–1 and 2–2).

We will spend our first five chapters describing and teaching these techniques and goals, with the caveat that supportive psychotherapy as we conceive and teach it is an eclectic therapy that does not limit itself to just the techniques and goals of the therapy in those tables. Whether or not you consider the add-ons from other techniques, supportive therapy is by no means simple or simplistic, and it does require exacting and complex skills of its practitioners. For the very reason that supportive therapy is indicated—such as for patients in crisis, in psychotic decompensation, or with low level of social functioning—its provision often taxes the clinician's abilities to offer empathy, understanding, and benevolent direction. Thus, it is ironic that trainees on inpatient units are often given the most impaired patients to treat, and those who are most in need of support, even before they have completed a basic course in psychotherapy.

Supportive Psychotherapy as an Eclectic Therapy

Many psychotherapists consider themselves "eclectic," either informally or in a certain technical sense, which we will discuss later. Nontechnically, *eclectic* refers to using different methods or drawing selectively from different sources, and the word presumes a positive connotation. Eclectic therapists use a reportory of techniques drawn from different sources, such as supportive, cognitive-behavioral, psychodynamic, interpersonal, and humanistic.

In the first edition of our book, we advocated for supportive psychotherapy as an eclectic therapy that draws on empirically supported methods. To avoid a misunderstanding, we would correct this slightly now to emphasize that supportive psychotherapy does have its own group of distinctive techniques, but that supportive *psychotherapists* should feel free to supplement their repertory with techniques from other psychotherapies. In our previous edition, the main source of techniques external to supportive psychotherapy was cognitive therapy. The other "external" set of techniques referred to were those of psychodynamic psychotherapy, which we said were used infrequently in supportive work but still had their place.

In looking at resources to expand your repertory of techniques, you will find many that present collections of techniques from various therapies, listing "the best" exportable techniques. You might wonder, however, how it is possible to be eclectic at all. Doesn't that require embracing incompatible theories of personality, mind, or behavior? We think there is considerable controversy over that question and no simple answer. Thus, if you are a strict behaviorist and do not believe in unconscious mental processes, you might find it difficult to use psychodynamic techniques. But what is it that you must accept to endorse some of the methods of dialectical behavior therapy, interpersonal psychotherapy, or mentalization therapy? Each of these therapies does have an underlying "fundamental belief." For example, a proponent of mentalization therapy may believe that failure to mentalize leads to the impulsive and self-destructive behaviors of borderline personality. In the first edition of our book, which was written before mentalization was developed, we referred to failure to self-soothe as one of the defects of borderline personality and suggested some of the therapeutic techniques developed under that assumption. We also hoped that supportive psychotherapy could utilize empirically validated techniques (which predated the current focus on what are called evidence-based methods), which were relatively atheoretical (e.g., those that simply worked without making the user feel bound to accept a deep scientific theory of human behavior as the justification for the use of that therapy). Some therapies such as eye movement desensitization reprocessing, or EMDR, are being used because the therapists believe they work even though they are not entirely sure of the reason why they work or the supposed reason they work (i.e., the reprogramming of rapid eye movements from dreaming). Similarly, there is a group of the aforementioned eclectic theorists who describe and advocate a "transtheoretical" approach to therapy.

We wish we had space to elaborate, but that will be left to you. Use your academic resources and talk to your teachers, mentors, and colleagues to find out how they arrived at their own orientations to doing psychotherapy. There are specific resources designed to help you develop a personal theoretical orientation to psychotherapy. For example, Halibur and Vess Halibur (2015) summarize six major schools of thought and discuss some different meanings of eclecticism. (By the way, these are the psychodynamic, behavioral, humanistic, pragmatic, constructivist, and family approaches.) Another reference provides a primer of techniques that are categorized as belonging to nine different theoretical orientations (Erford 2015). For example, most therapists are familiar with reframing, thought stopping, guided imagery, and journaling. Some therapists feel comfortable switching theories, and others find that paradoxical but feel comfortable switching techniques. We urge you to learn from such guidebooks and from your patients as you find out what works and does not work so well, building your own library of techniques and putting aside the ones you do not find useful.

Although we have mentioned supportive therapy as existing for 2,000 years, when it was discussed by the psychoanalytic therapists, it frequently obtained the character of being a subset of a full set of psychoanalytic techniques, used with the most impaired patients who were not suitable for psychoanalysis. Clearly, this is not how we or other advocates of supportive psychotherapy conceive of it. In fact, as we mentioned, *some* supportive techniques are common to most forms of psychotherapy, including psychoanalytic. Therefore, supportive psychotherapy is more like the keystone in all psychotherapies, and without it the structure would collapse. (And continuing the analogy, you can build some very different arches having the same keystone.) Other writers describe it similarly as a base of the letter Y, illustrating common competencies and techniques in teaching psychotherapy (Plakun et al. 2009).

Therefore, as a guide for your own future development, we outline the repertory of a typical supportive psychotherapist in Table 1–1.

Table 1–1.   Repertory of a typical supportive psychotherapist

- Occasional techniques that might be useful but presume other theories of the mind and interpretations (e.g., dream interpretation)

- Isolated techniques that the therapist has found effective (e.g., the empty chair technique borrowed from Gestalt therapy)

- Frequently used techniques without theoretical assumptions (e.g., journaling, thought stopping, guided imagery, progressive muscle relaxation)

- Core techniques of supportive psychotherapy

- Therapist's favorite techniques but from other psychotherapies (e.g., inter-personal, mentalization-based, emotion-focused, Rogerian, motivational interviewing)

- Techniques from cognitive-behavioral therapy

- Techniques from psychodynamic therapy

- Techniques from psychoanalytic therapy

- Techniques from humanistic therapy

- Techniques from family therapy

How Effective Is Supportive Psychotherapy?

The effectiveness of supportive psychotherapy was well established 25 years ago, but the number of positive studies and applications to mental diagnoses has proliferated since then. However, there are still some problems and issues in documenting the effectiveness in specific studies. One problem is the "traditional" use of supportive psychotherapy as a control or comparator in psychotherapy studies conducted by researchers with the desire to prove the effectiveness of some other type of therapy. This has resulted in some negative studies as well as many surprisingly positive outcomes for supportive psychotherapy. Supportive psychotherapy also ends up being a "pseudo placebo" in some studies, sometimes even by being outrageously unsupportive or negative. However, we emphasize that the evidence that supports supportive psychotherapy has grown tremendously in the past 25 years.

Can Supportive Psychotherapy Be Harmful?

Therapists also wonder if they should warn their patients that therapy could be harmful to them, and there are indeed ethical obligations from the major professional organizations to do just that in obtaining a formal consent to begin therapy. Reassuringly, many researchers on effectiveness also looked in this direction and concluded that historically there are relatively few "therapies" that have proven to be outright harmful (Wampold and Imel 2015). One example was CISD, or critical incident stress debriefing, and in a similar vein the use of certain grief counseling in subjects undergoing normal bereavement reactions. Also, familiar to all therapists with some years of experience were certain therapies uncovering memories of childhood abuse, which later was shown to not possibly have occurred.

A much-discussed study (Schermuly-Haupt et al. 2018), however, discussed the negative outcomes in cognitive psychotherapy. Based on a survey of cognitive therapists, it was thought that about a quarter of their patients had negative side effects from the therapy, such as worsening condition and family stress. However, it was not implied that therapy was not itself a worthwhile decision for a person seeking help. Given that the survey was sent to experienced and presumably ethical therapists, the risks of psychotherapy are much more likely to be enhanced with inexperienced or unethical therapists, and anyone who has practiced in the field knows that from having reengaged with patients from such therapists. Therefore, therapy could certainly end up being minimally or marginally effective and hence a waste of time and money and possibly a cause of lost opportunities to get better faster. A good comparison, in our opinion, is with a highly effective, low-risk surgical procedure such as an appendectomy or cholecystectomy. You are usually much better off having such a procedure than not. Then there are moderate benefit–moderate risk surgeries such as back surgery and finally dangerous surgeries such as brain aneurysm repairs. However, we think that psychotherapy is analogous to the first group.

It would also be wrong, we think, to use supportive therapy when there is a more effective therapy available that the therapist is skilled to perform or for which the therapist can make a referral. For example, if a patient with fear of flying really seems to need exposure therapy and the therapist does not do that, the patient would need a referral. So we hope that none of our readers will end up doing ineffective or ineffectual therapy when something clearly better is possible.

In the history of psychotherapy effectiveness research going back as far as 1936 and the work of Saul Rosenzweig, however, there has been a major theory that many therapies are equally effective, presumably because of nonspecific factors in their psychotherapeutic methods (see Duncan 2002). This has been called the "dodo bird effect," after a fictional race in Chapter 3 of Lewis Carroll's *Alice's Adventures in Wonderland* (an analogy to politics), in which the Dodo claims that "everyone has won, and all must have prizes." (A thorough yet fairly brief history of both sides of the issue may be found in Wikipedia [2019].) In the last few decades, however, we have seen some therapies that do seem to rise a cut above the pack, such as cognitive-behavioral therapy. So when we propose the use of supportive therapy for specific diagnoses in this book, we are careful to note the limitations on patient selections and techniques, and do make mention of some of the other therapies.

We all wish, as do major authors in the field, that supportive psychotherapy will continue its development as an evidence-based treatment (Hellerstein and Markowitz 2008).

Core Supportive Techniques

Definition and the Place of Theories and Concepts

The supportive psychotherapist plays an active and directive role in helping the patient to improve his social functioning and coping skills. The emphasis is on improving behavior and subjective feelings rather than achieving insight or self-understanding. We believe there is a core of supportive techniques in many of the hundreds of psychotherapies, most of which provide patients with support, improve defenses, reduce anxiety, and so forth.

Supportive psychotherapy also differs from most other psychotherapies in its epistemological basis to the extent that it does not require a deeply theoretical concept or theory of the mind. Thus, a good definition of supportive psychotherapy is as follows:

> Supportive psychotherapy is a form of psychotherapy that uses techniques that are *empirically and/or evidence based*—that is, techniques that have been ob-

served to work—to achieve the following aims: 1) promote a supportive therapist-patient relationship; 2) enhance the patient's strengths, coping skills, and capacity to use environmental supports; 3) reduce the patient's subjective distress and behavioral dysfunctions; 4) achieve for the patient the greatest practical degree of independence from his or her psychiatric illnesses; and 5) foster the greatest possible degree of autonomy in treatment decisions for the patient.

Supportive Therapy Is Empirically Based and Patient Driven (Rather Than Theory Guided)

The therapist's activity at any point in the therapy is determined by the patient's current state and the therapist's selection from a repertory of proven techniques without theoretical bias. In addition, the supportive psychotherapist may change techniques as the therapy proceeds, based on observations of what is effective with given symptoms of the patient's illness. Concepts such as *transference* and *defense mechanisms* are frequently invoked, but theories as to the supposed cause of the patient's disorder are not required. Even those therapists committed to certain theories can use supportive psychotherapy principles at those times when they determine that any single theory is inadequate to explain the complexity of behavior or to form the basis for intervention. Supportive psychotherapy is, to use a term defined by Beitman et al. (1989), *technically eclectic*, in that it does not presuppose a particular theory of psychopathology; it can draw as needed from particular schools of psychotherapy, including psychodynamic, cognitive-behavioral, interpersonal, and experiential. It is also eclectic in that it may address different symptoms with potentially different therapeutic methods (Kramer 1989).

Goals of Supportive Psychotherapy

Potential goals of supportive psychotherapy, based on our definition, are presented in Table 1–2. These goals can be divided into those that are frequently chosen and those that are usually given less emphasis. Specific goals are reached by the therapist's active selection of priorities and emphases on the content of therapy sessions. Some of these goals (e.g., strengthening defenses) may even appear contradictory to reciprocal goals (weakening defenses), but this is a matter of relative emphasis and selection of particular defenses, as will be described later in our chapters on technique.

Table 1–2. Goals of supportive psychotherapy

Frequent goals	Infrequent goals
Reducing behavioral dysfunctions	Enhancing insight and self-understanding
Reducing subjective mental distress	Exploring interpersonal experiences
Supporting and enhancing the patient's strengths and coping skills, and his or her capacity to use environmental supports	Exploring inner experiences
	Understanding childhood determinants of adult personality
Maximizing treatment autonomy	Resolving intrapsychic conflicts
Achieving maximum possible independence from psychiatric illness	Restructuring personality

Examples

Resolving acute crises—for example, bereavement, trauma, disaster, suicide attempt, and crises associated with medical illness

Promoting adherence to treatment plans

Decreasing inappropriate behavior

Decreasing dysphoric thought processes and content

Improving coping skills

Improving social skills

Resolving external conflicts

Preventing relapse, deterioration, or hospitalization

Enhancing self-esteem

Improving reality testing (of patient, others, and the world)

Strengthening healthy defenses

Weakening maladaptive defenses

Maximizing family and social support

In a patient-driven, symptom-focused, or empirical therapy, you must address the treatment with the relative goals in mind. A patient who is experiencing a psychotic breakdown probably needs to be asked about his medication; no therapist of any school would wait for the patient to bring up the topic, if ever he did. Similarly, the high-functioning executive brought in by her family for depression requires a directive interview with attention to suicidal intent. She may benefit from long-term characterological change, but that is not the most important goal of therapy at this moment.

Supportive psychotherapy is often described in negative terms as a therapy suited for patients who cannot benefit from, afford, or engage in the time-consuming, long-term psychodynamic forms of therapy. This negative approach toward definition does not do justice to the fact that supportive therapy is probably a preferred mode of treatment for the majority of mentally ill persons (Dewald 1971). However, the negative bias against supportive therapy is an intellectual one that assumes that treatment with psychoanalytic methods is perhaps more interesting or rewarding to the clinician. Such bias is reflective more of the lack of knowledge of supportive therapy and of how to conduct it.

Supportive therapy does not presuppose low function, psychosis, or chronic mental illness, although these characteristics are likely to make it a preferred mode of treatment. The methods and goals of supportive therapy are equally applicable to high-functioning patients in crisis or with limited access to more intense therapies. It is not a linguistic accident that supportive therapy has developed along a parallel track as part of the biopsychosocial treatment of bereaved, suicidal, or traumatized patients as well as of acutely, chronically, or terminally medically ill patients, regardless of their preexisting psychopathology, if any. For these reasons, such supportive interventions are included in the spectrum of topics in this manual, for these constitute the same form of treatment and not just disparate ones with the same name.

Evidence for Effectiveness

Traditionally, supportive psychotherapy has been considered the treatment of choice (often in conjunction with medication) for patients in crisis or for those with very chronic medical or psychiatric illnesses. Many studies, however, including some with surprising or counterintuitive outcomes, have established the wide applicability and efficacy of supportive psychotherapy. As we said even in the first edition of this book, it is not even possible to discuss all the positive studies that have been published. However, as in the past, we will emphasize the groundbreaking studies with the addition of some more recent research. (Note: More recent studies are often given in the diagnosis-specific chapters of the book.)

In the Boston Psychotherapy Study (Gunderson et al. 1984), a sample of 95 persons with schizophrenia were treated with either a reality-adaptive, supportive (RAS) form of psychotherapy or an exploratory, insight-oriented (EIO) type. Two-year outcomes showed minimal differences in only 3 of 10 areas of assessment, with RAS treatment slightly superior in reducing hospitalizations and improving occupational function, and EIO treatment modestly superior in improving ego functioning. Given the cost of hospitalization, the RAS treatment was clearly more cost-effective, pending the development of specific treatment strategies for patients. One review of outcome studies (Krauss and Slavinsky 1982, pp. 230–232) emphasized the generally positive results but noted that the stimulation of group settings could worsen symptoms, especially in unmedicated patients. In addition, the provision of group socialization in clinic settings may be a substitute for community activities that does not aid in the patient's adjustment in the community. (For additional discussion, see Goldberg et al. 1977; Hogarty et al. 1974, 1979.)

A later study of first-episode psychosis also reported positive findings (Rosenbaum et al. 2005). However, the most comprehensive analysis of supportive psychotherapy has since been reported by the Cochrane Collaborative and is readily available (Buckley et al. 2015). There are actually three downloadable documents, consisting of a brief summary, a moderate-sized report (150 pages), and a detailed analysis of individual studies (250 pages). The Collaborative's conclusions are that the quality of evidence is poor for reasons we suggested earlier in the chapter: that supportive therapy is often used as a control condition, weak comparator, and so on, and in studies with the purpose of proving the superiority of other types of psychotherapy. So the greatest benefit is actually found in their analysis of individual studies showing which ones report a positive trend for supportive psychotherapy.

Supportive psychotherapy was shown to be as effective as behavior therapy in the treatment of phobias (Klein et al. 1983; Zitrin et al. 1978). A subsequent study (Barrowclough et al. 2001) found that its effectiveness was broadly equal to that of cognitive-behavioral therapy for several anxiety disorders.

The usefulness of supportive psychotherapy in depression was established in the National Institute of Mental Health's Treatment of Depression Collaborative Research Program (Elkin et al. 1989), which compared the effectiveness of four 16-week treatment conditions, two of which utilized a clinical management (CM) component that was described as approximating a "minimal supportive therapy" because it included support, encouragement, and direct advice along with medication management and a review of the patient's condition. For a severely depressed subgroup of patients, the imipramine-CM treatment was superior to (in order of lessening superiority) interpersonal psychotherapy, cognitive psychotherapy, and placebo CM. For a less depressed subgroup, no other treatment was more effective than the placebo-CM condition. This study attested not only to the therapeutic efficacy of medication combined with supportive psychotherapy but also, as the authors themselves suggested, to the effectiveness of supportive therapy alone for less severely depressed patients. Although there was no isolated placebo treatment, for ethical reasons, Elkin et al. (1989) suggested (on the basis of previous placebo-alone studies) that placebo and CM combined would be a more effective treatment than placebo alone.

In addition, a review of 26 articles, most of them studies of supportive-type therapies for depression and related problems, concluded that "there is evidence to suggest that the group of therapies often referred to as supportive are effective, and equally as effective as selected other therapies, in the treatment of adult depression" (Jacobs and Reupert 2014, p. 2). The therapies identified in this article include many with methods and techniques more limited than those of the therapy we advocate in this book (e.g., supportive and nondirective counseling).

Many other studies have been conducted in various types of depression and different samples such as adolescents assigned to cognitive, family, or supportive psychotherapy (Renaud et al. 1998), and supportive psychotherapy was found to be superior for mild depression but not as much for severe. As for bipolar disorder, both supportive therapy and mentalization-based therapy were found to be effective in treatment (Meyer and Hautzinger 2012).

We previously mentioned the availability of treatment manuals for substance abuse and mentioned Luborsky's (1984) supportive-expressive psychotherapy. It should be pointed out that supportive therapy for cocaine abusers was found to be effective but was not the superior treatment in a large National Institute on Drug Abuse study of 400 patients and four treatment arms (Crits-Christoph et al. 1997).

Studies involving medical conditions abound. One of the earlier controlled studies was that of Mumford et al. (1982), which showed multiple benefits in patients receiving ancillary supportive psychotherapy after myocardial infarctions and surgery (e.g., increased adherence, increased speed of recovery, fewer complications and days in hospital). Sjödin et al. (1986) reported a controlled study of patients with peptic ulcer disease showing favorable results in those who had supportive psychotherapy added to their medical treatment. (For newer references, see Chapter 12, "The Medically Ill Patient.")

Quite fascinating and still worth emphasizing are the results of the Menninger Foundation's Psychotherapy Research Project, a long-term (1956–1972) naturalistic study of expressive and supportive psychoanalytic psychotherapy with 42 patients. The initial findings in this complex study showed that "the modality of treatment by itself did not have significant effect on the outcome; however, successful supportive treatments require a higher skill in the therapist than the expressive treatments" (Burstein et al. 1972, p. 79). A major variable that did correlate positively with treatment outcome was ego strength. Based on the finding that patients with initially low ego strength benefited more from expressive than supportive treatments, Kernberg (1984) was led in his interpretation of the study to prescribe a somewhat limited role for supportive psychotherapy in the treatment of severe personality disorders. In sharp contrast, subsequent analysis by Wallerstein (1989) led the latter to draw what might seem (to some) to be radical conclusions:

- Treatment results for both methods tended to converge rather than diverge.
- All courses of treatment embodied a greater number of supportive elements than originally intended, and these elements accounted for more of the changes than was anticipated.
- The changes (regardless of the treatments used to achieve them) "often seemed quite indistinguishable from each other and equally represented structural change in personality functioning" (Wallerstein 1989, p. 205).

It is the last statement, which argues for the effectiveness of supportive psychotherapy in producing long-term personality change, that shows most clearly the ability of supportive psychotherapy to achieve one of the treatment goals often ascribed to psychoanalysis alone. (For additional discussion, see the original data, Wallerstein's arguments, and his monograph based on the Menninger project [Wallerstein 1986].) More recently, Kernberg (2018) has addressed the role of supportive psychotherapy in treating severe personality disorders, given that the resources for more psychodynamic treatments are not available (e.g., are too expensive or time consuming, or trained therapists are not available to perform them).

Other studies on use of supportive psychotherapy in treating personality disorders have also been reported. Brief supportive psychotherapy was found equally effective as short-term dynamic psychotherapy in high-functioning outpatients with personality disorder (Hellerstein et al. 1998). General equivalences were found between transference-focused therapy, supportive psychotherapy, and dialectical behavior therapy in outpatients with borderline personality disorder (Clarkin et al. 2007), and supportive-expressive psychotherapy was found to be as effective as psychodynamic therapy in outpatients with Cluster C personality disorders (avoidant, dependent, obsessive-compulsive) (Vinnars et al. 2005). Both mentalization based and supportive psychotherapy were found to be highly effective in treating patients with borderline personality disorder (Jørgensen et al. 2013), and mentalization-based treatment and a fairly minimal therapeutic method called *structured clinical management* were both found to be effective in treating borderline personality disorder (Bateman and Fonagy 2009). And supportive psychotherapy has been found to be as effective in treating bipolar disorder as cognitive-behavioral therapy (Pedersen 2018).

Historical Background to Supportive Psychotherapy

Supportive psychotherapy has a long and varied history dating back to the ancient Greeks, who conceived of methods of treating the mentally ill humanely as well as the more specific approaches of counseling and support for persons in crisis (Ducey and Simon 1975).

Various methods of dealing with the irrational in man can be found in Plato, Aristotle, Hippocrates, and other classical authors (Dodds 1951). Many of these techniques (e.g., emotional catharsis, education) have direct applicability to supportive psychotherapy. For example, Gorgias, the Sicilian Greek sophist of fifth century B.C.E., and Antiphon, an Athenian Greek sophist of approximately the same era, both had reputations for curing certain illnesses through verbal methods (Lain Entralgo 1970). Gorgias was the brother of the physician Herodicus of Leontini but did not identify himself as a physician. The Platonic dialogue *Gorgias*, in which Socrates debates the aged Gorgias, illustrates the latter's reputation for persuading patients to take their medicine when physicians themselves could not so persuade them. (It appears that some issues remain cogent, even after 2,500 years.) In this dialogue, Plato has Gorgias say: "I have often, along with my brother and with other physicians, visited one of the patients who refused to drink his medicines or submit to the surgeon's knife or cautery, and when the doctor was unable to persuade them, I did, by no other art but rhetoric" (Hamilton and Cairns 1961, p. 239). An elaborate discussion of this example ensues. Included in the argument of Socrates is the conclusion that the person who uses verbal methods to cure must also know medicine.

Additional elements of supportive psychotherapy technique can be found in Greek tragedy and the Asclepian temple healing procedure (Gorelick 1987). Further examples can be cited for philosophers such as Cicero or medieval physician-philosophers such as Avicenna (Shafii 1972). Indeed, the various components of supportive psychotherapy in use for many centuries have often been the province of philosophers, poets, political leaders (Williman and Kvarnes 1984), religious practitioners (Finucane 1973), and indigenous healers, rather than a part of the armamentarium of the medical profession.

The first systematic organization of these principles as part of the overall field of medicine was put forth by the German physician Johann Christian Reil (1759–1813), who was also the first to use the word *psychiatry.* His 1803 book, *Rhapsodien über die Anwendung der psychischen Curmethode auf Geisteszerrüttungen* ("Rhapsodies on the Application of the Psychic Cure Method to Mental Disorders"), outlined a complete method of psychotherapy for the treatment of mental disorders (Reil 1803, cited by Ellenberger 1970). Reil emphasized security, stimulation, and comfort accomplished through talking, rest, appropriate physical work, massage, music, education, occupational therapy, art therapy, and even a form of psychodrama. Based on the systematization of his ideas and their integration into a comprehensive view of mental disorders and medical treatment, such that verbal methods are part of a total treatment plan, Reil has been called the founder of rational psychotherapy (Colp 1989), and perhaps he may also be considered the modern-day founder of supportive psychotherapy.

Most psychotherapies, and especially supportive psychotherapy, have a humanitarian thrust. Philippe Pinel's (1745–1826) unchaining of the psychiatrically ill of Bicêtre in 1792 and of the Hôpital Salpêtrière in Paris in 1794 is generally regarded as the beginning of the modern era of humanitarian treatment. This action, frequently depicted dramatically in art, is often seen as the beginning of the medical model of mental illness (Van den Berg 1987). It was not merely this decision but his development of treatment guidelines (including productive activities for the mentally ill) that established Pinel's place in history.

In the United States, this current of reform was continued by the founder of American psychiatry, Benjamin Rush, a signer of the Declaration of Independence. In addition to his many biological treatment innovations, Rush counseled direct advice, educational efforts, healthy employment or productive activities, and temperance—approaches that can be seen as forerunners of supportive psychotherapy (Rush 1809/1972).

In a more modern context, Freud, who had himself elaborated and then abandoned the use of direct suggestion and hypnosis in lieu of associative psychoanalytic technique, predicted that "the large-scale application of our theory will compel us to alloy the pure gold of analysis freely with the copper of direct suggestion" (Freud 1919[1918]/1955, p. 168). Subsequently, supportive psychotherapy was defined by a succession of clinicians with respect to its differences from psychoanalytic technique. Alexander and French (1946), in a reaction to nondirective analytic technique, conceived the notion of the "corrective emotional experience," which was tailored to provide the missing components of a patient's nurturing and a relearning of assumptions about interpersonal relationships. Their work spawned lines of development in behavioral therapies and focused brief psychotherapy.

The focused, limited, and non-insight-oriented aspects of Alexander and French's method were developed further by Gill (1951), who proposed that the usual interpretations of defenses could not be applied to patients with low ego strength, who risked regression and could not handle the anxiety. Such patients needed differential support of behaviors that expressed adaptive defenses. A similar conception of supportive interventions, derived by Draper et al. (1968) from Heinz Hartmann's "regressive adaptation" (Hartmann 1958), defined "adaptive psychiatry" as a technique to mobilize ego strengths so that the patient remained functional. A key tenet of Draper et al.'s treatment was to support psychological defenses—even overt, pathological ones such as paranoid delusions. This formulation of supportive therapy concerned its role in the strengthening and inculcation of a patient's individual coping and socialization skills.

And here are some additional views of supportive psychotherapy:

- Knight (1954) describes it as a "superficial psychotherapy" that utilizes inspiration, reassurance, suggestion, persuasion, counseling, reeducation, and other techniques for patients who are too psychologically fragile, inflexible, or defensive for exploratory devices.
- Bloch (1979) stresses sustenance and maintenance rather than suppression and repression as the focus of supportive psychotherapy.
- Werman (1984) sees supportive psychotherapy as a substitutive form of treatment that supplies the patient with those psychological functions that he or she either lacks entirely or possesses insufficiently.
- Wallerstein (1988), following Gill (1951), defines supportive psychotherapy as one that strengthens defenses and represses selected symptoms (in favor of exploring others), using means other than interpretation or insight to achieve these goals.
- Pinsker and Rosenthal (1992) describe individual supportive psychotherapy as "a dyadic treatment characterized by use of direct measures to ameliorate symptoms and to maintain, restore, or improve self-esteem, adaptive skills, and psychological function. To the extent necessary to accomplish these objectives, treatment may utilize examination of relationships, real or transferential, and both past and current patterns of emotional response or behavior" (p. 21).

Rockland (1989, pp. 22–39), in his excellent review, has traced the development of supportive psychotherapy, the key points of which are as follows. In 1912, Ernest Jones wrote that suggestion depends on the patient's positive transference to the healer. Edward Glover, in 1931, developed the concept of "inexact" interpretations.

In 1938, Paul Schilder wrote that supportive psychotherapy consisted of the following:

- Discussion
- Advice
- Persuasion
- Appeal to willpower
- Hypnosis
- Suggestion
- Relaxation and concentration
- Hospitalization

In 1942, Maurice Levine added to Schilder's list the following:

- Medications
- Reassurance
- Occupational therapy
- Daily routine
- Hobbies
- Authoritative firmness
- Education
- Provision of acceptable outlets for aggressiveness
- Provision of acceptable compensations for fears and feelings of inferiority
- Ignoring certain symptoms and attitudes
- Satisfaction of neurotic needs
- Opportunities for healthy identification
- Confession and ventilation
- Desensitization

In 1946, Alexander and French wrote of two techniques that have since become part of supportive psychotherapy: 1) corrective emotional experience and 2) varying frequency and length of sessions.

Gill, in 1951, identified three basic principles of supportive psychotherapy:

1. Support and praise ego activities in which adaptive defenses are combined with gratifications.

2. Never undermine defenses that are absolutely necessary to the patient's continued functioning.
3. Set up an "artificial neurosis" to achieve partial discharge of instinctual drives.

Bibring, in 1954, noted that psychotherapy includes suggestion, abreaction, manipulation, clarification, and interpretations, and that supportive psychotherapy differs from psychodynamic psychotherapy only in not using interpretations.

In the 1960s, Tarachow (1963) stressed that a core difference between psychoanalysis and supportive psychotherapy is that in the former the transference is treated as an unreal relationship, whereas in the latter it is treated as real. He also contended that an acceptable technique is to supply the patient with displacements, projections, and introjections when these contribute to the patient's stability.

In 1969, Schlesinger noted that although support is an essential aspect of all therapies, a psychotherapy that excludes all exploration is not a psychotherapy at all.

In 1971, Dewald suggested that supportive psychotherapy has aspects of the early parent-child relationship and proposed that therapists using this modality encourage secondary process thinking. In 1984, Pine introduced the concept of "striking while the iron is cold."

The first two books devoted exclusively to supportive psychotherapy were written by Werman (1984) and Rockland (1989). Both described psychodynamically oriented supportive psychotherapy. Rockland's book more specifically addressed the historical roots that we just summarized and more clearly demarcated a definition of psychodynamically oriented supportive psychotherapy. Rockland et al. (1992) investigated supportive psychotherapy of patients with borderline personality disorder. (This work was the first book to deal with supportive psychotherapy of an individual disorder.)

Finally, as mentioned earlier, extensive work on supportive psychotherapy was done at the Mount Sinai Beth Israel medical center in New York by Henry Pinsker's team. These investigators developed a number of manuals and have presented supportive psychotherapy training programs that have enhanced the prestige of supportive psychotherapy. The second edition of their primer on supportive psychotherapy is now being prepared. They and others (e.g., Bedi and Vassiliadis 2010) discuss the training issues and skill sets involved in teaching supportive psychotherapy. It is clear that supportive psychotherapy has evolved tremendously over the last few thousand years, and it will continue to develop in the future. In fact, one historical account (Sjöqvist 2007) divides its development into four stages: a prehistory (1900–1950), phase of definition (1950–1960), phase of establishment (1960–1990), and integrative phase (1990–2007, the date of the article). Is that where we are now?

Conclusion

We close this chapter not with a summary, but with a lesson to inspire you to read the rest of this book. Supportive psychotherapy is the most commonly used therapy by therapists and is the treatment of choice for many persons and many illnesses (Hellerstein et al. 1994). Learning it gives you the core competencies for doing other psychotherapies. Put pithily and paradoxically by Markowitz (2014): "[I]f you cannot do this, the rest of psychotherapy does not matter...[and] if you can do this, the rest of psychotherapy does not matter."

Key Points

- Supportive psychotherapy is an evidence-based, eclectic mode of treatment suitable for most patients who need psychotherapy.

- Supportive psychotherapy is the most commonly used therapy by therapists and is the treatment of choice for many persons and many illnesses.

- Supportive therapy has a long history going back to the ancient Greek philosophers.

- A supportive relationship and supportive techniques are common to most of the popular and familiar "named" psychotherapies, including cognitive-behavioral, psychodynamic, and even psychoanalytic psychotherapies. However, there are well-defined, manualized psychotherapy treatments that rigorously define supportive psychotherapy for its use in specific populations or for research purposes.

- Developing skills in supportive psychotherapy should be a goal for all psychotherapists.

References

Alexander F, French TM: Psychoanalytic Therapy: Principles and Applications. New York, Ronald Press, 1946

Barrowclough C, King P, Colville J, et al: A randomized trial of the effectiveness of cognitive-behavioral therapy and supportive counseling for anxiety symptoms in older adults. J Consult Clin Psychol 69(5):756–762, 2001 11680552

Bateman A, Fonagy P: Randomized controlled trial of outpatient mentalization-based treatment versus structured clinical management for borderline personality disorder. Am J Psychiatry 166(12):1355–1364, 2009 19833787

Bedi N, Vassiliadis H: Supervised case experience in supportive psychotherapy: suggestions for trainers. Advances in Psychiatric Treatment 16(3):184–192, 2010

Beitman BD, Goldfried MR, Norcross JC: The movement toward integrating the psychotherapies: an overview. Am J Psychiatry 146(2):138–147, 1989 2643360

Bibring E: Psychoanalysis and the dynamic psychotherapies. J Am Psychoanal Assoc 2(4):745–770, 1954 13211442

Bloch S: Supportive psychotherapy, in An Introduction to the Psychotherapies. Edited by Bloch S. New York, Oxford University Press, 1979, pp 196–220

Buckley LA, Maayan N, Soares-Weiser K, et al: Supportive psychotherapy for schizophrenia. Cochrane Database Syst Rev 14(4):CD004716, 2015 25871462

Burstein ED, Coyne L, Kernberg OF, et al: Psychotherapy and psychoanalysis I: the quantitative study of the psychotherapy research project: psychotherapy outcome. Bull Menninger Clin 36(1):1–85, 1972 5030799

Clarkin JF, Levy KN, Lenzenweger MF, et al: Evaluating three treatments for borderline personality disorder: a multiwave study. Am J Psychiatry 164(6):922–928, 2007 17541052

Colp RJr: History of psychiatry, in Comprehensive Textbook of Psychiatry, 5th Edition, Vol 2. Edited by Kaplan HI, Sadock BJ. Baltimore, MD, Williams & Wilkins, 1989, pp 2132–2153

Crits-Christoph P, Siqueland L, Blaine J, et al: The National Institute on Drug Abuse Collaborative Cocaine Treatment Study: rationale and methods. Arch Gen Psychiatry 54(8):721–726, 1997 9283507

Dewald PA: Psychotherapy: A Dynamic Approach, 2nd Edition. New York, Basic Books, 1971

Dodds ER: The Greeks and the Irrational. Berkeley, University of California Press, 1951

Draper E, Daniels R, Rada R: Adaptive psychotherapy: an approach toward greater precision in the treatment of the chronically disturbed. Compr Psychiatry 9(4):372–382, 1968 5665470

Duccy C, Simon B: Ancient Greece and Rome, in World History of Psychiatry. Edited by Howells JG. New York, Brunner/Mazel, 1975, pp 1–38

Duncan B: The founder of common factors: a conversation with Saul Rosenzweig. J Psychother Integr 12:10–31, 2002

Elkin I, Shea MT, Watkins JT, et al: National Institute of Mental Health Treatment of Depression Collaborative Research Program: general effectiveness of treatments. Arch Gen Psychiatry 46(11):971–982, discussion 983, 1989 2684085

Ellenberger HF: The Discovery of the Unconscious. New York, Basic Books, 1970

Erford BT: 40 Techniques Every Counselor Should Know, 2nd Edition. New York, Pearson, 2015

Finucane RC: Faith healing in medieval England: miracles at saints' shrines. Psychiatry 36(3):341–346, 1973 4270304

Freud S: Lines of advance in psycho-analytic therapy (1919[1918]), in The Standard Edition of the Complete Psychological Works of Sigmund Freud, Vol 17. Translated and edited by Strachey J. London, Hogarth Press, 1955, pp 157–168

Gill MM: Ego psychology and psychotherapy. Psychoanal Q 20(1):62–71, 1951 14834272

Goldberg SC, Schooler NR, Hogarty GE, et al: Prediction of relapse in schizophrenic outpatients treated by drug and sociotherapy. Arch Gen Psychiatry 34(2):171–184, 1977 843177

Gorelick K: Greek tragedy and ancient healing: poems as theater and Asclepian temple in miniature. Journal of Poetry Therapy 1:38–43, 1987

Gunderson JG, Frank AF, Katz HM, et al: Effects of psychotherapy in schizophrenia, II: comparative outcome of two forms of treatment. Schizophr Bull 10(4):564–598, 1984 6151246

Halibur DA, Vess Halibur K: Developing Your Theoretical Orientation in Counseling and Psychotherapy, 3rd Edition. New York, Pearson, 2015

Hamilton E, Cairns H (eds): The Collected Dialogues of Plato. New York, Pantheon, 1961

Hartmann H: Ego Psychology and the Problem of Adaptation. New York, International Universities Press, 1958

Hellerstein DJ, Markowitz JC: Developing supportive psychotherapy as evidence-based treatment. Am J Psychiatry 165(10):1355–1356, author reply 1356, 2008 18829888

Hellerstein DJ, Pinsker H, Rosenthal RN, et al: Supportive therapy as the treatment model of choice. J Psychiatr Pract Res 3(4):300–306, 1994 22700197

Hellerstein DJ, Rosenthal RN, Pinsker H, et al: A randomized prospective study comparing supportive and dynamic therapies: outcome and alliance. J Psychother Pract Res 7(4):261–271, 1998 9752637

Hogarty GE, Goldberg SC, Schooler NR: Drug and sociotherapy in the aftercare of schizophrenic patients, III: adjustment of nonrelapsed patients. Arch Gen Psychiatry 31(5):609–618, 1974 4374156

Hogarty GE, Schooler NR, Ulrich R, et al: Fluphenazine and social therapy in the aftercare of schizophrenic patients: relapse analyses of a two-year controlled study of fluphenazine decanoate and fluphenazine hydrochloride. Arch Gen Psychiatry 36(12):1283–1294, 1979 227340

Jacobs N, Reupert A: The effectiveness of supportive counselling, based on Rogerian principles: a systematic review of recent international and Australian research. Melbourne, PACFA, 2014. Available at: https://www.pacfa.org.au/wp-content/uploads/2012/10/PACFA-Supportive-Counselling-literature-review-May-2014-Final.pdf. Accessed February 19, 2019.

Jørgensen CR, Freund C, Bøye R, et al: Outcome of mentalization-based and supportive psychotherapy in patients with borderline personality disorder: a randomized trial. Acta Psychiatr Scand 127(4):305–317, 2013 22897123

Kernberg OF: From the Menninger project to a research strategy for long-term psychotherapy of borderline personality disorders, in Psychotherapy Research: Where Are We and Where Should We Go? (Proceedings of the 73rd Annual Meeting of the American Psychopathological Association, New York, March 3–5, 1983.) Edited by Williams JBW, Spitzer RL. New York, Guilford, 1984, pp 247–260

Kernberg OF: Treatment of Severe Personality Disorders: Resolution of Aggression and Recovery of Eroticism. Washington, DC, American Psychiatric Association Publishing, 2018

Klein DF, Zitrin CM, Woerner MG, et al: Treatment of phobias, II: behavior therapy and supportive psychotherapy: are there any specific ingredients? Arch Gen Psychiatry 40(2):139–145, 1983 6130751

Knight RP: A critique of the present status of the psychotherapies, in Psychoanalytic Psychiatry and Psychology. Edited by Knight RP, Friedman CR. New York, International Universities Press, 1954, pp 52–64 [First published in Bull N Y Acad Med 25:100–114, 1949]

Kramer PD: Moments of Engagement: Intimate Psychotherapy in a Technological Age. New York, WW Norton, 1989

Krauss JB, Slavinsky AT: The Chronically Ill Psychiatric Patient and the Community. Boston, MA, Blackwell Scientific, 1982

Lain Entralgo P: The Therapy of the Word in Classical Antiquity. Translated by Rather LJ, Sharp JM. New Haven, CT, Yale University Press, 1970

Leichsenring F, Leibing E: Supportive-expressive (SE) psychotherapy: an update. Curr Psychiatry Rev 3(2):57–64, 2007

Levine M: Psychotherapy in Medical Practice. New York, Macmillan, 1942

Luborsky L: Principles of Psychoanalytic Psychotherapy: A Manual for Supportive-Expressive Treatment. New York, Basic Books, 1984

Markowitz JC: What is supportive psychotherapy? Focus 12(3):285–289, 2014

Meyer TD, Hautzinger M: Cognitive behaviour therapy and supportive therapy for bipolar disorders: relapse rates for treatment period and 2-year follow-up. Psychol Med 42(7):1429–1439, 2012 22099722

Mumford E, Schlesinger HJ, Glass CV: The effects of psychological intervention on recovery from surgery and heart attacks: an analysis of the literature. Am J Public Health 72(2):141–151, 1982 7055315

Pedersen T: CBT, supportive therapy equally effective for bipolar. August 8, 2018. Available at: psychcentral.com/news/2012/07/08/cbt-supportive-therapy-equally-effective-for-bipolar/41324.html. Accessed February 19, 2019.

Pine F: The interpretive moment: variations on classical themes. Bull Menninger Clin 48(1):54–71, 1984 6692050

Pinsker H, Rosenthal R: Beth Israel Medical Center Supportive Therapy Treatment Manual. Corte Madera, CA, Social and Behavioral Sciences Documents, 1992; quoted in Pinsker H: The supportive component of psychotherapy. Psychiatr Times 15(11), November 1, 1998

Piper WE, Joyce AS, McCallum M, et al: Interpretive and Supportive Psychotherapies: Matching Therapy and Patient Personality. Washington, DC, American Psychological Association, 2002

Plakun EM, Sudak DM, Goldberg D: The Y model: an integrated, evidence-based approach to teaching psychotherapy competencies. J Psychiatr Pract 15(1):5–11, 2009 19182560

Reil JC: Rhapsodien über die Anwendung der psychischen Curmethode auf Geisteszerrütungen. Halle, Germany, Curtsche Buchhandlung, 1803

Renaud J, Brent DA, Baugher M, et al: Rapid response to psychosocial treatment for adolescent depression: a two-year follow-up. J Am Acad Child Adolesc Psychiatry 37(11):1184–1190, 1998 9808930

Rockland LH: Supportive Psychotherapy: A Psychodynamic Approach. New York, Basic Books, 1989

Rockland LH, Braun D, Perry S, et al: Supportive Therapy for Borderline Patients: A Psychodynamic Approach. New York, Guilford, 1992

Rosenbaum B, Valbak K, Harder S, et al: The Danish National Schizophrenia Project: prospective, comparative longitudinal treatment study of first-episode psychosis. Br J Psychiatry 186:394–399, 2005 15863743

Rush B: Medical Inquiries and Observations (1809). New York, Arno Press, 1972

Schermuly-Haupt ML, Linden M, Rush AJ: Unwanted events and side effects in cognitive behavior therapy. Cognit Ther Res 42:219–229, 2018

Schilder P: Psychotherapy. London, K. Paul, Trench, Trubner & Co, 1938

Schlesinger HJ: Diagnosis and prescription for psychotherapy. Bull Menninger Clin 33(5):269–278, 1969 5345953

Shafii M: A precedent for modern psychotherapeutic techniques: one thousand years ago. Am J Psychiatry 128(12):1581–1584, 1972 4554405

Sjödin I, Svedlund J, Ottosson JO, et al: Controlled study of psychotherapy in chronic peptic ulcer disease. Psychosomatics 27(3):187–191, 195–196, 200, 1986 3961091

Sjöqvist S: On the history of supportive therapy. Nordic Psychology 59(2):181–188, 2007

Tarachow S: An Introduction to Psychotherapy. Madison, CT, International Universities Press, 1963

Van den Berg JH: The rise and fall of the medical model in psychiatry: a phenomenological analysis, in Psychiatry and Phenomenology. Pittsburgh, PA, Simon Silverman Phenomenology Center, 1987, pp 1–24

Vinnars B, Barber JP, Norén K, et al: Manualized supportive-expressive psychotherapy versus nonmanualized community-delivered psychodynamic therapy for patients with personality disorders: bridging efficacy and effectiveness. Am J Psychiatry 162(10):1933–1940, 2005 16199841

Wallerstein RS: Forty-Two Lives in Treatment: A Study of Psychoanalysis and Psychotherapy. New York, Guilford, 1986

Wallerstein RS: Psychoanalysis and long-term dynamic psychotherapy, in Review of General Psychiatry, 2nd Edition. Edited by Goldman HH. Norwalk, CT, Appleton & Lange, 1988, pp 506–514

Wallerstein RS: The Psychotherapy Research Project of the Menninger Foundation: an overview. J Consult Clin Psychol 57(2):195–205, 1989 2708605

Wampold BE, Imel ZE: The Great Psychotherapy Debate, 2nd Edition. New York, Routledge, 2015

Werman DS: The Practice of Supportive Psychotherapy. New York, Brunner/Mazel, 1984

Wikipedia: Dodo bird verdict. February 12, 2019. Available at: https://en.wikipedia.org/wiki/Dodo_bird_verdict. Accessed February 19, 2019.

Williman JP, Kvarnes RG: A medieval example of psychotherapy. Psychiatry 47(1):93–95, 198, 1984 6366859

Winston A, Rosenthal RN, Pinsker H: Learning Supportive Psychotherapy: An Illustrated Guide. Washington, DC, American Psychiatric Publishing, 2012

Zitrin CM, Klein DF, Woerner MG: Behavior therapy, supportive psychotherapy, imipramine, and phobias. Arch Gen Psychiatry 35(3):307–316, 1978 31847

2

The Supportive Relationship

We consider the supportive relationship or therapeutic alliance to be so important that it warrants placement in our second chapter. Without an alliance the patient will not benefit and is likely to leave the therapy anyway. (We should add: If they have a choice; in many of the settings we discuss, the patients may be detained or residential, and at most they can refuse to see or be minimally cooperative with the therapist but may not have a choice of another therapist.)

The relationship between therapist and patient is often said to have three related but nevertheless distinguishable aspects:

- The real relationship
- The working (or therapeutic) alliance
- The transferential relationship

In supportive psychotherapy, the real relationship is typically the major source of support, and it provides the underpinnings for the development of the other two aspects.

The Concept of Support

All forms of psychotherapy involve supportive elements that play a role in the success of the therapy (Luborsky 1984, p. 71), but these elements are paramount in supportive therapy. Not only is the supportive relationship between therapist and patient a vehicle for exchange of information between patient and therapist, but the relationship itself is of therapeutic benefit in other, nonspecific ways. To see this, it is important to define *support* so as to avoid misconceptions. A supportive relationship is not a friendship but may involve elements found in a friendship. One approach is Jerome Frank's paradigm of psychotherapy, consisting of four "common features" of all therapies (Frank 1975, pp. 124–125):

1. A structured, "trusting, confiding, emotional" relationship that boosts the patient's morale
2. A treatment setting with an aura of safety and sanctuary
3. A conceptual scheme or explanatory model for the patient's problems that provides a rationale for the patient's treatment and relief
4. Therapeutic procedures consistent with the conceptual scheme that relieve the patient's anxiety and encourage new behaviors

The first two elements provide the basis for a supportive relationship, engendering the emotional activation necessary for behavioral change and even more straightforward cognitive learning. The nonspecificity hypothesis of psychotherapeutic change holds that it is these nonspecific relational elements, cultivating an expectation of change, that are important in fostering that change.

This hypothesis has variants. For example, some proponents of nonspecificity hold that psychotherapy works solely because of faith or a placebo effect. Others hold that communication per se is of therapeutic benefit, regardless of content (Kaiser 1965). The latter claim is made within the context that it is the communicative aspects of the *relationship* that are therapeutic. Thus, although communication is one of the essential components of the supportive relationship, all aspects of the relationship should be viewed as the basis for therapeutic change. Using Frank's paradigm, one can say that the nonspecific supportive relationship makes possible some quite specific strategies of change (Parloff 1986):

- Reality testing and the learning of new coping behaviors
- Cognitive and experiential learning
- Enhancement of self-esteem through mastery, competence, success in the setting of therapy, and actual success

Whether one can add "significant personality change" to this list is controversial. The role of the supportive relationship in treating personality disorders is described in Chapter 10, so you may decide for yourself.

Support, therefore, can be thought of as a matrix in which more specific techniques of therapy can be embedded. A supportive relationship with one's patient may be therapeutic by itself, and in addition makes it possible to implement other specific techniques. Indeed, each of the three strategies just mentioned will be elaborated in the chapters that follow.

The desirable (and necessary), possible, and undesirable elements of a supportive relationship are presented in Tables 2–1, 2–2, and 2–3, respectively. Many (but not all) of these elements are applicable to all forms of psychotherapy. For the proper elements of supportive psychotherapy to flourish, the therapist must actively promote the development of the relationship. For example, a therapist might express concern for the patient rather than assume it is understood. This is an aspect of supportive therapy that creates uneasiness in some therapists who find it difficult to support a patient whom they do not intrinsically like as they would like a friend. Indeed, it often seems to supportive therapists that they are being called upon to "like" their patients in a demanding way. But "liking" within the context of a professional therapy does not demand the more exacting characteristics of being a friend. It requires a regard for the patient as an independent being and a willingness to support his personal growth. Liking, in this context, does not require admiration, but one can (and must) enjoy talking and listening to patients about their lives. For instance, a severely narcissistic person may be boring as a friend but intensely interesting if the therapist plays the professional role of exploring the patient's self-centered world, without expecting the mutuality of a friendship.

Another aspect of the supportive relationship is nurturing of the patient's healthy adaptive efforts. Like Alexander's concept of the corrective emotional experience (Alexander and French 1946), this embodies D. W. Winnicott's (1965) concepts of "holding environment" and "good-enough mothering." The good-enough therapist, like the good-enough mother, will sometimes be

Table 2–1.   Desirable elements of a supportive relationship

The setting allows for

A moderate to high level of activity in both participants

Therapeutic structure

Two-way communication

Adjunctive use of medication

Adjunctive use of other treatments and therapies

The therapist shows

An involved, active attitude

Willingness to develop and contribute to a real relationship

An attempt to develop a positive transference

Empathy and concern for the patient

Nonjudgmental acceptance of the patient's current state (i.e., tolerance)

Support of the patient's healthy adaptive efforts

Noncondemning, nonmoralizing responses to the patient's failures

Willingness to understand

Respect for the patient as a human being

Genuine interest in the patient's life activities and well-being

An attempt to like the patient and sometimes express that liking

Maximum allowance of the patient's autonomy to make treatment and life decisions

The patient shows

Willingness to speak about life events

Acceptance of the therapist's supportive role

Willingness to participate in the therapeutic program and adhere to the therapeutic structure

Table 2–2.   Elements of a supportive relationship that must be carefully controlled if present

Friendship

Uncritical agreement with the patient's view of himself or herself

Acceptance of delusional material

Acceptance of the patient's rationalizations for behavior and other defenses

Socialized and shared activities (meals, games, walks—depending on level of patient's function)

Therapist's relationship to the patient's family

Therapist's judicious self-disclosure

Direct gratifications such as verbal praise, gifts, or food

Sympathy

Humor

Casual physical contact

Benevolent direction of the patient's interests

Promotion of the patient's dependency (only as much as necessary to achieve goals of therapy and within ethical guidelines)

critical and "bad" in the patient's eyes but in the long run acts to foster the patient's healthy development and growth. Confrontation and criticism are an important part of supportive therapy, but they are always offered within the context of support.

The Working Alliance

In the previous section we introduced the supportive relationship: a real relationship between patient and therapist based on mutual respect, communication, and emotional involvement. However, as we noted previously, the supportive relationship is not simply friendship; it requires that therapist and patient share attitudes regarding the goals of treatment and the roles each plays—for example, the therapist as helper and the patient as being helped—to achieve

Table 2–3.   Nonsupportive elements in a relationship

Inactive therapist

Unstructured relationship

Undue influence on the patient's life

Romantic or sexual involvement

Pity

True peer relationship

Humoring the patient or the patient's family

Talking down to the patient

Tacit collusion or mutual avoidance of areas that need to be explored

Receiving or giving gratifications that do not serve a therapeutic purpose

those goals. This aspect of the relationship has been called the *therapeutic alliance* (Zetzel 1956) or the *working alliance* (Greenson 1967).

You may be well versed in your role as helper, but your patient may be unable to appreciate it, especially in the midst of psychosis. For the patient to assume the corresponding role of being helped, some therapists think that a certain amount of abstractive or self-distancing ability is required. Therefore, such therapists think it is less likely for chronically ill patients with social skills deficits to sustain a therapeutic alliance. We need to remember, however, that all patients (as well as therapists) play multiple roles during therapy. You can, for example, remind a patient in the midst of a psychotic crisis of the working alliance: "I'm not trying to hurt you. I'm your therapist and I want to help." Similarly, psychotic patients in therapy may disregard reality in most of their transactions but still accept the physician's prescriptions and advice.

The therapeutic alliance has also been considered to be one of the so-called nonspecific factors in the success of therapy, and empirical measures of this alliance have even been used as predictors of success (Luborsky 1976, cited in Rockland 1989). For example, a study by Horowitz et al. (1984, cited in Rockland 1989) supports the correlation of positive therapeutic alliance and positive outcome in bereaved patients with low (and not in those with high) motivation, suggesting that an overly positive relationship may make it difficult for the patient to express negative affect. Such studies point to the need for flexibility both in establishing relationships with and in maintaining distance from patients. The therapeutic alliance is not necessarily a positive one but simply the understood sharing of the goals of therapy. This is one of the reasons that the therapist must be counseled against turning the supportive relationship into a friendship in which the patient gets the message that the therapist would like to "hear no evil."

Transference

Transference is defined as the process that leads to attitudes, assumptions, and feelings in the patient that are outgrowths of the patient's earlier relationships with significant others, especially parents. As a result of this process, which is mostly unconscious, the patient may also replay or re-create emotional relationships from the past, using the therapist as a new object. Because supportive therapy is especially apt to re-create a parent-child pair, it is likely to rekindle both good and bad aspects of the patient's previous relationships with parents. Transference, positive or negative, is an emotional reenactment of the past in the present, providing a here-and-now relationship for interpretation in psychodynamic psychotherapy. In supportive therapy, transference is active and cannot be ignored. Its management, however, is a matter of considerable skill and judiciousness, at times leading to no intervention by the therapist beyond his own recognition, at other times leading to interpretation, but most often calling forth a management without interpretation. This balanced, or "managed," transference is detailed below.

Extremes of positive and negative transference in supportive therapy can be dangerous and detrimental, because the patient may act upon them. Physical (including sexual) assault or displaced destruction of the therapist's property (e.g., office or car) or of hospital property can occur. At the other end of the scale, erotomania, rejection dysphoria, or dysfunctional dependence can result.

Transferences are sometimes very important to recognize when you are formulating the patient's difficulties. Although transference manifestations are not part of any DSM-5 (American Psychiatric Association 2013) criteria set, they can form a major understanding of the patient's disorder.

Table 2–4.   Elements of the managed transference

Adjustment without interpretation of the patient's extreme misperceptions

Regulation of distance between therapist and patient

Judicious self-disclosure

Generation of consistent expectations

It should be kept in mind that transferences are usually mixed emotions—and, by definition, are initially unconscious. Although a patient may be expressing only a positive transference, for example, there are likely to be some negative feelings. (For a classical discussion of this point, see Brenner 1982.) When the patient's transference is extremely negative or has some other very substantial anti-therapeutic thrusts, the therapist will have to use techniques that restore a therapeutic relationship, as described in the next section.

Managed Transference

The best approach to transference is to maintain a balanced, or *managed*, transference involving the following elements: 1) adjustment without interpretation of the patient's extreme misperceptions, 2) regulation of distance between therapist and patient, 3) judicious self-disclosure, and 4) generation of consistent expectations (Table 2–4). Extremes of positive and negative transference must always be addressed, although in general they must not be interpreted in relation to unconscious determinants. For example, "upwards interpretations" can be made of erotic feelings in the transference. It is often safe to leave a mildly positive transference entirely alone, but a negative one must be managed, although not interpreted. Management without interpretation involves recognizing, acknowledging, and addressing those feelings of the patient you believe are transferential and making necessary adjustments to restore the patient's sense of reality, without interpreting the patient's feelings as transferential per se.

Distance between patient and therapist must also be regulated to meet the former's needs. This involves being prepared to change the frequency of meetings and the duration of sessions. You must also avoid generating expectations of gratifications and then failing to follow up on them. If you say, "I'll always be available when you need me," and then go on a 6-week vacation, you may encounter upon return a highly disturbed patient. It is better to say, more accurately, "The clinic will always be here when you need it," drawing on the strength of the institutional transference (Grotjahn and Wells 1989). If you are in private practice, we hope you can assure the patient that there is always a competent therapist covering the practice in your absence. Some patients (especially those with schizophrenia) are threatened by a potentially close relationship. Others (especially some with borderline personality disorder) will use a close relationship manipulatively. Despite these pitfalls, the supportive relationship should be as close as possible. Although Bloch (1979) cites the turnover of therapists as a reason for maintaining a more distant relationship, in the practice of therapy in public clinics most of us establish a close and warm relationship (if appropriate to the patient), despite its ultimate termination and the constant threats of disruption and discontinuity inherent in the clinic setting.

Sometimes you may find it desirable to appear, as Freud put it, as a "blank screen" that the patient can fill with imagined characteristics or fantasies. More often, some self-disclosure is called for to burst the bubble of transference fantasies and is useful in the management of the extremes of transference such as when deflating an idealized transference. However, self-disclosure has its own dangers and fails to create the desired effect in many patients with impaired thinking. For example, knowing the therapist is married may not make her less of an erotic object, and it may create dangers to the therapist's family instead. Therapist self-disclosure must therefore be carefully controlled and based on the patient's history of reality testing, not the therapist's current assessment of the patient, who could temporarily be functioning very well. In general, details of the therapist's personal relationships should be avoided. Some shared knowledge is useful. Talking about common interests such as sports, hiking, movies, books, and the weather can maintain the relationship without making it too personal.

Psychotic Transference

Broadly defined, psychotic transferences occur when patients develop delusional beliefs about their therapists. A psychotic transference may occur when a patient loses her sense of reality and experiences the therapist as identical to some real or imagined significant other. One can often, but not always, anticipate such developments. For example, a cognitively intact but psychotic patient may ask a new therapist, "Weren't you my doctor before?" or remark that the doctor looks like a relative or lover. In such cases, the therapist can empathetically acknowledge the patient's perception without agreeing with implications of this perception. "Perhaps I look like a doctor you used to know. What was his name? How did he treat you? But I'm not that same doctor, because I wasn't working at this office last year." Implicit in the patient's question is a wish or fear about the current treatment. The expression of a delusion may be a covert request to be told what is real or a request for assurance that the fears represented by that delusion are illusory. The therapist must exercise skill in choosing a response (Searles 1963). Although psychotic transferences are often positive, they are all potentially dangerous in that they involve the loss of reality testing.

Some patients, usually those with severe schizophrenia or dementia, cannot form any relationship, real or transferential. However, even some supposedly "unreachable" patients can develop a treatment relationship with their caregiving institution, as discussed in the next subsection.

Institutional Transference

Institutional transference has been defined as the patient's transference to the corporate or collective treating institution. It is considered a transference because it involves a parental personalization of the institution, and like other transferences, it may be positive or negative.

If positive, it provides continuity for a patient being seen in a setting with frequent therapist turnover. The treating institution is abstract and general enough that the patient often uses it projectively, as will be discussed below. At one extreme, the institutional transference (and the patient's relationship with her impersonal therapist) can be so sustaining as to support a clinic model, in which the patient is seen by a different therapist every time (Bloch 1979; Daniels et al. 1968). The patient's perception of the institution as almost omnipotent but impersonal can be beneficial for grandiose patients who identify with sources of power, as well as those who cannot acknowledge dependence on an individual therapist (Safirstein 1968). The stability of care in the hospital system can also be emphasized when therapy with an individual therapist must be terminated.

The therapist will often hear patients say that they hate the clinic but like the therapist, or vice versa. Opinions about the clinic (or other treating personnel) may represent splitting or a safer displacement of negative attitudes toward the therapist onto others in the clinic. Given the aforementioned dangers of a negative transference to the therapist, it may be best to leave negative institutional transference uninterpreted. Negative transference to specific staff, however, must be explored (not interpreted) at face value because it can pose a danger.

Managing Dependency and Entitlement

Dependency and entitlement occur in all forms of psychotherapy and can be problematic in supportive psychotherapy because of the emphasis on the real relationship between therapist and patient. Dependency, however, is less objectionable and may be unavoidable and permanent, as in an impaired patient who requires indefinite therapy. All dependency is not undue dependency, and it may be the necessary vehicle by which the patient learns the meaning of trust and a model for future trusting relationships (Mendel and Green 1967).

Entitlement, on the other hand, connotes the expectation of attention and services that are inappropriate. Yet therapists should not believe that any dependency, once granted, will turn into an entitlement. Indeed, patients, like children, can be pampered or spoiled, but they also require nurturance at appropriate times in order to grow up or out of therapy. Therefore, the therapist should expect to regulate the amount of dependency or expressed entitlement as the patient progresses or regresses in therapy. It is by no means impossible for the therapist to wean the patient from already claimed entitlements and "special privileges" when the patient is ready for it, explaining the rationale in terms of the patient's further growth.

Countertransference

Countertransference has a number of specific meanings arising from psychoanalytic theory. Originally, it was used to denote the therapist's projections onto the patient of unconscious attitudes and feelings. However, we will use the term in its common, broad definition today, by which it denotes *all* the therapist's feelings toward a patient. These feelings bear scrutiny; close examination not only may avoid substantive impediments to the therapeutic process but also may suggest the patient's interpersonal pathology. Properly attended, counter-transference yields insight into the patient's experience. For example, repugnance can be helpful in assessing the antisocial or sadistic nature of a patient's behavior. A depressed patient makes you feel sad. Feeling manipulated often suggests personality disorder and especially borderline traits. There is also a particular recognition of bizarreness and unrelatedness that clinicians have called the "praecox feeling," suggestive of *dementia praecox* (i.e., schizophrenia) (Rümke 1960). Such feelings, although tentative, can often be validated by reference to other staff treating the patient. Finding that many staff have had the same reaction to a patient can, at times, be extremely important in the management of the patient.

Case Vignette

A therapist found that he did not want to see a smart, well-meaning, depressed accountant and that others in the clinic did not like the patient either. Everyone working with the patient, it turned out, found his circumstantial and controlling style very annoying. Eventually, this observation turned out to be more useful to the patient than the information that had led to his diagnosis of dysthymia, because it was the patient's controlling style of behavior and the problems it caused him that were behind the development of his depression.

Thus, it is useful in supervision or in team meetings to openly discuss one's feelings about the patient. In these discussions, one needs to take an objective, nonjudgmental approach that assumes everyone has feelings that are useful, not shameful.

Finally, it is worth mentioning a kind of comprehensive way to use your countertransference to determine the goals of therapy. "What would the therapist do if he or she were in the patient's body, exactly in his or her present position, but with the therapist's capacity to assess the situation and the knowledge of what he or she could do to improve it?" (Kernberg 2018, p. 134).

All countertransference feelings are relational, but for clarity of exposition they can be divided into those that are predominantly caused by factors within the therapist, the patient, or the therapy itself (see Table 2–5).

Table 2–5. Causes of countertransference

Within the therapist

Different cultural background from patient ("mainstream" therapist/minority patient or minority therapist/"mainstream" patient)

Mutual blind spots shared with the patient (arising from similar personal or cultural assumptions)

Romanticizing of mental illness in general

Idealized perception of role as healer and helper

Inadequate understanding of the patient's disease process

Transferential elements in the therapist's past (patient evokes relationship with significant others in the therapist's past)

Resentment if patient pays low or no fee

Pity

Unresolved issues in the therapist's life (especially death and disability)

Overidentification and sympathy in place of empathy

Within the patient

Symptomatic behavior

Primitive affect

Criminal behavior or other antisocial traits

Lack of insight

Repetitive failures in coping

Intelligence and verbal ability different from therapist's

Lack of motivation

Noncompliance with medication

Noncompliance with other prescribed therapies

Failure to follow therapist's advice

Hurtful behavior toward family members

Dependent traits (see below)

Poor hygiene and self-care

Patient's use of public funds

Table 2–5.   Causes of countertransference *(continued)*

Within the therapy

Dependency on the therapist

Anger and/or hostility toward therapist

Paranoid or threatening behavior

Manipulation

Splitting

"Acting out" in the therapy

"Acting out" outside the therapy

Time demands on the therapist (e.g., the "difficult" patient)

Stress in the therapeutic session

Real relationship with the therapist that is too intense

Countertransference includes such rational reactions as fear when a patient becomes threatening and satisfaction when a patient gets a new job. Other reactions are understandable but detrimental to the therapy. For example, a young therapist who feels like a child with an older patient (who has assigned the therapist that role) will assume a less active and more acquiescent stance that makes it difficult for the patient to experience the therapy as supportive. When the therapist feels he is experiencing feelings beyond the scope of the supportive relationship as it has been defined, a general approach is to consult Table 2–5 after such sessions for suggestions as to the source of these countertransference feelings. Nearly every issue listed in the table can be addressed by the therapist's insight or as an intervention at the next session.

It is difficult, of course, for a therapist to appreciate countertransference patterns that are primarily unconscious and developmental in origin. However, paying attention to one's *behavior* toward patients will bring many such patterns to light, as when one notices that one is replaying patterns of juvenile competition or sadistic relationships with siblings.

Countertransference factors originating primarily in the patient include the patient's symptomatic behavior itself, particularly the display of irrational cognitive processes or the range of primitive affects that the therapist may encounter (Wallace 1983, p. 346). The therapist can expect to witness affects expressive of aggression (murderous rage, derision, contempt), sexuality (seductiveness, sexual advances, and various autoerotic behaviors such as masturbation), and dependent/oral behaviors. If the affect is threatening to the therapist, she must understand why. Often, the uneasiness arises because such affects, were they to occur in the therapist's ordinary social relationships, would be signals for permanent breakdown of the relationship. They do not, however, necessarily have that meaning in a therapeutic relationship.

A somewhat less threatening affect, boredom, arises frequently in all types of therapy, but the supportive psychotherapist might be tempted to attribute it to the supposedly mundane or prosaic nature of the work. Rarely is this the case. Often boredom is generated because the patient is avoiding productive therapeutic work and/or obscuring feelings in a wealth of detail, as might the depressed accountant mentioned above. Or the therapist may be bored because he is at the limits of his abilities and cannot move the therapy onward. Most understandable and yet most serious, we think, is boredom that arises from the therapist's attempt to distance himself from the patient's suffering so as to take an uninvolved and "Who cares?" attitude that will certainly not improve the therapy.

Burnout

Burnout is a complex syndrome that can affect all workers in the helping professions. The somatic factors of burnout have even been characterized in a manner that sounds like a DSM-5 disorder: exhaustion, fatigue, irritability, gastrointestinal upset, insomnia, dysphoria, anxious feelings, cynicism, and lack of curiosity (Caton 1984). Burnout is a major issue for all clinicians, but especially for nurses and physicians, whose burnout rate is twice as high as that in other professions (Babyar 2017). If use of electronic medical records is part of the reason, you can point out to your hierarchy the huge drop (53% to 13%) in the sense of burnout when staff are hired to focus on record management, leaving clinicians more time to do therapy (Wright and Katz 2018). We consider burnout, less somatically, to be *the loss of meaning or pleasure in the experience of one's helping capacity*. Specific attitudinal countertransference problems and approaches to avoiding burnout in each of these cases are given in Table 2–6. Burnout, however, is not necessarily a countertransference syndrome, and its causes appear to reside in broad system factors that influence both physician wellness and patient care (Pollock 2018):

These include the following physician factors:

- Learning/practice environment
- Organizational factors
- Regulatory business and payer environment
- Sociocultural factors

These factors include the following more specific factors:

- Health care role
- Personal factors
- Skills and abilities

Burnout from the system needs to be addressed with changes in that system. Predisposing factors include excess patient loads, overwork with an excess zeal, and the neglect of personal growth. Some staff claim burnout but use it as an excuse for failure to address possible avenues of change. They may be involved in such work for the wrong reasons. Associating with "burned out" staff can easily defeat the enthusiasm of the beginning therapist. Unfortunately, staff may be burned out from and "burned up" at the structural, bureaucratic aspects of their work. Systemic problems may seem unchangeable for the psychiatrist treating the patients. In these circumstances, the best morale booster may be to create a climate of professional growth for oneself: "I have an impossible task, but I am learning skills that will serve me well in the future."

Burnout from the content of therapy may be addressed through considering countertransference issues. For example, in working with schizophrenia patients, the following reactions may contribute to burnout (Minkoff and Stern 1985):

- Devaluing patients with chronic disease
- Overvaluing the effectiveness of therapy, either psychotherapy or pharmacotherapy
- Attributing the illness and lack of progress to the patient
- Attempting to effect an acute cure
- Experiencing difficulty empathizing with hopelessness

Table 2–6. Avoiding countertransference burnout

Attitude	Approach to solution
"I must personally cure my patient."	Although it is a genuine pleasure to be solely responsible for someone's cure, neither cure nor total credit for it is possible in most supportive work. The therapist must accept his or her role on a treatment team offering long-term interventions.
"My chronic patients do not appreciate me."	This is likely to reflect poor therapeutic technique. Patients in supportive therapy are usually extremely appreciative of help, and the greater reality of the relationship offers the therapist satisfactions that are not available in psychoanalytic work.
"Supportive therapy is not real psychotherapy."	Supportive therapy encompasses many psychodynamic methods but also includes behavioral, cognitive, and educational techniques.
"I don't know what to do."	Supportive methods have not been as widely taught as psychodynamic technique. Therapists may feel uneasy at first to offer advice, direction, and education.
"Despite all my work, my patients do not change. I am a failure."	Significant change occurs in all therapies. However, there has been a historical tendency to overvalue insight at the expense of behavioral change.
"It's depressing to deal with all these hopeless patients all day."	Developing a better "patient mix" can provide variety for the therapist. In addition, the therapist must have significant time with colleagues.
"My supervisor doesn't devote any attention to the chronic patients."	The therapist may need to experiment with different supervisors until one is found who can impart enthusiasm as well as specific strategies for supportive work.
"My patients do not want to get well."	It depends on the patient. Many patients in psychoanalysis also have a great resistance to improvement. The therapist must appreciate that mental illness can affect the ability to make even self-interested judgments.

Table 2–6.   Avoiding countertransference burnout *(continued)*

Attitude	Approach to solution
"When I lose a patient, it hurts too much."	All therapy involves significant emotional investment that must be balanced by professional detachment and flexibility. But the therapist who can make such investments is rewarded by having genuine encounters with other people.

Source.   Information based in part on Minkoff and Stern 1985.

These reactions are not limited to schizophrenia, of course, and can often be dealt with through better preparation of staff and trainees regarding the realistic prognosis of patients.

The American Psychiatric Association (2019) has a resource site addressing burnout, especially as it affects psychiatrists.

Key Points

- It is important to review the desirable (and necessary), possible, and undesirable elements of a supportive relationship.

- A supportive relationship has a real aspect, transferential qualities, and a therapeutic alliance.

- Transference is the process that leads to attitudes, assumptions, and feelings in the patient that grow out of the patient's earlier relationships with significant others.

- The supportive therapist must use skill in deciding whether or not and when to interpret the transference so as to create a balance or managed transference.

- Countertransference denotes all the therapist's feeling toward the patient.

- Burnout is a common problem when therapists lose their enthusiasm, efficiency, and ability to cope with the requirements and stresses of performing psychotherapy.

References

Alexander F, French TM: Psychoanalytic Therapy: Principles and Applications. New York, Ronald Press, 1946

American Psychiatric Association: Diagnostic and Statistical Manual of Mental Disorders, 5th Edition. Arlington, VA, American Psychiatric Association, 2013

American Psychiatric Association: Well-being and burnout. Available at: https://www.psychiatry.org/psychiatrists/practice/well-being-and-burnout. Accessed March 14, 2019.

Babyar JC: They did not start the fire: reviewing and resolving the issue of physician stress and burnout. J Health Organ Manag 31(4):410–417, 2017 28877620

Bloch S: Supportive psychotherapy, in An Introduction to the Psychotherapies. Edited by Bloch S. New York, Oxford University Press, 1979, pp 196–220

Brenner C: The Mind in Conflict. New York, International Universities Press, 1982

Caton CLM: Management of Chronic Schizophrenia. New York, Oxford University Press, 1984

Daniels R, Draper E, Rada R: Training in the adaptive psychotherapies. Compr Psychiatry 9(4):383–391, 1968 5665471

Frank JD: General psychotherapy: the restoration of morale, in American Handbook of Psychiatry, 2nd Edition, Vol 5: Treatment. Edited by Freedman DX, Dyrud JE (Arieti S, editor in chief). New York, Basic Books, 1975, pp 117–132

Greenson RR: The Technique and Practice of Psychoanalysis, Vol 1. New York, International Universities Press, 1967

Grotjahn M, Wells PH: Schizophrenogenic trends in therapy. Voices (reprinted from Voices, Vol 3, no 2, 1967). Journal of the American Academy of Psychotherapists 25(1–2):47–50, 1989

Horowitz MJ, Marmar C, Weiss DS, et al: Brief psychotherapy of bereavement reactions: the relationship of process to outcome. Arch Gen Psychiatry 41(5):438–448, 1984 6721669

Kaiser H: The universal symptom of the psychoneuroses: a search for the conditions of effective psychotherapy, in Effective Psychotherapy: The Contribution of Hellmuth Kaiser. Edited by Fierman LB. New York, Free Press, 1965, pp 14–171

Kernberg OF: Treatment of Severe Personality Disorders: Resolution of Aggression and Recovery of Eroticism. Washington, DC, American Psychiatric Association Publishing, 2018

Luborsky L: Helping alliances in psychotherapy, in Successful Psychotherapy. Edited by Claghorn JL. New York, Brunner/Mazel, 1976, pp 92–116

Luborsky L: Principles of Psychoanalytic Psychotherapy: A Manual for Supportive-Expressive Treatment. New York, Basic Books, 1984

Mendel WM, Green GA: The Therapeutic Management of Psychological Illness: The Theory and Practice of Supportive Care. New York, Basic Books, 1967, pp 36–44

Minkoff K, Stern R: Paradoxes faced by residents being trained in the psychosocial treatment of people with chronic schizophrenia. Hosp Community Psychiatry 36(8):859–864, 1985 4029911

Parloff MB: Psychotherapy outcome research (Chapter 11), in Psychiatry, Revised Edition, Vol 1. Edited by Michels R, Cavenar JO Jr, Brodie HKH, et al. Philadelphia, PA, JB Lippincott, 1986

Pollock D: Broad system factors influence physician wellness, patient care. Psychiatric News 53(6):4–5, 2018

Rockland LH: Supportive Psychotherapy: A Psychodynamic Approach. New York, Basic Books, 1989

Rümke HC: Contradictions in the concepts of schizophrenia. Compr Psychiatry 1:331–337, 1960 13744709

Safirstein SL: Psychiatric aftercare in a general hospital: a system of prevention in the community. Psychother Psychosom 16(1):17–22, 1968 4304940

Searles HF: Transference psychosis in the psychotherapy of chronic schizophrenia. Int J Psychoanal 44:249–281, 1963 13987538

Wallace ER: Dynamic Psychiatry in Theory and Practice. Philadelphia, PA, Lea & Febiger, 1983

Winnicott DW: The Maturational Process and the Facilitating Environment: Studies in the Theory of Emotional Development. London, Hogarth Press/Institute of Psycho-analysis, 1965

Wright AA, Katz IT: Beyond burnout—redesigning care to restore meaningful sanity for physicians. N Engl J Med 378(4):309–311, 2018 29365301

Zetzel ER: Current concepts of transference. Int J Psychoanal 37(4–5):369–376, 1956 13366506

3

Principles of
Supportive Technique:
Explanatory Techniques

In this chapter we introduce the principles of supportive technique, many of which are used in other therapies as well. Those that are used most frequently can be divided into two types: *explanatory* (Table 3–1) and *directive*. Explanatory techniques will be detailed here, and directive techniques will be covered in Chapter 4. Techniques used primarily in psychodynamic therapies and much less frequently in supportive therapy (see Table 3–2) are covered in standard textbooks and will receive minimal discussion here.

Spectrum of Explanatory Techniques

It can be helpful to think of different explanatory techniques as functioning at different depths, beginning at the surface and working at ever deeper levels. For our purposes, we have defined three levels of techniques. The first level encompasses *basic communicative techniques*. One of these, *managing the transfer-*

Table 3–1. Major techniques of supportive psychotherapy: explanatory techniques

First level: communication

Managing the transference[a]

Talking to the patient[b]

Listening to the patient[b]

Generating and conveying empathy[b]

Helping the patient to test reality

Reassuring (its cognitive aspects)

Observing

Expressing interest and concern

Echoing

Tracking

Commenting

Restating

Eliciting current life reports (here-and-now emphasis)

Encouraging ventilation and expression of affect (balance with control of affect, a directive technique)

Second level: confrontation

Directing attention to inconsistencies in behavior

Directing attention to conflicting goals and motivations

Third level: clarification, explanation, and interpretation

Clarification (of information available to the patient but of which he or she is not aware)

Explanation (of mechanisms responsible for patient's behavior)

Benign projections and introjections

Table 3–1. Major techniques of supportive psychotherapy: explanatory techniques *(continued)*

Third level: clarification, explanation, and interpretation *(continued)*

Interpretations

- Defenses

- Limited and on the surface

- Inexact, incomplete, and upwards

- Avoided, delayed, softened, and controlled

- Displaced, universalized, generalized, normalized, and metaphorical

- Of transference (limited)

- Of dreams (limited)

Association of past to present activity (genetic and pseudointerpretations)

Miscellaneous explanatory techniques

- Psychodynamic life narrative

- Induced dichotomy of personality

^aDiscussed in Chapter 2. ^bDiscussed in this chapter.

Table 3–2. Techniques of supportive psychotherapy that are for limited or occasional use

Anonymous therapist	Deep interpretations
Abstinence, neutral attitude	Anxiety-provoking interpretations
Therapeutic or "technical" neutrality	Weakening of defenses
Total professional detachment	Encouragement of fantasy
Blank screen	Daydreams
Uninvolved, inactive attitude	Free association
Deep or genetic interpretations of transference	Relationship of current to unconscious content
Dream associations or analysis	Encouragement of regression

ence, was discussed in Chapter 2. Managing the transference has been classified as a communicative technique because it involves conveying attitudes and information to the patient to maintain a positive relationship. For example, one of the ways the transference is managed is by the therapist's judicious self-disclosure to prevent the development of fantasies by the patient. Other communicative techniques will be discussed throughout this chapter.

As you begin to deal with inconsistencies in your patient's behavior and to make your patient aware of discrepancies between his stated goals and actions, you may employ the second level of technique, that of *confrontation.* At the third level, you offer *clarification, explanation, and interpretation* of your patient's behavior. These two deeper levels of technique will be discussed later on in this chapter.

As in selection of therapeutic goals, use of a technique should not be an all-or-none decision, but instead a matter of relative emphasis. Not all techniques will be used with any one individual, but apparently contradictory techniques (e.g., the expression of affect and the control of affect) could be used at different times depending on the context. However, long-term supportive therapy is likely to utilize, at some time or other, a majority of the techniques discussed in this chapter and in Chapters 4 and 5.

To use explanatory (*or* directive) techniques successfully, you must be aware at all times of the goals of therapy for the particular patient. Such goals will differ and evolve with each treatment plan, but you should recall the general definition of supportive psychotherapy given in Chapter 1 and the more specific goals of this approach (see Table 1–2). Many of these goals, such as maximizing the environmental supports of medication and family, are covered in separate chapters. To show how techniques are adapted to goals, however, we shall turn now to several concepts fundamental to supportive psychotherapy.

Fundamental Concepts in Supportive Technique

Reality Testing

The philosophical question What is reality? has no obvious answer, but it *is* obvious that we each perceive and understand the world in different ways. For example, we know all too well that events that have been observed by many witnesses will be interpreted differently, even when the individuals are under oath.

Similarly, the worlds of our patients are different from our world as therapists. Indeed, in traditional psychiatric classifications, the hallmark of psychotic illness is disturbance in reality testing, manifested by alterations in perception (hallucinations) and belief (delusions) that cannot be validated by independent observers of the same culture. However, this distinction, although valid, is not absolute. Most psychiatric problems, including neurotic behavior, phobias, and depression, involve distortions in worldview. Pathological thought processes—those that do not follow accepted manners of reasoning and consideration of evidence—result in pathological beliefs, and, in recognition of this, many modes of therapy, such as cognitive therapy for depression, presume that a patient can change the inferences and conclusions he reaches based on basic perceptual experience.

If the patient's world is pathologically distorted, you should help to correct his view and possibly help him understand how the distortion came about. This means that you may have to compensate for his deficits, either temporarily or indefinitely. This function involves helping the patient to test his own version of reality, correcting it as necessary. In psychoanalytic terms, this aspect of therapy can be considered to be "lending ego." For example, one may need to validate or disagree with specific perceptions of the world and their consequences (Werman 1984).

Sometimes, this reality-enhancing work is simply a matter of supplying the patient with missing information. A patient who is fearful of riding the bus, for example, may simply need some help in learning what the fare is and what stops to use. Another patient, burdened by a major depression, may be helped by knowing that there is a likelihood that medication will relieve it.

A further step is to involve the patient in activities that lead to greater opportunities and satisfactions in life. She may need guidance or encouragement in the following:

- Learning new skills
- Trying out new behaviors and experiences
- Overcoming avoidant or phobic behaviors toward feared situations
- Giving up dysfunctional behaviors
- Thinking about herself in more positive terms

Defenses

So far, your role might seem simple and limited to that of educator, teacher, and guide, and you should perform such functions when needed for the patient's progress. But a few hours (or even minutes) of therapy invariably reveals obstacles to such progress, because patients' existing adaptations to reality are, ironically, resistant to further adaptation. Patients are often unwilling to learn new ways of perceiving, believing, and behaving, because they are defended against doing so.

Psychological defenses are usually portrayed as unconscious mechanisms of thought or action wielded to ward off internal or external threats causing dysphoric affect (e.g., anxiety, sadness). To tackle defenses in supportive psychotherapy without invoking the rest of the traditional Freudian structural apparatus of ego, id, and superego might seem inappropriate. In justifying this approach, one can point out that defenses are less theoretical entities than the Freudian structural components and can be sufficiently appreciated as interpersonal adaptations rather than intrapsychic ones (see, e.g., Swanson 1988). All "normal" individuals employ complex patterns of defenses that can be observed in their verbalizations and other behaviors. Defenses have even been empirically validated and placed in a hierarchy (Vaillant 1988; see Table 3–3), which provides an indication, if only probabilistic, of relative dysfunctionality. Dysfunctionality, however, is often a matter of degree. Highly functional and well-adapted people are not without their moments of denial, projection, splitting, and regression—defenses in the low-functioning constellation. Similarly, humor can be cruel and sadistic or gentle and provocative. Rationalization, a defense in the middle constellation, can flout the laws of logic in a psychotic individual or be scholastically compelling in the obsessive-compulsive person. So the dysfunction expressed and created by a defense varies considerably and should be assessed from a perspective that encompasses the patient's overall functioning. Because most defenses involve repression (i.e., exclusion from conscious awareness), the nature of the repressed content usually affects the seriousness of the defense. Thus, a patient who forgets her own identity has chosen (if unconsciously) a more significant object than the patient who forgets his anniversary.

The wholesale reconstruction of psychological defenses, involving no doubt a Herculean renovation of character and personality, is clearly too daunting a

Table 3–3. Psychological defenses: a convenient classification

Mature defenses	Low-level defenses
Altruism	*In beliefs*
Affiliation	Splitting
Self-assertion	Dissociation
Self-observation	Projective identification
Suppression	Somatization
Sublimation	Rationalization
Humor	Autistic fantasy
Intermediate defenses	*Action*
Obsessional	Passive aggression
Intellectualization	Repression of major memories
Isolation	Running away, stopping the
Isolation of affects	input, leaving the therapy
Undoing	session, or terminating
	therapy
Other so-called neurotic	*Negating and delusional*
Repression of minor memories	Psychotic denial
Reaction formation	Delusion
Dissociation	Denial (of external reality)
Displacement	Major distortion (of external reality)
Narcissistic	Fabrication
Omnipotence	Pathological lying
Idealization	
Devaluation of others	

Source. Based on Di Riso et al. 2011, p. 62; the 7-level Defense Mechanism Rating Scale (Perry 1994); and Vaillant 1988, p. 203. We have added some of the lowest-level defenses seen in supportive therapy patients.

task for any therapist. However, the supportive therapist can certainly improve a patient's defensive structure, even if by some judicious sweeps under the rug. Moreover, you need not expect your patient to rearrange his defenses through intellectual insight or through a sudden grasp of understanding that results in quick change. Rather, you can assist by modifying his defenses and behaviors a little bit at a time. Patience and repetition, as in so many aspects of supportive psychotherapy, are required here as well. Even highly psychotic individuals, who are besieged by an internal barrage of perceptions, feelings, and desires, do not engage in continuous, unrestrained sexual and aggressive activity. They retain, as everyone does, a variety of defenses to support their self-esteem and maintain appropriate behaviors, and these defenses can be improved. For example, a person who has been acting defensively and fearfully against a nonexistent threat can learn, in time, to give up that defense or substitute a less disabling one.

We mention this because some practitioners of supportive psychotherapy would not engage in any work whatsoever on psychological defenses. That is a more limited conception of the therapy than the one we use. One mental health provider, actually the medical director of a large medical system, urges community mental health providers not to give up on the interpretation of defenses but to understand that insight might take a laborious process with a lot of oscillation back and forth between the external world and inner awareness (Hoffman 2002).

Later in this chapter we discuss more specific techniques to use when faced with a patient who has substantially dysfunctional defenses. However, you should know now what to do when you notice a dysfunctional defense. Your initial goal should be to *learn more* about the patient's general pattern of defenses, rather than to criticize the specific defense. Because attacking (or even appearing to attack) defenses creates anxiety that is disturbing to patients whose defensive structures and personalities are already deficient, criticisms as well as interpretations of defenses must be offered carefully to blunt their full force. Defenses can sometimes be changed piecemeal, but you will need a holistic view of the patient's defensive patterns backed up by an in-depth understanding of psychological defense processes. In the initial psychiatric assessment and sessions that follow, you must construct in your own mind a view of the patient's adaptive hierarchy of defenses (Wallace 1983, pp. 349–350).

Distortions of Reality

A major issue with many patients concerns the distortions of reality that take the form of ideas of reference and delusions as well as other distortions that cannot quite be placed under these two rubrics. Although we describe the management of these distortions in subsequent chapters on specific psychiatric disturbances (e.g., schizophrenia in Chapter 6), there are some general aspects to the process that should be known in advance.

The distortions of patients can apply to themselves, to others, or to the surrounding world. For example, people frequently misinterpret natural events for defensive purposes, and their most significant distortions involve interpretations of human action. We make errors in the attribution of motives to ourselves and others because making such attributions is difficult, even in ideal circumstances for a disinterested observer. Startling cases of false attribution of motives in normal individuals can be created by posthypnotic suggestion. For example, Aronson (1988, p. 114) describes an individual who follows a hypnotist's suggestion to buy a bottle of liquor at a distant store and then offers various rationalizations for the action even though the person had no such motives at the time. Despite the contrived nature of hypnosis, such an example can be used to argue that self-justification processes are often highly irrational and biased by personal need, in particular the need to appear to others as a consistent, rational person! As nature is said to abhor a vacuum, we cannot tolerate our own irrationality and fill it with motives, often spurious and ad hoc. Frequently, delusions arise after the fact—that is, as post hoc explanations of events that cannot be assimilated by other explanations.

Just as motives attributed to oneself can be mistaken, attributions to others are frequently distorted, often in the transferential relationship to the therapist. A patient may attribute motives to the therapist that are blatantly irrational but powerfully felt. For example, the patient may feel that the therapist is sexually interested in her if the therapist criticizes the patient's spouse. If the therapist has to leave a session early for an emergency, the patient may assume the therapist was bored. Whenever the therapist observes an attribution of motives to self or others (including the therapist), he has the opportunity to help the patient correct any distortion of reality by offering alternative explanations that are closer to the therapist's sense of what is occurring. This strategy is especially helpful with paranoid patients.

Paranoid distortions of reality are usually caused by the pathological operation of projection. The attribution of evil motives to others may be interpreted as an operation of the patient's projection of her own aggressive drives onto others. However, it is also partly the result of illogical generalization from a history of abuse and mistreatment. It is hard for the patient to trust, and often this is for good reasons. When the patient attributes motives or reasons for action to others, at first it is usually advisable not to weaken the defensive operation (i.e., projection) but to approach it as a cognitive error, suggesting that other motives might be operational.

Case Vignette

A paranoid woman complains bitterly of her mistreatment at work. She is not appreciated by her boss. In fact, there are two people who give her work and claim to be her boss. She confronts one of them and asks for a raise. In return, the raise is denied, but she gets a written review in which she is praised, and she is asked to defer her request until her review date. The patient feels discriminated against. The therapist discusses the patient's feeling of overwork and the lack of authority, and addresses the boss's position: The boss has been willing to praise the patient in writing in her permanent personnel record. Surely this carries more weight than the boss's evil thoughts, if any. Perhaps the patient is mistaken in thinking that her boss hates her, and if her boss likes her, the patient's constant complaining may make the situation worse.

A deep interpretation might eventually explain this behavior as the projection of the patient's own hatred onto her boss, but in supportive therapy the approach is to focus on an appreciation of the negative consequences of her actions. Also stressed is the patient's power to do well and get the raise or to antagonize the boss and get fired. Her paranoid helplessness is countered by a realistic appraisal of her power.

Case Vignette

A paranoid patient thinks that others are talking about him on the bus. Instead of immediately challenging the patient's perception, the therapist points out that no one has hurt the patient and no one has said anything to his face, and that the patient has the power to ignore them, a power that would illustrate his strength and self-control. Meanwhile, the therapist can continue to explore the reality of the delusion. The therapist does not agree with the delusion but simply explores its consequences and defuses the threat it represents.

Coping Behaviors

The term *coping behaviors* refers to the most observable type of defenses. Often, but not always, these defenses are appropriate to the situation or threat that evokes them. We will continue to use the term in this way, without implying a major distinction between the purposes of defenses and coping behaviors. One copes with an impending hurricane, for example, by purchasing supplies, boarding up the windows, and taking refuge inland with family. One may cope with a deep chest pain by attributing it to indigestion—often a fatal defense— yet denying the seriousness of one's heart attack after one is in the intensive care unit may serve to improve survival. Just as in an understanding of defenses, the therapist's appreciation of coping behaviors in context is vital to the modification of these behaviors in therapy.

A survey of schizophrenic outpatients, for example, classified coping behaviors into nine categories (Cohen and Berk 1985). Methods used appeared to vary with social and demographic variables such as sex, employment, and whether the patient lived alone. The results (Table 3–4) give the therapist much to consider. Certainly, these data show that patients are not indifferent to their symptoms and can be enlisted as willing allies with the therapist in acquiring more effective coping behaviors. (As we shall see in Chapter 9, the use of alcohol and drugs occurs much more frequently than this survey would imply, and one should expect that patients' answers to such surveys are biased by the need to appear socially acceptable.)

Reassurance and Enhancement of Self-Esteem

We have seen that psychological defenses, such as the posthypnotic rationalization mentioned earlier in this chapter, act to preserve and improve self-esteem. However, more direct bolstering of self-esteem is often necessary in supportive therapy, for the following reasons:

1. Improved self-esteem and its consequence, self-confidence, are recognized as factors that promote adequate performance (e.g., see Beck and Emery 1985, p. 76). A patient who gains in *realistic* self-esteem can therefore overcome previously disabling unrealistic fears.
2. "Disbelief in oneself" is a self-fulfilling prophecy of failure that in turn leads to even lower self-esteem.

Table 3–4. Coping behaviors in a sample of 86 outpatients with schizophrenia

Coping response	Percentage reporting
Fights back (trying to overpower unwanted thoughts)	25.4
Accepts symptoms and lives with them	17.5
Uses isolated diversion (e.g., TV, radio, eating, smoking)	16.5
Feels helpless	13.1
Naps, sleeps, meditates	7.9
Seeks medical assistance	7.8
Seeks social diversion	5.7
Uses prayer	4.5
Uses street drugs or alcohol	1.3

Source. Adapted from Cohen and Berk 1985.

3. The cognitive *anticipation of failure* can generate excess anxiety that impairs performance.

Self-esteem is probably altered in all illness—acute and chronic, physical and mental. Some patients, such as depressed or bereaved persons, have an obvious deficit in self-esteem, evidenced by their own self-deprecating remarks. Others, such as the grandiose manic or paranoid schizophrenic individual, express a highly inflated and delusional sense of self-worth. If one examines these expressions more closely, however, one often finds that they are compensations for lowered self-esteem at a deeper level. The grandiosity implicit in being the KGB's (now the FSB's) prime target is not as salient as the manic person's overt claim (and the narcissist's covert claim) that he is the smartest person in the world, but these claims have in common a distortion in self-image that needs realistic correction. Therefore, it is not contradictory to offer self-esteem-enhancing interpretations to grandiose patients. What these patients need is a new definition of self-esteem. They need the message that they are worthwhile human beings who do not need delusions in order to have that worth.

Enhancing self-esteem is therefore a general strategy for improving the patient's adaptation to her world. *Reassurance* involves more specific statements about the patient's beliefs and behaviors. It is an amalgam of reality testing and suggestion, which is why we have considered it to be both explanatory and directive. For example, reassurance may involve simply pointing out that the patient has been an effective parent, despite a recent setback. Usually it involves an emphasis on positive or hopeful elements in the patient's life that she may have neglected. This might include emphasis on the good prognosis for a physical illness or downplaying the duration of hospitalization or of mental or physical anguish. The therapist can provide what the patient lacks: the longer time perspective that makes suffering more endurable and happiness more tenable.

Reassurances are needed when a patient expresses a fear as an overgeneralization, such as in the following:

- "I'm going crazy."
- "I'll never leave the hospital."
- "Nobody will ever help me."
- "What in the world have I done with the last 10 years of my life?"
- "I'll be in pain forever."
- "My family will never forgive the crazy things I did."
- "My life will never return to normal."

The therapist must assess 1) the factual validity of the fear, which may range from imaginary to entirely justified; 2) its consequences, which may be overblown; and 3) its emotional validity, which should be acknowledged but not necessarily accepted at face value, either, because it may represent a displacement from another fear. For example, a patient may focus on physical complaints when the fear is not of the pain itself but of disfigurement from the operation. The therapist who responds too readily to the patient's stated fear may miss the unstated one.

Proper reassurance can reduce guilt for encountered loss. This is important in working with the schizophrenic patient who blames herself for her illness; it is equally important in the physically ill patient, even when by some measures the patient has contributed to his own illness, as in lung cancer and accidents that have resulted from intoxication. Alleviation of guilt raises self-esteem. It is proper to do so when dwelling on the past makes the patient worse.

Reassurances, as a function of reality testing, must of course be realistic, but they also should capitalize on the suggestive element and the expectation of positive outcome that were discussed earlier. When there is uncertainty in outcome, you may wish to emphasize the positive, rather than agree with your patient's stark appraisal of the facts. You should not offer hope against hope, but you can go a long way toward righting your patient's skewed apprehension of reality.

The utility of an informed reassurance cannot be overemphasized. However, bland reassurances, not based on an understanding relationship with the patient, are bound to be taken as insincere.

Self-esteem is ultimately enhanced through feedback to patients about their behavior as they are guided into increasingly productive and rewarding activities. This is the rationale behind the graded approach to community work through vocational skills training, industrial therapy assignments, and sheltered workshops. Competence, mastery, and success raise self-esteem more effectively than talk. One writer (who is a major proponent of supportive psychotherapy) uses the term *plussing* to refer to the positive comments and acknowledgments and points out, "Most patients with low self-esteem have defects in the ability to nurture or forgive themselves ('self-soothe')" (Battaglia 2007, p. 32). We also mentioned this defect (of self-soothing) in Chapter 1.

Explanatory Techniques

Communicative Techniques

How can you improve your patient's self-esteem and reality testing? This question brings us back to a discussion of the first level of supportive psychotherapy technique: communicative techniques. This begins by listening to the patient.

Personal listening begins by learning about a patient's life from his point of view and by beginning to develop feelings and reactions to the patient. One might compare this process to listening to a symphony without any knowledge of music theory.

Perhaps a component of personal listening would be what Harari (2014) calls "*emotionally attuned listening:* the doctor listens to the patient's story, the feelings the patient expresses and nonverbally communicates, and the doctor's own 'gut' responses. The unsaid is also important; thus, a medically ill patient who complains endlessly about treatment may be avoiding the frightening question 'am I going to die?'" (p. 440).

Professional listening consists in applying structures and categories to the patient's statements, just as a professional musician would discern the underlying themes and orchestration of a musical composition. Because a major task of supportive therapy is to strengthen and restructure the patient's defenses and coping behavior, you must begin to categorize (and formulate future questions about) the patient's defenses and coping styles. Your initial impression may have to change, but you should begin to see if the patient's defenses are, in general, primitive or sophisticated and more specific. Is the patient overly intellectual and indecisive, or impulsive and heedless of consequences? How does she explain or rationalize her behaviors? What motives does he attribute to others (using the defense mechanism of projection)? Although introductory texts often warn against premature interpretations, it should be emphasized that the professional work of listening is the basis for future targeted interventions, and it is what makes supportive therapy more than a succession of friendly chats.

It can be incredibly difficult simply to keep the communication going, but focusing on *current life reports* with a here-and-now emphasis can help. To ask the supportive therapy patient "What's been happening in your life?" is definitely better than silence and usually better than the anxiety-provoking "How shall we use the time today?"

Communicative techniques were discussed and developed in depth by Carl Rogers, who built his theoretical approach on the concepts of understanding his patients and their circumstances and establishing a relationship with them. His theory of communication can be described as *active listening*, which he applied to therapy as well as managerial and other interpersonal communications. With active listening, the therapist is listening to the words, the intonation, and the meaning behind the patient's statements as well as attending to the understanding the therapist has gained through the therapeutic process and progress made in the therapy (modifying and reassessing along the way as needed) (Rogers 1961, p. 21). One of the hallmarks of active listening is to provide the patient with evidence that the therapist is invested in the relationship and understands the patient's point of view without challenging the patient's defenses. As enumerated by Rogers and Farson (2015, pp. 9–13), active listening includes

- Listening for total meaning: the content and feeling in what is being said.
- Responding to feeling as well as content.
- Noting all cues, verbal and non-verbal.
- Testing for understanding by getting feedback from the patient and testing your own responses by rephrasing the meaning and discussing it with the patient.

Beginners in psychotherapy do often wonder how much of their own personalities should infuse or inform the therapy. They may sometimes hear the admonition "Be yourself," but that might be immediately qualified by "depending on what kind of a self you have." Reviewing what that self is takes a high level of unbiased self-examination or therapeutic supervision. The importance of supervision in this respect is discussed further by Douglas (2008), and we urge you to avail yourself of supervision of your skills if you are in a position to do so. If not, however, you may consider joint therapy sessions with colleagues who can provide you with honest feedback about your technical and emotional performance in a therapy session.

You build upon the basic techniques of empathic/*active* listening and talking by *observing* your patient. How is he dressed? How are his feelings and moods related to the conversation? To encourage communication, *expressing interest and concern honestly* is fundamental. *Echoing* the patient's statements, in the same or slightly altered words, is the simplest form of acknowledgment. Emotions, too, can be echoed empathetically. *Tracking* is a way of indicating, by words or gestures, that you are following the patient's account. *Commenting* on the patient's behavior (as in, "You seem really anxious today") may simply convey understanding, or it may be part of a more thoughtful plan to relate different aspects of the patient's behavior in a later interpretation.

A particularly important type of communication, *restatement*, which involves reformulation of the patient's remarks, is the beginning of the process in which the therapist uncovers hidden aspects of the patient's situation or infers thoughts that the patient is unable or unwilling to express.

Case Vignette

A patient tells his therapist about interruptions from the patient's mother when he is watching TV. The therapist infers and restates, "You would like to have more privacy." The patient agrees and expresses his underlying frustration: "There's nowhere I can go, except the bedroom, but I don't have my own TV." The therapist can now continue to explore the limitations, real and imagined, of the patient's ability to meet his perceived needs.

Although in the preceding example the therapist made inferences about the patient's needs, simpler restatements may be equally powerful in helping patients to understand themselves both as individuals and as social beings. Many chronically mentally ill patients lack basic communication abilities; others are quite verbal but frequently *mis*communicate their intentions and, as we have already discussed, both types of patients lack the ability to communicate to others in a realistic way so that their needs can be met by social negotiation. The therapist's ability to restate such needs, even without embellishment, reflects back to the patient the therapist's understanding.

Such techniques provide feedback to the patient that the therapist is listening attentively and trying to understand, thus serving that variant of the nonspecificity hypothesis, which holds that communication per se is of therapeutic value. Although this thesis has been challenged for more highly functional patients and the need for exploration has been emphasized (Shapiro 1989, pp. 151–153), we believe that communication per se is basic to supportive psychotherapy.

Restatement and echoing also serve to convert affects into words, a helpful technique for a patient who is expressing extremes of affect such as hatred, rage, anxiety, or depression and helplessness. This technique can be likened to the process of attunement described by Pine (1985) (discussed in Rockland 1989, p. 50). For example:

PATIENT: I'm not coming back here again. This isn't doing me any good. I still don't have a job.
THERAPIST (*restating*): So, you don't think your therapy is working?
PATIENT: No, I just can't wait all morning to see you.

Even if cognitively mistaken about the patient's reasons for leaving, the therapist has initiated a fruitful discussion. The act of restatement itself, rather than its accuracy, begins the process. Whether the therapist should echo the patient's emotion of anger or counter with a soothing process depends on the patient's style and level of affect. Actually, the therapist in all cases needs to establish some overlap with the patient's affect. Thus, with the bereaved patient, the therapist must echo some of the sadness and stress in her own response, because overly cheerful injunctions would be insincere. In this regard, some therapists have found that audiotapes provide useful feedback to patients who have communication difficulties or problems in perceiving themselves and their therapists objectively. Replaying the tapes at home, patients can experience the therapist's words without the concomitant anxiety of having to respond in the session (Satel and Sledge 1989).

When either affect or cognitive information needs to be expressed but is not forthcoming, the therapist may need to *encourage ventilation of feelings and expression of affect.* Indeed, the rediscovery and expression of isolated or repressed affects are central to psychoanalytic abreaction. However, this process must be used judiciously, particularly in patients with poor reality testing or poor self-control. *No* therapist should indiscriminately encourage a patient to "express all your feelings." Rather, the therapist must selectively encourage the expression of some affects and the suppression of others based on his knowledge or on what the patient can handle.

Confrontation

Psychotherapy is a never-ending exploration of another person's life. As we talk about managing the therapy (Chapter 5), you will begin to explore surface issues in initial sessions. As you explore below that surface of what a patient relates willingly and often effortlessly, talk shifts to matters that generate anxiety and resistance. This is the area of *confrontation.*

Confrontation implies the existence of conflict. Some therapists limit the term to a forceful or insistent presentation of painful truths to the patient. Others believe that the patient must be confronted with behaviors and self concepts that he or she finds unacceptable or has long ago disowned. Such direct confrontations may also involve opposition to the patient's current plans, beliefs, or ideas. For example, you may say, "You can't continue cutting your arms when you go home at night." This type of confrontation is often necessary with patients who must be restrained from committing destructive acts, and you must not shy away from such directness when the patient needs to be told the truth immediately. However, absolute bluntness, in the style of "You're wrong about that," is rarely effective in day-to-day therapeutic interaction. For instance, in patients with acute paranoia or even paranoid personality disorder, such directness may actually be dangerous.

Most of the time it is preferable to think of *confrontation* in its other meaning of "comparison" (or its etymological meaning of "facing together"). This is because the patient needs to feel that she and the therapist are facing the problem together.

Confrontation is often best used to talk about discrepancies in the patient's behavior or statements. Psychodynamically, these discrepancies may be indicative of underlying conflicts in psychic structure, but the confrontation need not refer to them directly, as in the following examples:

- "You told me 5 minutes ago that I was the best therapist you'd ever had, and now you just said I'm not worth a damn." [This confronts the patient's rapid change of attitude from idealization to anger, possibly leading to further exploration of primitive defenses such as splitting.]
- "I know that you would like to have your daughter back home with you, but I wonder if you are able to take care of her as well as you would like to." [This confronts the patient's denial of illness and incapacity.]
- "You said that you were going to spend your paycheck on a winter coat, but instead you spent it on cocaine." [This confronts the patient's rationalization of drug use.]

It will be helpful for you to distinguish between *primary* confrontations, which involve a discrepancy between an acknowledged goal and the patient's behavior, and *secondary* confrontations, which involve discrepancies between aspects of behavior, none of which is clearly acknowledged as superior. A typical primary confrontation points out a patient's resistance to a therapy or treatment that he has voluntarily sought, as exhibited in absences or failure to pay. Further discussion may reveal that the patient is uncommitted to the acknowledged goal and that it is time to reaffirm or restructure the goals of treatment. In a secondary confrontation, involving, say, a patient's difficulty in choosing between two romantic relationships, you must allow the patient's own choices to unfold.

Case Vignette

A 27-year-old woman with schizophrenia has been living in a group home for 5 years. Every spring she declares that she is going to get a job, and she is observed busily perusing and marking the want ads. Each year she goes to one interview in a disheveled state, at which she is rejected with apparent relief. After noting the pattern, the therapist points it out to the patient and asks for her reasons. This confrontation may lead to an understanding of the patient's fears about work, of problems with her self-presentation and interview skills, or of motives such as trying to please the therapist.

Clarification, Explanation, and Interpretation

As the therapist begins to discover more hidden aspects and motivations of the patient's behavior, she explores aspects of the patient's self that may be unknown to the patient, finding both positive and negative behaviors, hidden skills, and strengths, as well as self-destructive tendencies.

A *clarification* is a relatively superficial interpretation that reveals unknown or unacknowledged aspects of the patient's life without delving deeply into the patient's hidden motives, fears, wishes, or defenses. Often this involves capturing a thought that has been fleeting and brushed aside by the patient; the therapist restates it and underlines its importance.

Explanation is the most general term for interventions in this category. It refers to the offering of causes, contributing factors, motives, reasons, mechanisms of action, and processes behind or antecedents to the patient's feelings, thoughts, and behaviors.

In the psychoanalytic tradition, *interpretation* relates the patient's current feelings, thoughts, and behaviors to past or present psychological processes or events, which are generally unconscious. However, we shall use *interpretation* more generally to refer to any explanation that is specific to the patient. Both explanations and interpretations may be genetic (which in psychotherapy includes early life and family influences, not just influences involving genes) or contemporary (i.e., explaining one current process by another one). They are useful agents of therapeutic change, not necessarily via insight, but because they result in changes in the patient's self-esteem, feelings, and repertory of behaviors.

The following example shows the way in which a therapist may choose how deeply to explain or interpret a single event:

> PATIENT: My mother yelled at me because I didn't change my clothes from yesterday, so I went into the shower. I just didn't feel like cleaning up afterward, so I left the towels on the floor.

THERAPIST: You've often told me that you get angry at your mother when she criticizes you. People often mess things up when they are angry. Maybe you were angry and that has something to do with the way you left the bathroom.

PATIENT: No, like I said, I just didn't feel like cleaning up the place.

THERAPIST: Still, it sounds to me as if you were angry at her.

In this example, the therapist uses a variety of techniques. The therapist *confronts* the patient's denial of anger and offers the *clarification* that the patient was angry. An *interpretation* is made that the messiness of the bathroom was an expression of the patient's anger. These techniques are designed to help the patient both learn and acknowledge the role of anger in motivating his actions. The therapist has also offered an *explanation*—in this case universalizing that other people often act the same way—to blunt the critical force of the clarification. The therapist might even go on, in a reality-testing mode, to point out that the towels on the bathroom floor may anger the mother further, noting with the sympathetic comment: "We know how your mother is about things being clean." The therapist does not at this stage suggest what would be another *interpretation* (i.e., that the patient harbors chronically aggressive feelings toward his mother). The therapist has, however, introduced the concept that the patient is responding to criticism with anger that, while understandable, is only making the situation worse.

Principles of Supportive Interpretation

We have introduced important principles above: the *level* of an interpretation is kept superficial, and, in general, the *force* (or critical import) needs to be blunted in a number of ways. The *pacing* and *timing* of interpretations are also crucial. Premature interpretations may be erroneous and therefore unhelpful and misleading. Even when correct, a premature interpretation may be ineffective or disregarded. Worse yet, it may anger the patient, create anxiety, and disrupt the therapy. In classical analysis, incorrect interpretations have been known to cause weeks of silence on the patient's part (and undoubtedly weeks of self-analysis or supervision on the therapist's part). Your position in supportive therapy is in some respects even more precarious. You may work with fragile patients, who can be frightened by premature or deep interpretations. Knowing this, you may be tempted to "tread lightly" and make the time pass without doing any effective work whatsoever. Fortunately, this understandable sensitivity can be counteracted by a repertory of techniques to utilize interpretations in the most effective way.

Inexact interpretation is the most general term that applies to interpretations that are partly true but not entirely so. For example, in listening to an apparently heterosexual male patient's account of going swimming with a male friend, the therapist may decide that the patient has felt an obvious homosexual attraction to the friend. Rather than interpret this directly, the therapist may address the patient's longings for friendship, which the patient would find perfectly reasonable. Inexact interpretations, as Glover (1931) noted, can also provide substituted and displaced behaviors and explanations that afford the patient relief of concerns and dysphoric feelings. Such interpretations, for example, may divert the patient from sources of anxiety or fruitless courses of action. This is not to say, however, that inexact interpretations are merely temporary palliatives. Rather, activities that are initially diversions from other desires provide rewards through competency and mastery of the environment, and the diversions may eventually become ends in themselves.

Biologically inexact interpretations can refer to what is typical in the disease and can offer reassurance and understanding, as in, "It's typical for hallucinations to get worse at bedtime." Or, as Torrey (1986) suggests to the patient who claims his food is poisoned: "It's quite common in schizophrenia for food to taste different from the way it usually does, but that does not mean that it is poisoned."

In the remainder of this chapter we will present a variety of techniques, almost all of which may be called inexact interpretations, limited in content or depth to prevent anxiety or a regressive response.

Using Interpretations Wisely

Fred Pine, who has already been mentioned for his work in relating supportive comments to affect attunement, has also addressed the use of supportive interventions in the therapeutic context (Pine 1986). His most memorable principle is to "strike while the iron is cold." Whereas psychodynamic therapists may strive to interpret experience when there is fresh (newly evoked) affect, the supportive therapist may prefer to wait until the patient is emotionally cool about the experience. This blunts the potentially critical or humiliating impact of the interpretation. For similar reasons, Pine advises the therapist to limit or close off the patient's associations to the interpretation, to introduce interpretations tentatively, to give the patient the opportunity to stop the discussion, and to prepare the patient for the interpretation by letting him or her know earlier in the session that the subject will be discussed later. This packaging of the interpretation allows for its effect to be anticipated (Pine 1985), which is a mature defense. Pine also emphasizes that interpretations can be softened by increasing the "holding aspects" of the therapeutic environment.

Another important principle is to open the door to future interpretations by stating one's readiness to talk about a difficult subject: "I know it's painful to talk about your drug use, and I see that you don't want to talk about it now. So let's put this off for a while until you feel ready." A statement like this is preferable to an unstated collusive bargain in which the topic is simply avoided.

When a group and its therapist address one patient's problems, the entire group benefits. Analogously, interpretations can be delivered effectively (though not as a regular practice) by directing them to someone other than the patient. Overheard remarks of the therapist (whether or not the patient was intended to hear them) can be profoundly effective or destructive, and the therapist should be aware that he is always "in role" when conducting a semiprivate conversation.

Even when delayed, temporarily avoided, packaged, softened, or blunted, interpretations require *repetition* to be effective, and the therapist must be creative enough to put old wine in new bottles without constantly reminding the patient that it tastes the same.

In the preceding discussion, although mixing metaphors, we have stated many important guidelines for the delivery of interpretations. These guidelines are summarized in Table 3–5, using our favored "door" metaphor.

Upwards Interpretations

The student of psychoanalysis is familiar with genetic interpretations that relate current conflicts to problems in early childhood and to retained and repressed infantile wishes. Such interpretations, even when the therapist is sure of their accuracy, are rarely used directly in supportive therapy. However, it is possible to use genetic interpretations as inexact interpretations that lessen the patient's guilt or blame for his or her condition. In fact, this is typically how

Table 3–5.   A metaphorical look at interpretations as doors

Rule	Rationale
Do not open a hot door.	There may be a fire behind it: the patient may be unable to handle the resulting emotional activation and may be unable to assimilate the cognitive component of the interpretation.
Don't open it wide.	Limiting associations to the material preserves most of the patient's defenses.
Open it cautiously and be prepared to close it.	The immediate effects may tell the therapist that the interpretation is premature, too deep, or too threatening.
Let the patient know you are going to open it.	This allows the patient to build anticipatory defenses.
Allow the patient to open and close it himself or herself.	Giving the patient control over the discussion of sensitive material allows him or her to maintain defenses.
Sometimes you must close it when the patient wants to open it.	The therapist must also be prepared to limit discussion if the patient decompensates or regresses.
Make the room comfortable.	Interpretations must be presented in a supportive environment.
Open the door repeatedly.	Interpretations must be repeated to overcome resistance.
Open the door for someone else.	The patient is more likely to appreciate the interpretation when not personally threatened by it.
If the door seems to be welded or cemented shut, it may not be worth the effort to open it.	If the defense is that strong, that suggests that the patient is not ready to handle the content that is concealed.
And maybe you can find another door that leads to the same place?	It makes sense to see if the desired insight or knowledge can be obtained through another means.

patients with character disorders defensively invoke such interpretations to protect themselves from responsibility (Arlow 1981). In the supportive therapy patient who has lesser control over characterological change, however, an inexact genetic interpretation can strengthen needed defenses. For example, the tendency of some patients with schizophrenia to blame their parents may serve a defensive function of warding off depression (Arieti 1974, quoted in Lamb 1982, p. 138). Because the supportive therapist, unlike the psychoanalyst, frequently has the opportunity of meeting the patient's family and comparing her own perceptions with the patient's, it may be possible to do further work with this defense when the patient is able to relate more realistically to his family.

The displacement of an interpretation from past origins to a current incident is what Loewenstein (1957) calls *upwards reconstruction*. Similarly, *upwards interpretations* provide inexact (usually intellectualized) explanations of less acceptable material. This metaphor has a physical meaning. In the symbolism of dreams, for example, Freud noted that parts of the face (i.e., nose, lips) are often symbols that have been displaced upwards from the genitals. The example given earlier, interpretively translocating a homosexual urge as a friendship need, is one of the most common.

Displaced Interpretations

Just as it is safer, proverbially speaking, to kick the dog instead of one's boss, it is safer to talk about one's problems in displacement. The therapist can take advantage of such displacements in many ways.

Vicarious discussion is familiar to all therapists as the use of topics that have personal relevance to the patient's pathology. Psychotic patients can talk about violence and aggression in current events, which invariably include an admixture of war and/or sports. The displaced discussion may by itself serve a ventilatory purpose, but the therapist can further relate the external issues to the patient's feelings and fears, as by noting: "It's a pretty scary world out there, with all those wars going on," or "It must be nice to be famous like one of those basketball stars."

Generalizing (or universalizing) serves to displace an interpretation from a specific person (usually, but not necessarily, the patient) to a group.

Case Vignette

A patient who will soon be placed in the community claims that he is having no problems or anxiety about it, but the therapist senses otherwise and wants to explore the issue. The therapist observes: "Many other patients find it difficult to leave the hospital after a long stay." The patient, consulted as an expert on hospital/community transition, responds eagerly: "Yes, the other patients worry about what it's going to be like. And you see Arthur over there? He was out for only 2 weeks and he came back. You kind of get used to the routine. Like, there's someone to play cards with. It takes you 2 years to get to this point and then they boot you out." He begins, without feeling conned or tricked, to talk about his own problems more openly.

The therapist could have phrased a similar question more personally and less certainly: "Don't you think that it's difficult for patients to leave the hospital?" Or the statement could have been transformed into an open question: "Do you think it's hard for patients to leave the hospital?"

Interpretations can also be *displaced to another specific person*. This is a frequently used technique in group psychotherapy, where it is hoped that other group members will benefit when the group focuses on the problems of one of its members. However, this technique can also be used in individual psychotherapy. We have frequently found it useful to discuss the stories in the public press regarding the mental illness or substance abuse problems of celebrities. One can also use anonymous examples, such as "I had a patient last year who was embarrassed about not knowing how to read, but he went to the literacy program and did really well." (Unfortunately, such examples, even when they are quite generic, can worry patients that their own confidentiality will be violated.)

The patient's response to displaced interpretations can be very helpful in determining future therapeutic maneuvers. Thus, it will be significant if the patient mentioned in the preceding vignette attributes Arthur's failure in the community to a problem in Arthur or a problem of the mental health system.

Defense Interpretations

In psychodynamic therapy, defenses are identified and interpreted in relationship to fears and unacknowledged unconscious wishes. From this process, the patient learns—both consciously and unconsciously, and emotionally and cognitively—that certain defenses are dysfunctional. Put simply, these defenses have outlived their usefulness and are generating more problems than they are worth. Defense interpretations, as used here, include the psychodynamic variety but also refer to the offering of interpretations that strengthen or modify the identified defense, or that substitute another defense in its place. Some therapies focus on interpretation of defenses as a frequent goal. In supportive psychotherapy, however, you may decide that the patient will be well served by some defense mechanisms such as intellectualization, sublimation, rationalization, suppression, and humor. Thus, you may want to interpret an idea of reference or delusion in such a way that the patient will substitute, for example, intellectualization for the idea of reference or delusion.

The rationale for defense interpretations of this sort should be understood in light of the patient's pathology, which is an outgrowth of dysfunctional defenses. For example, intellectualization may reduce a patient's anxiety, and the giving of hope may indirectly foster denial. Even delusions can often be approached as defenses in which the patient organizes the frightening and disruptive mental events generated by the biological substrate of the illness. The content of a delusion is not biologically determined but elaborated in response to individual memory and cultural factors. Borderline personality traits are ingrained, but they are also developmental outgrowths of coping behaviors that reflect inadequate early caregiving and affective instability. Through painstaking and careful work, both delusions and ingrained personality traits can be shaped or modified so that they become less disruptive to the patient's life while retaining their defensive functions.

A special type of defense interpretation is called *unlinking*. This approach allows the patient to maintain a given defense while changing the actions that follow from it. For example, a patient might be allowed to maintain a specific defense (e.g., denial of illness) and yet to carry out an action that was originally prohibited by the defense (e.g., writing a will). Similarly, by offering specific defenses (e.g., the rationalization that "the roads were slippery, and the accident couldn't be avoided"), the therapist might help avert a depressive reaction to an accident (e.g., "I injured somebody, and I am a bad person").

Defenses can even be explained by other defenses. Such "displaced defense interpretations" might include explaining grandiosity (a defense against the feeling of worthlessness) as a need for recognition, or a personal vendetta against the political system as an attempt at political reform. Usually these are intended as transitional interpretations, serving to identify underlying needs that can then be addressed more productively.

Poetry and Metaphor

Metaphor, the figure of speech in which one object substitutes for another in unstated symbolism, and *simile*, in which the analogy is openly stated, provide the basis for another set of interpretations that have especial use in supportive therapy (Berlin et al. 1991). Metaphor (which is derived from the Greek word for "transfer" and its constituents meaning "bearing next to") is another form of displaced interpretation. It is a step beyond upwards interpretation, because the literal message may not be apparent and may be effective just *because* it is not apparent.

You will have frequent occasion to relate stories and examples to the patient in supportive therapy. Myths, biblical stories, fables, the classics of literature, historical precedents, examples from popular entertainment, Broadway musicals, and comic strips may often be used to illustrate the patient's predicament. Fairy tales, for example, deal with universal human problems and situations, primitive feelings, and existential dilemmas; they often foster strong identification with the main characters (Bettelheim 1976). Even "pseudodisclosures" about the therapist or his friends can be used, provided they do not imply violation of confidentiality.

It is also possible to interpret a patient's own belief metaphorically. You can agree with the patient that her belief is important, and in a sense true, but only metaphorically so. Some therapists use proverbs or supply their patients with metaphorical objects (which can come to symbolize the patients' needs). However, use of well-worn proverbs (such as "You can't cry over spilled milk" when the patient reports a setback) usually makes the therapist appear superior and all-knowing rather than sympathetic. If proverbs are used, therefore, we suggest that you turn to more interesting ones (see, e.g., Fergusson 1983) and tailor them to patients who will respond positively to the wisdom or humor displayed.

The utility of metaphorical communication in "highly functioning" patients is attributed to the ability of metaphor to speak to patients' unconscious while bypassing their defenses against direct criticism or manipulation. But in patients who tend to think concretely, one may wonder if the symbolic power of the story is lost. In such patients, the generalized meaning of the story can be explained. To do so to patients with a high capacity for abstract thinking would seem patronizing, but we have found that more concrete patients will continue to perceive it consciously as a story and not a criticism.

Use of sophisticated metaphorical or literary devices requires an adept therapist who is comfortable in the role. The therapist interested in this area might wish to consult the lucid presentation by Barker (1985). Each therapist will develop his or her favored approaches using metaphor and should make note of which ones work with certain patients.

Dream Interpretations

The role of dreams in supportive psychotherapy is problematic. Because the interpretation of dreams may involve the decoding of manifest content into latent content, the latter involving censored wishes and desires, it may be undesirable to voice such interpretations to the patient. In supportive therapy with chronically mentally ill patients, most therapists prefer to divert attention from dreams. In general, that is the correct attitude to take. Showing interest in a dream and spending time on its explanation will, by simple reinforcement, result in more dream reports. So it is often best to use a dismissive, inexact interpretation of the dream process itself, pointing out that dreams are difficult to interpret and of uncertain relevance to the patient's life. However, in supportive work with certain patients, and occasionally with all patients, dreams are reported and useful to the therapy. Sometimes, in fact, they are significant communications to the therapist.

In Freudian theory, dreams represent attempts to deal with unconscious infantile wishes, disguised by condensation, displacement, and secondary revision. Many dreams of supportive therapy patients, however, belong to the category of anxiety dreams, which remained problematic to Freud. Some such dreams are supposed to represent the dreamer's failure to disguise successfully the unacceptable wish, generating anxiety in the dream itself.

Others seem to represent a compulsion to repeat traumatic events, perhaps in an attempt to master, after the fact, the events' unanticipated assault on the senses. The latter kind of interpretation—that the patient's dream is a positive attempt to master a problem—is more appealing than talking about unacceptable wishes. We have found that repetitive nightmares should be treated as part of posttraumatic stress disorder with behavioral methods (Krakow 2002).

Overtly erotic dreams about the therapist may be brought up as queries or disguised seductions or fears. The therapist, in such cases, should be noncondemnatory and should also be realistically responsive with the upwards interpretation that these dreams represent wishes for closeness with the therapist, but that erotic contact will not occur.

If you were to have a record of all the patient's dreams between therapy sessions, you might develop a useful resume of the patient's defensive processes. As all therapists learn, however, dream reports are unpredictable. Many factors govern the repression, forgetting, and recall of dream material. In a highly functional patient, presentation of dreams may represent a desirable advance in the transference. In the less functional patient, the opposite may be true, because dreams may represent a resurgence of repressed material. In either case, the dreams may tell you something important that should not be shared with the patient, such as that you are being overly sadistic or seductive, or at least are being perceived as such. Thus, the patient's early dreams in the therapy are especially important because they can represent potential problems before a stable supportive relationship has solidified.

Case Vignette

A young woman in her 20s (about the same age as her therapist) with borderline personality disorder reports a dream in the third week. In it, she sees from behind someone in a "Dick Tracy trench coat" who is female and who vaguely resembles the therapist. Because the therapeutic alliance is still uncertain at this stage, the therapist briefly explores the associations. Does the trench coat mean that the patient views the therapist as a detective, ferreting out clues about the patient's crimes? Does it represent the mystery of the therapist's personal life? Why is the therapist/detective walking away from the patient? Is it because the patient would like the therapist to walk out of her life? The therapist says reassuringly that it is natural to have such curiosity and such wishes. She uses the therapy as a springboard for discussion but does not investigate other possibilities such as the patient's sexual feelings toward the therapist or the wish that the therapist were male.

Guidelines for dream interpretation in supportive psychotherapy are summarized in Table 3–6.

Other Displacements: Externalization, Projection, and Counterprojection

Externalization of blame, a dysfunctional defense frequently used by patients with personality disorders, involves the attribution of causes or responsibility

Table 3–6. Guidelines for handling dreams in supportive psychotherapy

Pay close attention to early dreams, which may represent the therapist's initial appearance to the patient and the patient's initial expectations and fears.

Use upwards interpretations of the dream and the dream process.

Do not reward the presentation of a dream unless you want to hear another one.

Pay attention to the report of the dream because it may tell you something about the transference.

Remember that interpretation of the dream may reveal more about you than about the patient.

Keep in mind that a dream may not be a dream; it may be the patient's way of reporting a wish, fantasy, or hallucination.

Consider repetitive nightmares and traumatic dreams to be failed attempts to master a past trauma, and treat with behavioral methods (see text for reference).

for actions to others. This defense may be as obvious and self-serving as in, "They left the key in the car, so I stole it," or as subtly demeaning as in, "I can't work, because nobody likes me." Working with the patient's externalizations of blame requires a sensitive approach. Often the therapist needs to substitute one externalization for another rather than demolish the defense entirely. For example, the person above who says, "Nobody likes me," may be citing that as a reason for failing at the job. If other reasons can be found, such as a specific unsympathetic boss, the patient can recover from failure but be encouraged to try again.

You may also use *projection* as a variation of the displaced interpretation. The therapist may need to agree that there is some truth to a patient's paranoid projections when these do not interfere with function ("Yes, the streets are very dangerous."). One can even use "benign projections and introjections" that blame the patient's problems on her family (i.e., pseudogenetic) or on the disease itself (i.e., pseudobiological) (Rockland 1989).

Counterprojection, an advanced technique, takes things further, with the therapist saying in effect that "things are even worse than you [the patient] think." The therapist (without officially agreeing) elaborates the patient's delusions even further than does the patient. This is an attempt, suitable for the adept therapist, to enter the psychotic patient's world and, through empathic communication, lead him out of it.

Case Vignettes

A middle-aged man thinks that a certain senator on the finance committee controls the world's entire military and economic system. The therapist does not question this, but observes, "There are certainly some powerful men in the Senate, and that seems to bother you. [This is close to reality.] I don't know much about these politicians, but maybe they have more control than I realize. [Projection] Maybe they control this hospital as well! [Counterprojection] What do you think?"

A woman who works in a department store and also has schizophrenia laments that her brother has gone to college and that she has not been able to. The therapist says, "But you have schizophrenia. It's like having diabetes. [Benign introjection] It's not your fault. It's going to limit you somewhat, but we'll try our best to manage it. Your family has got to understand that, and they should stop demanding so much of you and criticizing you. No wonder you feel bad much of the time." [Externalization of blame]

Drawing parallels between a psychiatric illness and diabetes sometimes requires going beyond the approach used with a patient with schizophrenia. For example, in working with persons who abuse substances, it is important to point out to patients that they must avoid that first drink, that first pill, and so forth, so as not to set off the physiological craving for the substance.

Although we do not recommend its use unreservedly, the disease model often frees the patient (and family) from blame for the mental illness and underscores the need for appropriate treatment. It should not, however, be used as an excuse for dependency, inactivity, and failure. To the patient who says, "I am mentally ill so I can't help myself," you must give the balanced message "You have a mental illness, but you must still try to act responsibly and get help to control it."

Miscellaneous Explanatory Techniques

Two other techniques are worth mentioning. The *psychodynamic life narrative* (Slonim and Hodges 2000; Viederman 1983) is promoted as a way of fostering responsibility for the present. The patient's telling of her own story is, of course, the starting point for the therapist's empathic understanding of the situation. Moreover, the patient's reflection on her own life story is an opportunity for integration of meaning and direction.

Induced dichotomy of personality (Ermutlu 1977) is the attribution of the patient's conflicts to "sick" and "healthy" parts. Therapy proceeds through three phases: identification, rejection, and organization. In the first phase, the patient identifies almost totally with the sick part. In the second, he is taught to identify more closely with the healthy or adult part and to reject the sick part. In the third, the patient learns to accept the sick part. Dichotomized interpretations can be used in the way that Ermutlu (1977) proposes, but can also be introduced without value judgments—for example, "It seems that a part of you would still like to stay at home, and another part would like to move out."

Key Points

- Explanatory techniques are divided into three levels: communication, confrontation, and the offering of clarifications, explanations, and interpretations.

- Communication techniques include personal and professional listening and require certain skills of active listening, a concept developed by Carl Rogers.

- Communication becomes more skillful and complex when reassuring, observing, tracking, commenting, making restatements, and encouraging ventilation and expression of affect.

- Confrontation involves directing attention to inconsistencies in behavior and conflicting goals and motivation.

- Therapists work with patients' psychological defenses, which can be view nontheoretically as interpersonal adaptations rather than as unconscious psychological mechanisms of motivation.

- The timing of interpretations is critical, and the same interpretation can fail or succeed simply on the timing by which it is offered.

- In additional to controlling their timing, therapists can modify the content of interpretations by making them inexact or displacing the object of the interpretation.

- Therapists should make use of supervision in order to improve their technical skills and to understand their emotional responses to their patients.

References

Arieti S: Interpretation of Schizophrenia, 2nd Edition. New York, Basic Books, 1974

Arlow JA: Theories of pathogenesis. Psychoanal Q 50(4):488–514, 1981 7302039

Aronson E: The Social Animal, 5th Edition. New York, WH Freeman, 1988

Barker P: Using Metaphors in Psychotherapy. New York, Brunner/Mazel, 1985

Battaglia J: 5 keys to good results with supportive psychotherapy: evidence-based technique gains new respect as a valuable clinical tool. Curr Psychiatr 6(6):27–34, 2007

Beck AT, Emery G: Anxiety Disorders and Phobias: A Cognitive Perspective. New York, Basic Books, 1985

Berlin RM, Olson ME, Cano CE, et al: Metaphor and psychotherapy. Am J Psychother 45(3):359–367, 1991 1719829

Bettelheim B: The Uses of Enchantment: The Meaning and Importance of Fairy Tales. New York, Knopf, 1976

Cohen CI, Berk LA: Personal coping styles of schizophrenic outpatients. Hosp Community Psychiatry 36(4):407–410, 1985 3997104

Di Riso D, Colli A, Chessa D, et al: A supportive approach in psychodynamic-oriented psychotherapy: an empirically supported single case study. Research in Psychotherapy 14(1):49–89, 2011

Douglas CJ: Teaching supportive psychotherapy to psychiatric residents. Am J Psychiatry 165(4):445–452, 2008 18381914

Ermutlu I: Induced dichotomy of personality as a technique in supportive psychotherapy. Psychiatric Forum 7:19–22, 1977

Fergusson R (ed): The Penguin Dictionary of Proverbs. London, Penguin Books, 1983

Glover E: The therapeutic effect of inexact interpretation: a contribution to the theory of suggestion. Int J Psychoanal 12:397–411, 1931

Harari E: Supportive psychotherapy. Australas Psychiatry 22(5):440–442, 2014 25183321

Hoffman RS: Practical psychotherapy: working with a patient's defenses in supportive psychotherapy. Psychiatr Serv 53(2):141–142, 2002 11821542

Krakow B: Turning Nightmares Into Dreams. Authorized audio series and treatment workbook for new dream therapy. The New Sleepy Times, 2002. Available at: https://www.sleeptreatment.com.

Lamb HR: Treating the Long-Term Mentally Ill. San Francisco, CA, Jossey-Bass, 1982

Loewenstein RM: Some thoughts on interpretation in the theory and practice of psychoanalysis. Psychoanal Study Child 12:127–150, 1957

Perry JC: Defense Mechanism Rating Scale, in I meccanismi di difesa: teoria clinica e ricerca empirica. By Lingiardi V, Madeddu F. Milan, Rafaello Cortina, 1994, pp 117–198

Pine F: Developmental Theory and Clinical Process. New Haven, CT, Yale University Press, 1985

Pine F: Supportive psychotherapy: a psychoanalytic perspective. Psychiatr Ann 16:526–529, 1986

Rockland LH: Supportive Psychotherapy: A Psychodynamic Approach. New York, Basic Books, 1989

Rogers CR: On Becoming a Person. Boston, MA, Houghton Mifflin, 1961, pp 4–27

Rogers CR, Farson RE: Active listening. Mansfield Center, CT, Marino Publishing, 2015

Satel SL, Sledge WH: Audiotape playback as a technique in the treatment of schizophrenic patients. Am J Psychiatry 146(8):1012–1016, 1989 2750972

Shapiro D: Psychotherapy of Neurotic Character. New York, Basic Books, 1989

Slonim R, Hodges B: The use of psychodynamic life narrative in crisis supervision. Am J Psychother 54(1):67–74, 2000 10822780

Swanson GE: Ego Defenses and the Legitimation of Behavior. New York, Cambridge University Press, 1988

Torrey EF: Management of chronic schizophrenic outpatients. Psychiatr Clin North Am 9(1):143–151, 1986 2870477

Vaillant GE: Defense mechanisms, in The New Harvard Guide to Psychiatry. Edited by Nicholi AM Jr. Cambridge, MA, Harvard University Press, 1988, pp 200–207

Viederman M: The psychodynamic life narrative: a psychotherapeutic intervention useful in crisis situations. Psychiatry 46(3):236–246, 1983 6622599

Wallace ER: Dynamic Psychiatry in Theory and Practice. Philadelphia, PA, Lea & Febiger, 1983

Werman DS: The Practice of Supportive Psychotherapy. New York, Brunner/Mazel, 1984

4

Principles of Supportive Technique: Directive Interventions

In this chapter we discuss a second type of supportive technique: *directive interventions* (see Table 4–1). To advise, suggest, direct, guide, command, or prohibit another person to do things is to exercise a responsibility that must have as its basis a patient's trust as well as the knowledge that giving one's advice is better than letting the patient go it alone. The ethical questions this raises—such as the imposition of values in therapy—will be acknowledged further in Chapter 17. Here we shall assume that directive interventions have been therapeutically justified as part of the treatment plan.

For example, when you tell a distraught patient in no uncertain terms to call you or the clinic before acting on a suicidal plan, you are acting in the patient's interests, because the agreed-upon purpose of your supportive relationship is to prevent suicide. Similarly, directive interventions in less pressing circumstances are guided by the rules of meeting the treatment objectives. Many supportive psychotherapy patients, with impaired judgment and motivation, cannot be expected to act on their own volition. You must assist. The follow-

Table 4–1.   Major techniques of supportive psychotherapy:
directive interventions

Suggestion

Advice and guidance

• Permission giving

• Reassurance (its guiding and encouraging aspects)

Explicit direction

Limit setting

• Inside the therapy

• Outside the therapy

Control of affects and impulses

Education

Social skills training

Work and work skills

Scheduling activities

Cognitive restructuring/behavioral and experiential learning

Modeling and identification with the therapist

Homework

Diversions, substitutes, and paradoxical interventions

Reinforcement of desirable behaviors

Provision of medications and other empirically based psychiatric treatments

Problem solving

Environmental interventions (e.g., encourage use of outside supports)

ing rationale explains when to offer direction and to what extent: Offer *what* the patient needs *when* the patient cannot provide it himself. (But note that in certain settings, as discussed in Chapter 14, we minimize or avoid use of directive interventions, or use them with considerable qualification.)

Suggestion

In the ordinary sense of *suggestion*, you can suggest new strategies, behaviors, or activities to the patient to meet her needs: "Have you talked to your mother about getting a new TV?" "Have you ever thought about coming to Job Club on Wednesdays?" Such suggestions are nothing more than guarded advice. But other suggestions also work unconsciously, as evidenced by their historical use in hypnosis. You can suggest that somatic symptoms will disappear, as is often done in the treatment of psychosomatic paralysis: "The type of weakness you are experiencing usually goes away by itself in about a month. Of course, we will keep treating you and following your condition meanwhile." This suggestion does not unearth the patient's presumed unconscious conflict generating the conversion symptoms, but it allows the patient a way to improve without embarrassment. Similarly, you may suggest that a patient's initial anxiety in working at a new job is likely to go away by itself after she gets used to the new surroundings, or that she will find it more pleasant in her community residence after she gets used to the routine. Such suggestions work because of the transference and because of the healthier adaptive dispositions they inculcate. Suggestion need not be limited to the supposedly impressionable individual or person of low intelligence, because it is equally effective in depressed and anxious patients in psychiatric clinics and hospital wards. As a therapist you should never forget that you wield the power to instill realistic hope and confidence in your patient to dispel pessimism and despair. We should also mention that *reassurance*, which was introduced as an explanatory technique, also encompasses suggestive aspects that combine both meanings of suggestion.

Advice and Guidance

Advice can be more obvious and directive, providing tremendous benefit to patients who cannot properly make decisions in their own interests. But it creates an inherent paradox: patients who do not need it will ask for it, and patients who do need it will resist it. For example, a patient may report a severe setback at work and announce his intention to quit immediately. In the time allotted, you need to explore the situation: the details of the incident, the patient's vulnerability to criticism, his personal feelings about the supervisor, and so forth. But at some point, time will run out. As therapist, you can leave the issue unresolved (with the patient likely to quit) or take a stand. You can, of course, delay the issue or schedule an extra session to consider the issue. If you feel that quitting the job would be a major setback in the patient's treatment, you should consider whether a carefully worded piece of advice is in order. It might just tip the balance of the indecision in the right direction.

Permission giving is a useful form of advice. For example, you might want to give a decompensating patient permission to quit her job if it is felt that she is too embarrassed to admit that the job is not working out: "It does seem that the problems have become overwhelming at work, and I'm more worried about your health at this point than your loss of income. I certainly wouldn't criticize you if you quit, and in fact I'm proud of you for having worked for so long." More generally, you can use permission giving to alleviate the effect of negative influences and allow the patient to express appropriate needs and desires: "You haven't spent much of your savings this year, and it doesn't seem extravagant for you to buy a small TV." Often you must give patients permission to be angry, to be depressed, or to grieve a loss. At other times you must withhold permission to quit, to give up, or to commit an injury. It is possible to phrase directions in various forms depending on the patient's best interests (see Table 4–2). Knowing which form to use is a skill and an art, yet it is based on our earlier proviso: use the strongest form that the patient needs.

Explicit Direction

Some patients need explicit direction or apparent commands, as in, "You must see me next week. You've missed two appointments this month, and I will not tolerate any more absences." Such directness would drive away many people and should be selected only when there is a high probability of success. Often explicit directness can be limited to situations in which the patient's behavior threatens the integrity of the therapeutic process (see the next section on limit setting). However, therapists should appreciate that there is a wide role for explicit direction with many patients who have impaired judgment or skills.

Limit Setting

Limit setting, or the outright, nonnegotiable prohibition of certain types of behavior, is often necessary in supportive work. Violence, sexual assault, and dis-

Table 4–2.   The many faces of direction in dealing with a patient considering leaving a job

Direct advice	"Don't quit your job."
"Objective"	"You have got to keep working."
Generalization	"It often helps for people to stay on the job during times like this."
Suggestion	"I know you feel like quitting right now, but I would suggest that you stick with it."
Probabilistic but specific to the patient	"You'll probably feel better if you go back and work out the problem."
Using therapist's influence	"I really think you need to stay on the job." (Implicitly: "Trust me, you'll thank me later for this.")
Hands off	"I can't make your decisions for you."
Exploration and interpretation	"It seems that you want me to make the decision for you."
Rhetorical question	"Don't you think it's better to hang on to the job and your income? You really need it now."
Open question	"Do you think you should be quitting work? What will you do?"
Paradoxical	
Indecisive	"I wonder if it would help to quit now."
Oppositional	"You can keep working if you want, but I don't think you can handle it!"
Permissive	"It's okay to quit if you feel that's best. I know you've been under terrible stress lately."
Delay	"Keep working a little longer, and we'll talk about your decision next week."

ruption of the treatment site are more likely if you fail to heed the warning signs of escalating behavior or respond to such behavior inappropriately. Limit setting also serves other important purposes:

- It can be used to shape the patient's behaviors into more appropriate and rewarding ones.
- It conveys your concern for the patient's well-being.
- It registers your own rights and the patient's need to respect them.

A major reason why many therapists fail to set limits is a desire to be liked or loved. The therapist may feel uneasy in setting limits for the same reason that a parent does not wish to discipline a child. Such hesitancies need to be examined in the therapist's countertransference. In fact, limit setting often improves the therapeutic relationship, making it safer and more predictable. It will reassure those patients who have difficulty controlling primitive rage and who fear that their rage will destroy the therapist (Adler 1982). Limit setting shows these patients that the therapist is not frightened but instead is capable of containing their behavior. Similarly, a patient who knows, as a result of limit setting, that the relationship will always be a nonerotic one can feel safer in expressing positive or dependent feelings toward the therapist.

Although we emphasize that limit setting should not be delayed by a fear of "loss of love," it is true that the therapist's ability to set limits is enhanced by a preexisting positive relationship with the patient. Otherwise, the limits are more likely to be disregarded. In addition, you should attempt to give the patient an opportunity to exercise self-control before issuing an absolute prohibition. This can be accomplished by making the patient aware of the consequences of an action before forbidding the action itself.

Limits Within the Therapy and Clinic Must Be Firmly Set

Limits must be absolute for physical abuse and threats of it. If the patient begins to lose control, the session may be terminated; if necessary, the therapist should leave the room first or call for help after the patient leaves. The limits of verbal abuse are somewhat more flexible. Every therapist has his own personal reactions to verbal abuse. It is important to ask whether a high tolerance of abuse serves a therapeutic purpose. It is also important to distinguish verbal abuse, which is a *substitute* for action, from threatening abuse, which is a *prelude* to violence. You may set flexible limits for the former and absolute limits to the latter.

Limits Outside the Therapy Can Also Be Flexible

A patient should be able to violate outside limits and talk honestly about the violations, which is difficult to do if the therapist is unyielding about them. Nevertheless, absolute prohibitions must remain for violence and life-threatening actions. The selection of limits outside the therapy should depend on the patient's response and needs. Some patients will respond to limits self-destructively; others will feel safer and contained. In deciding to set limits such as not leaving a job, not walking out on family or spouse, not using drugs, or not getting into fights, the therapist serves as an external restraint. As Lamb (1982, p. 129) notes, the patient may adhere to limits to please the therapist, but the limits can then be internalized by identification with the therapist, and adherence to the limits provides a sense of competence and mastery.

The following is a list of do's and don'ts of limit setting. You may also wish to consult the monograph by Green et al. (1988).

- **DO** distinguish between absolute (i.e., nonnegotiable) and relative (i.e., negotiable) limits of the therapy. The reasons for the difference should be made clear to the patient.
- **DO** convey the limits to patients both verbally and nonverbally. A serious limit must be conveyed in a serious manner rather than as a dry rule.
- **DON'T** give mixed signals (e.g., verbally prohibit, nonverbally encourage). Your verbal and nonverbal statements and attitudes, respectively, should be in concordance. You should not be smiling when you say, "I really cannot tolerate your drug abuse."
- **DO** examine the countertransference implications of limit setting (e.g., manipulative, punitive) or failure to set limits (e.g., reaction formation, being overly nice, desire to appear permissive, need to be loved).
- **DON'T** assume that it is sufficient to tell the patient once. Although some obsessive-compulsive or overly dependent patients will quickly respond to a limit (and often overreact to it), most patients who need limits have obviously had difficulty in setting their own, and the therapist must have some tolerance of noncompliance to most limits.

- **DO** examine the patient's responses to limit setting and be willing to change your limits. For example, if a limit is experienced (and reported) as punitive, consider the possibility that it was inappropriate and be willing to change. You may explain the basis for change as that your understanding of the patient has changed and the reason for the earlier limit is no longer valid.
- **DON'T** set arbitrarily different limits for different patients in groups or public clinics; they will soon discover the differences and you will have to justify them.
- **DON'T** take on the job of limit setting when it belongs to someone else. This situation frequently arises when patients have multiple therapists or separate therapists and medicators. The medicator, for example, should not tell the patient that he is calling the therapist too often; that is the therapist's job. (The issue can be *explored* by the medicator, but he should not set the limit.)

Limit Setting Implies That There Will Be Limit Testing

Limit testing is exhibited by patients with a variety of diagnoses and for a variety of reasons. The manic patient, because of impaired judgment and inflated self-esteem; the dependent patient defining the limits of her role; the borderline patient who is trying (unconsciously) to find an omni-tolerant parent—each will find ingenious ways to test your resolve. Therapists, especially at the beginning of treatment, often feel they must be overaccommodating to establish rapport with the patient. Indeed, early treatment is a time of mutual exploration of the therapist by the patient and vice versa. But limits can be reassuring as well as constraining, and most therapists discover that patients appreciate limits even if they complain vociferously when these limits are initially set. This includes limits regarding session times and frequency. The therapist must be willing to make *some* accommodations (e.g., when a patient arrives late) but must also generate a clear-cut expectation of *how* accommodating she will be and be consistent about it.

Control of Affects and Impulses

In addition to setting limits, you must also give the patient strategies for control of affects and impulses. Impulsive patients are frequently overwhelmed by painful, dysphoric, or angry affects. Quitting jobs, taking drugs, and fighting with family are typical outcomes of impulsivity; appropriate treatment depends on the patient's current level of insight. Some patients are literally unaware that their decision making is impaired, and they need to become aware that they have a problem. They may benefit if verbally rewarded for instances of good impulse control. Other patients are painfully aware of their impulsivity and its consequences, but are unable to control it. They have a different agenda: to modify the processes that lead to the generation of their affects.

Strategies for dealing with impulsive behavior are summarized as follows:

- Elaborate the unwanted and self-destructive consequences of impulsive behavior.
- Pit self-destructive consequences against equally powerful motivators.
- Note that condemnation only reduces a patient's self-esteem further.
- Address and empathize with the affect that generates the impulses.
- Find more appropriate ways to satisfy the need that generates the impulse.

Education

In matters large and small, the therapist serves to educate or provide factual and objective information about various matters to the patient. You may not be an expert in the matter under discussion, but you may be the only available educator, in which case you should not shirk the task if the request for information is genuine and not the patient's way of avoiding more emotionally charged issues.

As therapist, you are also an educator about mental illness itself. Receiving education about one's condition has increasingly been recognized as an important factor in medical compliance and cure. For example, inpatient educational programs have been shown to have an ameliorative effect on the negative symptoms of schizophrenia (Goldman and Quinn 1988) and on compliance in schizophrenia and mood disorders (Seltzer et al. 1980). We believe that a major benefit of education in such disorders is the ability to distinguish healthy from pathological feelings and cognitions. Patients can learn to recognize the danger signs of increased paranoia, delusional thinking, and expansive mood.

In our own practices, we frequently print out relevant information about a patient's condition from the Internet. We bookmark our favorite (and most reliable) sites and have some preprinted materials available. We urge you to pre-screen anything that you recommend personally and be prepared to discuss, agree with, or disagree with it. It is true that patients can selectively use statements from other sources to augment resistance to the therapy, or they may discover unorthodox or dangerous treatments and insist that these be undertaken instead of standard treatments such as medication. However, we feel that open discussion, with its benefits, is better than a one-sided approach. Finally, as all therapists are aware, there is a considerable amount of antimedication, anti-psychiatry, and anti-therapy material on the Internet, and your patients may have questions about those sites and the validity of their information.

Some patients spend many hours a day online and will research their own conditions. They may be more knowledgeable than you are about their illness, and that is just something you might have to admit one day. However, as for many patients in supportive psychotherapy, they will use the Internet to research side effects of medicine and to communicate with others in an anonymous way that is less threatening because they are paranoid or fearful, and so on. Some patients, however, are fearful of using the Internet to learn about their illness and may need to be encouraged (if you feel it is valuable). (For some current research based on patient surveys, see Schrank et al. 2010, 2014.) Resources for therapists are now widely available, so we will let you develop your own library.

Your major therapeutic questions will concern the extent to which specific types of information should be provided to a patient at a specific time. You may be concerned that education about the illness will not be understood or will generate stigma or irresponsibility (Bisbee 1979). The stigma of mental illness is indeed significant, and it is usually fruitless to directly attack delusions or denials of illness. Moreover, the consequences of ascribing a major diagnosis should be considered.

In addition to use of outside sources such as the Internet, we think that most therapists should make time to discuss mental illness in the therapy. Also, education for patients with chronic illness requires considerable time and repetition and is often best presented in standardized group programs. Educational materials, although subject to their own misinterpretation, carry independent authority. Most therapists can recount an experience in which their patients disagreed with them about some facet of their illness until they found corroboration in the popular press. Materials distributed by the clinic often add to the institutional transference and provide the patient with an emotional link to the clinic. They also help to dispel confusion over verbal statements of the therapist, since patients may misinterpret educational statements because of transferential reasons. For example, when you say, "I think your illness can be effectively treated," the patient may think that you are trying to be kind and understate a bad prognosis. For that patient, reading about effective treatments for the condition may be reassuring because the information comes from an "objective" source.

Social Skills Training

One type of education is worth special mention. Many chronically mentally ill patients have impaired cognition and judgment and lack basic social skills, the presence of which appears to increase survival time in the community (Linn et al. 1980). Social skills training, a modular, highly structured program of interpersonal skills training, has received extensive implementation and validation (Liberman 1988; Liberman et al. 1985). The program includes roleplaying, videotaped feedback, and the practice of skills in group and community settings. In the next chapter, we discuss an important program of self-management based on the work of Albert Bandura (see Fluent 2013).

The individual therapist can help to provide many of the items in formal social skills training, as shown in Table 4–3. Social skills should be addressed as needed in the therapy (such as when a deficit is revealed) or through specific training scenarios rather than as abstract lectures. One should not assume that all patients can learn the social skills they need; some researchers have questioned whether the training can overcome some of the apparently inherent deficits in schizophrenia, including deficits in affect recognition and sensitivity to negative affect (Bellack et al. 1989).

Work and Work Skills

Patients frequently ask for advice about work, and it is important for therapists to be able to talk about this topic appropriately. Here are some guidelines.

Table 4–3.   Important social skills to consider in therapy

Making eye contact	Standing up for one's rights (self-assertion)
Learning verbal intonation	Developing multiple approaches to presented problems
Learning social conversation	
Learning to give and accept compliments	Making appointments
Recognizing social cues	Applying for a job
Making appropriate self-disclosures	Using the telephone effectively
Rehearsing strategies for dealing with anticipated situations	Enjoying use of leisure resources
	Managing one's medications

Source.   Bellack et al. 1989; Liberman et al. 1985.

Work skills are not identical to social skills. For example, the self-absorption of many schizophrenic or depressed patients can be converted into task absorption, and persons with schizoid personalities often succeed admirably in isolated tasks focused on inanimate objects. On the other hand, the verbal adeptness or social viscosity of many patients with personality disorders and hypomanic patients may be incompatible with the attention required of work. A corollary is that the therapist should not be deterred from referring undersocialized patients for vocational training, and the vocational rehabilitation counselor should be consulted to arrive at the proper placement (Mackota and Lamb 1989). Although for legal purposes physicians are often called on to evaluate disability and work capacity, it is important to be aware that work skills are complex, and assessment may require extended evaluation (Massel et al. 1990).

Work has mostly positive connotations for patients with psychiatric disorders. Although work may connote drudgery and servitude for some patients who would envision a life free of it, work has positive connotations for most of us most of the time:

- It is a shared social enterprise.
- When remunerated, it can be converted into other positive reinforcements.
- It provides a subject matter to discuss with other workers, family, and the therapist.
- It conveys independence, self-sufficiency, and productivity.
- It creates an agency of self-mastery and a challenge that can be intrinsically rewarding and boosting to self-esteem.

Case Vignette

A regressed patient with a diagnosis of schizophrenia had a tendency to ramble excessively on abstruse philosophical topics, never getting to his point. Well educated, the patient had major interests in the works of G. K. Chesterton and Marcel Proust, and he was never seen reading a comic book or popular magazine. Nevertheless, the therapist discovered that he had previously spent 2 years commuting to a job as a dishwasher until his illness prevailed, resulting in the current hospitalization. It appeared that the patient had genuinely liked his job. He now wanted to continue in some productive capacity. Despite the therapist's heartfelt conviction that the patient could not complete the simplest of tasks without digressing, the patient was successfully placed in a clerical and filing position and received high evaluations for his consistent work performance. [Note that when a patient likes a "low level" job, the therapist may be disappointed or have other countertransference reactions.]

Ambivalence about work does not usually reflect a fundamental conflict of values, but instead the operation of understandable fears and anxieties about performance. Work is stressful, if only because it generates some social interaction that results in emotional relationships, decision making, and the ratings of success and failure. Therapy may be the only place a patient can express such fears and anxieties, because he may feel that such admissions to family or friends will be interpreted as weakness or laziness.

Quite different from the man in the preceding vignette is the patient whose work aspirations are patently grandiose and unrealistic. Sometimes the transferential implications are obvious, as in many individuals who express the desire to become doctors, and others who choose training programs in which they have no intrinsic interest as a defensive maneuver so that failure does not hurt their self-image. Still others may fail *in order* to prove their worthlessness. In such cases the therapist needs to defeat the maneuver by refusing to interpret failure in work as a personal failure—a task that might be difficult for the therapist to do in her own personal life.

Scheduling

Treatment planning comprises short-term goals that address specific problems, usually smaller, that can be approached in individual sessions or over a short period of time, and longer-term goals that seek to complete the objectives therapy. Ideally, the shorter-term goals are building locks to longer-term goals (Berman 2015).

When scheduling activities in treatment plans, you need to be sensitive to the individual with whom you are working, as well as any practical considerations of the length of the program itself. For example, individuals who have a lower level of functioning, such as the more severely mentally ill or those with intellectual disabilities will require more directive assistance in meeting goals in a timely and structured manner. Persons who are experiencing severe depression may have trouble with meeting scheduling goals, and patients who are manic may have trouble with organizational skills (Maruish 2002). As with all aspects of treatment, the assessment of progress and the achievement of goals will usually be more interactive than linear.

Cognitive Restructuring and Behavioral and Experiential Learning

Cognitive therapy has established itself as an effective mode of therapy for several disorders. A specific program of cognitive therapy involves more structured elements than will be discussed here, but many cognitive and behavioral techniques are already used successfully by therapists, and additional ones can be used without conducting a complete cognitive therapy program.

In Beck's theory of depression, the patient suffers a cognitive triad of negative self, world, and the future, created by underlying internalized, irrational belief systems (i.e., cognitive schemata) that are expressed in numerous cognitive distortions of events in the patient's life. Therapists will probably recognize many of these distortions immediately (see Table 4–4), although they may not have had names for them. (These cognitive distortions are discussed in many texts on cognitive therapy; see, e.g., Freeman 1987; Beck and Emery 1985; Wright et al. 2017.)

The patient's cognitive distortions are accompanied by typical response patterns. Patients with anxiety disorders, for example, are essentially "prisoners" to involuntary negative associations to events. Their automatic thoughts and images, which dwell on the harmful meanings and consequences of events, can be recorded and scrutinized with the help of the therapist. Examples of such negative responses are given in Table 4–5. Patients may also have generalized potentially harmful stimuli to include a wide range of events. For example, a person hearing a car horn may think of an accident. Unlike less

Table 4–4. Typical cognitive errors leading to depression or anxiety

Cognitive error	Example
Selective abstraction	"Something bad happened today, so my day is ruined."
Catastrophizing	"If I don't get this job, it will be the end of my career."
Arbitrary inferences (includes negative predictions and mind reading)	"My boss didn't talk to me this morning; he must be mad at me."
Homogenization	"Everyone's opinion of me counts equally."
Centering	"Everyone's attention is focused on me (and that makes me nervous)."
Absolutist (all-or-nothing) thinking	"If my work isn't perfect, it's not worth anything at all."
Overgeneralization	"That plane crash last week just proves that it's not safe to fly."
Disqualifying the positive	"Even though I hold two jobs and take care of six children, that doesn't mean I'm doing anything worthwhile."
Magnification or minimization	"My coworker is so much better than I am." (magnification applied to others) "I can never get any work done." (minimization applied to self)
Should/must/ought statements	"I should diet/exercise/work harder/be nice to people [etc.]."
Labeling and mislabeling	"I'm no good; I'm a failure."
Personalization	"It always rains when I plan a picnic."

Source. Categories are from Beck and Emery 1985; Wright et al. 2017. The examples are ours.

Table 4–5.   Typical automatic thoughts and images

"Oh boy. I should never have started this!"

"I can feel the plane crashing and I see the falling all around me."

"I'll never get this done on time!"

"Why do I always get myself into these predicaments? I should have stayed home."

"I can hear them laughing at me when I read the report in the meeting."

"If only I could figure out what to do! But I am so stupid!"

Source.   Modeled on statements in Beck and Emery 1985.

anxious people, anxiety-prone patients cannot adapt or habituate to stimuli that are known to be harmless (Beck and Emery 1985, pp. 31–34).

The cognitive therapist directs the patient's attention to the latter's automatic responses, both cognitive and behavioral, attempting to increase the patient's voluntary control. This requires repeated exercises in which the patient learns how his or her experiences are linked to cognitive distortions and develops alternative interpretations that are less threatening. Because the therapist explores these associations when the instigating situation has "cooled off" (or, as Pine [1986] would say, when the "iron is cold"), the connections can be seen more objectively. It is important for patients to realize that the actual anxiety-provoking situation increases irrational thinking. When patients recede from the actual situation, they often regain their objectivity and realize that it was not dangerous.

At a deeper level, when faced with potentially threatening stimuli, anxious patients typically activate a constellation of cognitive schemata that collectively is called a *vulnerability set*. At this level, the patient's basic assumptions are eventually spelled out and challenged. Some of these basic assumptions are given in Table 4–6. We have used some examples that seem most relevant to our practices. We must always have some evidence, however, that the assumption is maladaptive for that patient. Some people who believe "I'm nothing unless I'm loved" or some people who think "I have to be best at whatever I do" never have any substantial psychopathology, so one cannot assume that these assumptions are pathological in themselves.

Based on this admittedly limited presentation of cognitive therapy, some points should be recognized:

Table 4–6.   Some major assumptions that are usually maladaptive

"I have to please others."

"I always have to be good."

"People need to like me all the time."

"I always have to tell the truth."

"When people criticize me, it's because I am bad."

"If I fail in one thing, I'm going to fail in everything else."

"Money means everything."

"If I lose control once, I'll never regain it."

"If I let someone get close to me, they'll take over my life."

Source.   Modeled after Beck and Emery 1985.

- Cognitive therapy is not likely to be appropriate for patients whose illog-icality is far reaching, as in many patients with schizophrenia. (However, it has been successfully used with such patients and should not be ruled out.)
- Cognitive therapy requires a level of task orientation and motivation that many supportive therapy patients may not be able to meet.
- Cognitive therapists usually prescribe homework, which may be beyond the capabilities of many supportive psychotherapy patients.
- Many cognitive and behavioral techniques can, however, be employed di-rectly and can be buttressed by specific supportive interventions.

In patients with anxiety disorders, for example, these interventions include the fostering of positive but less restrictive basic assumptions that enhance the patient's self-esteem. For example, the patient needs to believe that "I am a good person even if I make mistakes," rather than "I am a failure if I make a single mistake." Improved self-esteem, in turn, affects the generation of auto-matic thoughts in anxiety-provoking situations. The patient is less likely to succumb to a mild threat if she is able to generate self-reinforcing responses to the threatening stimuli.

In Chapter 3, we introduced the notion of a defense modification called "unlinking." A form of this, *anticipatory unlinking*, may be especially effective in offering directive interventions. At the extreme, therapists such as Milton Erickson have specifically given patients a directive to fail so that the exposure can be decatastrophized once and for all. For example, Erickson's underachieving patient Harold was told to take and fail algebra (Haley 1986, p. 129).

Modeling and Identification With the Therapist

The therapist's role as a model for the patient has always been emphasized in psychotherapy. Even when emphasizing modeling, the therapist must still be alert to manifestations of transference.

Case Vignette

A woman who has just overcome her shock at the burglary of her apartment remarks, "I was wondering how a top-level male executive would have handled it." The therapist echoes, "A top-level male?" "Yes," replies the patient, "and actually I was thinking how *you* would have handled it."

The nature of supportive psychotherapy allows modeling and identification with the therapist. The patient may know many personal facts about the therapist, providing less room for fantasy. Social differences and the serious nature of the patient's crisis may also make the distance greater. However, the therapist can counter these tendencies and the distortions of transference by offering some examples of what she *would* do.

Homework

One proponent of supportive psychotherapy (whom we quoted at the end of Chapter 1) recommends against assigning homework (Markowitz 2014). The rationale is that the supportive psychotherapy patient does not have capacity to do homework and/or the damage to his self-esteem from failing the assignment outweighs any potential benefit from the homework. However, we believe that you can determine the desirability of using homework in the treatment. As with traditional school homework, we believe that homework in therapy may be assigned to provide opportunities for the patient to learn or generalize important skills. Doing, as opposed to listening and talking, can be an extremely important positive step in therapy. In social skills training, for example, the therapist might ask a patient to pick up a job application and bring it into the session to fill out, or ask a patient with a bipolar or panic disorder to chart daily variations in mood. Homework can also be based on known relationships between behavior and symptom amelioration. For example, exercise has an antidepressant effect and is a proper sublimation of aggression, and hobbies provide a feeling of mastery and stimulate intellectual and motor skills.

Homework is also a symbolic substitute for the therapist. It evokes an image of the therapist in the patient's mind and gives her a reason to return and report on it. The therapist should therefore ask the patient, "Did you get a chance to do that assignment?" This is better than letting it pass. It conveys the attitude that the therapist remembered the assignment and cares about the patient. Even if the patient did not do the homework, the therapist's concern will be remembered. Resources for homework are numerous, including the well-known series by Jongsma (2016).

Diversions, Substitutes, and Paradoxical Interventions

It is often helpful to prescribe *diversions*, as in the standard advice to "take a vacation," when there is no other means of facing a situation and a respite would be beneficial. *Substitutes* can also be offered for undesirable behaviors. Sometimes one must point out that talking is better than hitting. Coping behaviors that utilize one defensive strategy may be substituted for others that use less adaptive strategies. For example, intellectualization and reaction formation have helped many patients to move from denying their illnesses to becoming experts about them. Suppression, a mature defense, is also useful for both internal and external events. For example, therapists often feel helpless with patients whose disturbing hallucinations do not yield to medication; however, telling such a patient that he has the power to fight back against hallucinations or to "not pay attention" to the voices may result in actual suppression and a greater sense of self-control.

Providing defenses (such as rationalizations) *for social use* is also important, because peer group influence and the fear of losing peer group approval are responsible for many destructive behaviors. Fears or projections of peer group opinions may also be exaggerations of realistic concerns about acceptance, or defensive covering of deeper fears such as loss of control. The therapist should supply the patient with verbal ammunition to resist destructive influences, as by telling the patient whose drug-using "friends" accuse her of being a wimp: "Tell them you're working tomorrow, or you were up the previous night and have to go home, or that you're into organic foods. You can give them plenty of reasons why you won't use drugs, even if you just can't say 'No' straight out."

So far, we have been describing directive interventions in which the therapist offers something that he believes is in the patient's best interest. However, there are also *paradoxical interventions*, in which the therapist advises, prescribes, or encourages what appears to be the opposite of a desired result. For example, Bergman (1982) reports success with radical interventions such as telling one patient that he was a dog trapped in a human body and another that he was a spy from the state mental hospital. Some such interventions work by changing the reinforcements that patients receive for irrational behavior, which is not particularly paradoxical but a rather straightforward goal of therapy. For example, a patient who is asserting her independence by not attending therapy regularly might be told that she must stay away from the therapist as much as possible. In that way, she needs to change the behavior that she uses to assert her independence and start to attend the therapy.

Therefore, oppositional or obsessional patients, or those who tend to have negative therapeutic reactions, may benefit from paradoxical interventions, but such tactics must be used sparingly and require considerable skill. In all cases, such interventions should not be made with a dishonest premise. For example, a therapist who "prescribes" that the patient have as many temper tantrums as possible (in the hope of making the behavior less rewarding) should simply offer that as a procedure to be tried, without reframing the temper tantrum as a desirable behavior itself. For both practical and ethical reasons, we oppose the use of paradoxical interventions that generate false impressions of the therapist's beliefs and introduce deception into the relationship.

Reinforcement of Desirable Behaviors

Although we have given many examples of specific direction and advice, we shall close this chapter by emphasizing that the therapist should use the many available opportunities to reinforce desirable behaviors that are observed in or reported by the patient. Sincere praise and compliments can be very effective if properly applied. We emphasize this point because many therapists trained in psychoanalytic methods have become quite wary of direct praise (as well as perplexed about what behaviors are desirable). To praise is likely to play the parent, and this can create a negative transference as patients relive dependency and control issues from earlier years. The supportive therapist is not immune from this danger of being directive, but the typical supportive therapy patient needs direction much more than discussion. As with many other topics here, we cannot explore this one fully but will refer the reader to the finely wrought explication of reinforcement by Wachtel (1989), who observes: "Put simply, we say 'yes' and 'no' in far more ways than we are usually willing to acknowledge, and while these responses are by no means omnipotent, they are heard; and their impact is substantial" (p. 256).

Key Points

- Direct advice is especially suitable for patients who need supportive psychotherapy and can be very useful when used judiciously. This includes giving advice and offering specific guidance.

- Suggestions can be made in two ways: in the ordinary sense as a kind of "what if" inquiry and akin to a hypnotic suggestion in which saying it leads to the patient to be inclined to do it.

- Limit setting, or the outright, nonnegotiable prohibition of certain types of behavior, is often necessary in supportive work. Absolute limits, such as the prohibition of violence, must be set within the therapy, although it may be necessary to negotiate other limits outside of the therapeutic setting since the therapist cannot totally control them.

- Interventions in the therapy can be supplemented with education interventions, internet resources, and smart phone applications.

- Supportive psychotherapists should know the basic tenets of cognitive psychotherapy, which is one of a few well-validated therapies that can be used to supplement supportive techniques.

- The therapist's repertoire should include a variety of other interventions: these include modeling and identification with the therapist, homework (which some supportive therapists do not recommend, but we do), diversions, paradoxical interventions (to be used cautiously and sparingly), and reinforcement of desirable behaviors.

References

Adler G: Supportive psychotherapy revisited. Hillside J Clin Psychiatry 4:3–13, 1982

Beck AT, Emery G: Anxiety Disorders and Phobias: A Cognitive Perspective. New York, Basic Books, 1985

Bellack AS, Morrison RL, Mueser KT: Social problem solving in schizophrenia. Schizophr Bull 15(1):101–116, 1989 2655067

Bergman JS: Paradoxical interventions with people who insist on acting crazy. Am J Psychother 36(2):214–222, 1982 7102841

Berman P: Case Conceptualization and Treatment Planning: Integrating Theory With Clinical Practice. Los Angeles, CA, Sage, 2015

Bisbee CC: Patient education in psychiatric illness. Orthomolecular Psychiatry 8:239–247, 1979

Fluent TE: How best to engage patients in their psychiatric care. Curr Psychiatr 12(9):22–36, 2013

Freeman A: Cognitive therapy: an overview, in Cognitive Therapy: Applications in Psychiatric and Medical Settings. Edited by Freeman A, Greenwood VB. New York, Human Sciences Press, 1987, pp 19–35

Goldman CR, Quinn FL: Effects of a patient education program in the treatment of schizophrenia. Hosp Community Psychiatry 39(3):282–286, 1988 3356434

Green SA, Goldberg RL, Goldstein DM, et al: Limit Setting in Clinical Practice. Washington, DC, American Psychiatric Press, 1988

Haley J: Uncommon Therapy: The Psychiatric Techniques of Milton H. Erickson, M.D. New York, WW Norton, 1986

Jongsma A: Adult Psychotherapy Homework Planner, 5th Edition. New York, Wiley, 2016

Lamb HR: Treating the Long-Term Mentally Ill. San Francisco, CA, Jossey-Bass, 1982

Liberman RP (ed): Psychiatric Rehabilitation of Chronic Mental Patients. Washington, DC, American Psychiatric Press, 1988

Liberman RP, Massel HK, Mosk MD, et al: Social skills training for chronic mental patients. Hosp Community Psychiatry 36(4):396–403, 1985 3997101

Linn MW, Klett CJ, Caffey EM Jr: Foster home characteristics and psychiatric patient outcome: the wisdom of Gheel confirmed. Arch Gen Psychiatry 37(2):129–132, 1980 7352844

Mackota C, Lamb HR: Vocational rehabilitation. Psychiatr Ann 19:548–552, 1989

Maruish ME: Essentials of Treatment Planning. New York, Wiley, 2002

Markowitz JC: What is supportive psychotherapy? Focus 12(3):285–289, 2014

Massel HK, Liberman RP, Mintz J, et al: Evaluating the capacity to work of the mentally ill. Psychiatry 53(1):31–43, 1990 2320681

Pine F: Supportive psychotherapy: a psychoanalytic perspective. Psychiatr Ann 16:526–529, 1986

Schrank B, Sibitz I, Unger A, et al: How patients with schizophrenia use the internet: qualitative study. J Med Internet Res 12(5):e70, 2010 21169176

Schrank B, Sibitz I, Unger A, et al: Metadata correction: How patients with schizophrenia use the Internet: qualitative study. J Med Internet Res 16(7):e165, 2014 30583453

Seltzer A, Roncari I, Garfinkel P: Effect of patient education on medication compliance. Can J Psychiatry 25(8):638–645, 1980 6110471

Wachtel PL: Psychoanalysis and Behavior Therapy: Toward an Integration. New York, Basic Books, 1989

Wright JH, Brown GK, Thase ME, Basco MR: Learning Cognitive-Behavior Therapy: An Illustrated Guide, 2nd Edition. Arlington, VA, American Psychiatric Association Publishing, 2017

5

Managing the Therapy

In this chapter, we describe the management of therapy from the standpoint of mostly the beginning therapist as well as the new patient. If either therapist or patient has had considerable experience in therapy, the initial conditions will be altered.

Selection of Patients for Supportive Psychotherapy

Although supportive psychotherapy has a broad therapeutic range, one still must consider whether and when to use it, just as one must decide whether to use a medication with broad indications. One wants to avoid using this modality when it would be a waste of the patient's and the therapist's time or when there is an even more effective and appropriate therapeutic choice. For example, supportive psychotherapy is regarded as wasteful in the later stages of dementia and as less potent than psychodynamic psychotherapy in achieving self-understanding.

Supportive psychotherapy should not be selected routinely without thought. Too often in clinical settings there is an automatic decision to provide supportive psychotherapy without full consideration of the indications and contraindications. This decision is sometimes based on economic considerations: "It's all we can afford." Especially in treatment sites in which the vast majority of patients need medications, there is a tendency to consider only supportive psychotherapy among the psychotherapies. Although this choice is flattering to those of us who know of the potency of supportive psychotherapy, we would still plead that one always ask the same question of supportive psychotherapy as one would ask of any other therapeutic approach.

Supportive psychotherapy is applicable to a range of patients in both hospital and outpatient settings. As noted in Chapter 1, controlled studies have shown it to be at least equal in efficacy to other modes of treating depression, schizophrenia, and certain phobic disorders. Its effectiveness is further supported by case studies on a variety of diagnoses.

Indications for supportive psychotherapy according to diagnoses or other syndromes are listed in Table 5–1. Although by no means complete, this listing is meant to orient you to the growing field of research and practice in which supportive psychotherapy is used. As the last category indicates, supportive psychotherapy is still not for everyone. For example, it is ineffective for patients with short-term memory disturbances who cannot maintain the personal relationship necessary for the therapy. Such patients will benefit from supportive care and counseling but not psychotherapy per se. Substance abuse, either single or polysubstance, is not a contraindication to supportive psychotherapy, but active substance abuse requires treatment based on detoxification and abstinence. We have seen supportive psychotherapy used successfully in detoxifying patients during substance (including alcohol) withdrawal without concurrent medications. Although there may be times when supportive psychotherapy has to be used in these situations, we do not automatically recommend alcohol detoxification without medications (which is usually called *social detox*). Even after acute detoxification, if substance abuse is the patient's only problem, supportive psychotherapy may be a poor substitute for a better form of treatment. Many substance abusers will accept supportive therapy but refuse more focused drug treatment programs when available. The therapist must decide if the patient's denial can be addressed in the therapy or if continuing with therapy will actually fuel the denial by enabling the patient to rationalize that he is receiving active treatment (while continuing the substance abuse). In a similar vein, criminal histories are not contraindications as such and supportive psychotherapy is easily adaptable to convicted criminals

Table 5–1. Diagnostic indications for supportive psychotherapy[a]

Large controlled studies, meta-analyses, and well-designed studies

Depression

Schizophrenia

Phobic disorders

Borderline personality disorder

Bipolar disorder

Delusional disorder

Major substance use disorder, including marijuana, cocaine, and opioids

Small studies and case reports

Psychosocial factors affecting physical condition
   (psychosomatic disorders, including alexithymia)

Panic attacks

Social phobias

Terminal illness

Chronic and potentially life-threatening illness

• HIV infection

• Cancer

Chronic medical illness

• Asthma

• Diabetes mellitus

• Chronic obstructive pulmonary disease

• Posttransplantation adjustments

• Disfiguring ailments

Table 5–1.　Diagnostic indications for supportive psychotherapy[a] *(continued)*

Small studies and case reports *(continued)*

Acute medical illness

- Acute leukemia

- Myocardial infarction

- Spinal injury

Disasters (e.g., paraplegia following earthquake) (Fauzia and Sholihah 2013)

Bereavement

Suicidal crisis or postattempt

Adjustment to rape

Early stages of dementia

Intellectual disability

Substance use disorders (accompanied by peer group treatment)

Some, but not all, personality disorders, including antisocial personality disorder

Effectiveness unlikely or not proven[b]

Delirium

Drug intoxication

Later stages of dementia

Some mental disorders due to medical conditions

Any disorder in which short-term memory is seriously impaired

Note.　See also Conte and Plutchik 1986.
[a]These categories are not necessarily DSM-5 disorders but are the categories that have been used in the literature about supportive psychotherapy.
[b]See Chapter 6. Meta-analyses concluded that there is a lack of evidence in existing studies.

(Werman 1988); however, the more purely antisocial the patient is, the more likely it is that group psychotherapy is indicated.

Diagnosis is only one consideration in the selection of supportive psychotherapy, and other characteristics must be given considerable weight. There are a variety of criteria for patient selection. A typical profile of a patient suitable for long-term supportive therapy is given in Table 5–2. Often this patient has had several acute psychiatric hospitalizations. Some characteristics (those marked [a] in the table) are likely to make such a patient unsuitable for more insight-oriented therapy. However, many therapists will undertake psychodynamic therapy (rarely, psychoanalysis) with some patients who have characteristics such as severe narcissistic traits, so-called borderline personality, acting-out behavior, and/or poor social support. Age by itself is not a contraindication to supportive therapy.

Characteristics of patients who may require and benefit from supportive therapy, generally in the short term, are shown in Table 5–3. Also included are many characteristics of patients who would probably also benefit from long-term psychodynamic psychotherapy.

Those characteristics that tend to make patients unsuitable for supportive therapy are shown in Table 5–4. Patients can be divided, based on these exclusionary criteria, into three groups: 1) those who would best be prescribed another type of treatment, such as group or family therapy or behavioral management; 2) those who are not likely to respond to, or may even get worse in, therapy; and 3) those who cannot be engaged in the therapeutic process. Patients who have responded negatively to therapy in the past are at high risk for such responses again, and their treatment should generally be reserved for experienced therapists who are skilled in working with the patients' types of pathology. Such patients may have a masochistic need to be punished in the therapy, or they may engage in a narcissistic power struggle to oppose and defeat the therapist's apparent good intentions. The supportive therapist is also likely to encounter patients with borderline personality who rapidly develop destructive transference relationships. Following Frances and Clarkin (1981), no treatment is often the best choice for such patients unless they are in immediate danger that outweighs the risk of treatment, or unless the therapy can be circumscribed to a specific area that does not create the destructive transference. According to those authors, the no-treatment group also includes a few patients for whom the no-treatment recommendation thwarts the wish for dependency or regression or serves as a paradoxical technique to generate oppositional improvement despite the lack of treatment.

Table 5–2.   Patient selection for *long-term* supportive psychotherapy

Chronically deficient or acutely weakened coping skills[a]

A history of acting out

Chronic stress from environment, family, or illness

Low capacity for introspection (not curious about thinking, not psychologically minded)

Inability to contain or tolerate affect, especially negative affect[a]

Poor social support

Poor object relations

Strong dependency needs

Poor impulse control (primitive impulses)[a]

Primitive defenses

Poor reality testing[a]

Cognitive disorganization or impairment (but short-term memory should be intact)[a]

Lack of motivation for treatment[a]

Fears or suspicions of treatment[a]

A tendency to externalize causes of failure

A tendency to somatize or an inability to speak of emotions (alexithymia)[a]

Note.   Psychopharmacology will frequently be indicated as an adjunct to supportive psychotherapy with these conditions.
[a]Denotes characteristics that especially tend to contraindicate insight-oriented therapy.

Treatment Planning

Treatment planning is the assignment and phased implementation of resources to address the patient's problems. Most systems in current use are adaptations of the Problem-Oriented Medical Record designed by Lawrence Weed (1969) (also Ryback et al. 1981); one starts with a patient problem list, linking

Table 5–3. Patient selection for *short-term* supportive psychotherapy

Previously or usually strong coping skills

An acute crisis requiring temporary intervention

A sense of internal conflict

The ability to obtain symptom relief through understanding

The ability to contain or tolerate affect

Good social support or temporarily disrupted social support

Good object relations

Good impulse control

Good reality testing

Intact cognitive abilities

Trust of the therapist

Motivation for treatment

Mature defenses

Mature coping mechanisms

Psychological-mindedness

A tendency to internalize causes of failure

Ability to identify and speak of emotions

Note. Depending on their situations, patients with characteristics listed here may also be candidates for psychodynamic psychotherapy or psychoanalysis.

it to goals of treatment and specific interventions to meet those goals. The following are some brief admonitions relevant to treatment planning for patients who receive supportive psychotherapy. In developing the treatment plan, there are many useful texts (see, e.g., Adams and Grieder 2014; Makover 2016; Maruish 2002) and two that are especially useful in supportive work are those describing the symptom-targeted behavioral approach of Taylor et al. (1982) and the level-of-function treatment planning by Kennedy (1992).

Table 5–4.   Exclusion criteria for supportive psychotherapy

Better suited for another form of treatment

In crisis, but effectively utilizing social supports

Not in crisis and able to afford and benefit from insight-oriented therapy or psychoanalysis

Interested in therapy for self-enrichment or training

Primary problem of antisocial personality (better suited for group treatment)

Primary problem social or family related (depending on the problem, better suited for couples, group, or family treatment)

Not likely to respond, or may even get worse

Not requiring therapy of any modality (includes patient forced into treatment by family)

Dangerously hostile to treatment or therapist

Significant cognitive or memory impairment

Severe mental retardation

Malingering (e.g., to prove disability)

Factitious illness

Failed to benefit or worsened in previous supportive psychotherapy (includes dependent, therapy-addicted patients

Unable to engage in treatment

Treatment simply not wanted

Total denial of illness (you may have to work with such patients in institutions)

Note.   One might wonder how much leeway should be given the *patient* in selecting a therapy. Choice should certainly be allowed to patients who can give plausible criteria for their preference.

The process of treatment planning begins with assessment by the therapist and members of the treatment team and the patient's own perceptions of what she needs, then a negotiated plan is developed that includes practical steps to meeting those needs. The plan will stem from the experience of the therapist and team in identifying steps that have a good probability of success. The therapist and patient discuss possible approaches and negotiate the types of interventions and activities that will be used. As treatment progresses, changes will be made as each sees what works and new problems or approaches are identified.

Another important function of treatment planning is that when there is a team such as in a hospital or clinic setting, there is a game plan that the whole team can use in coordinating care across disciplines and providing the patient with a consistent understanding of what is going on.

Although the treatment plan is often institutional and necessarily bureaucratic in format and presentation, it is crucial in the supportive therapy approach that the plan begin from the point of view of welcoming and respecting the value of the patient as an individual who has the right to self-direction and decision making and helping him develop skills that enhance self-direction and a sense of self-direction (Adams and Grieder 2014, p. 55; Fluent et al. 2013).

Makover (2016) describes the function of treatment planning as a way to help therapist and patient make sense of the process, record progress, identify measurable outcomes, and enhance efficiency. The aim of therapy should be to resolve distress, restore function, and further progress toward goals and increase the patient's self-reliance and management of her illness. As therapy proceeds, the focus changes, as do treatment modalities and goals. Assessment as treatment proceeds will lead to adjustments and changes to the activities recommended.

Interventions Should Be Individualized

Few problems are unique, and standardized interventions can be described for almost any conceivable psychosocial problem. However, effective treatment planning still requires the adaptation of standard interventions to the specific patient. Understandably, it will be necessary to make major changes in the treatment plan as treatment progresses; nonetheless, overly simple plans with "generic" interventions such as "group therapy," "antipsychotic treatment," and "individual psychotherapy" will not provide adequate guidance. The therapist needs a more specific plan, even if it is not reflected in the formal treatment plan.

Interventions Must Be Phased In

For most patients, major interventions should be phased in stepwise instead of simultaneously. For chronically mentally ill patients, a good rule of thumb is to make only one change at a time, such as in medication or vocational training (Yee 1989).

Interventions Must Be Negotiated

Although the therapist's assessment of the problem may differ from the patient's, it is important to secure agreement with the patient on some of the goals of treatment, and it is even more important to be willing to negotiate the goals in the context of a doctor-patient relationship that is not one sided or authoritarian (Eisenthal et al. 1979). Fluent et al. (2013), building on the work of Albert Bandura (1977) and research on illness management, start from the premise that "[o]ptimal care is best achieved through a partnership between patient and provider" (p. 22). Examples of self-management skills that they believe should be incorporated into treatment planning include the following:

- Actively participating in treatment and learning to be responsible for monitoring and managing symptoms and progress
- Formulating goals and learning skills relevant to the patient's disease
- Identifying problems that can be addressed with targeted interventions
- Building medical and behavioral management skills such as adherence to medication, participation in therapy, and completion of homework assignments and other behavioral activities designed to promote health
- Adjusting to changes in responsibilities and expectations
- Learning to manage emotional responses to stressors and day-to-day living

Phases of Therapy

Initiating Therapy

As with opera overtures, initial meetings in supportive therapy have a special task: to set the mood and tone for the succeeding exposition. Just as an overture may contain themes of the work that follows, so do the initial meetings in therapy, but they have a different agenda. The opening agenda (see Table 5–5) must eventually cover the mechanics and business arrangements, but these should be worked into the session piece by piece.

Cost, Frequency, and Duration and Availability

Will there be a limited trial of therapy before the decision is made to continue? Will there be meetings once a day, week, or month, and will they be at a fixed time or during a span of clinic hours? Will the sessions be variable or fixed in

Table 5–5.   The opening agenda

Clarify the mechanics.

- Discuss time, cost, flexibility, and availability.
- Determine frequency of sessions.
- Determine trial vs. fixed plan.
- Determine fixed vs. variable duration.
- Discuss treatment contracts and contingent arrangements.

Listen to the patient personally and professionally.

Develop your own impression.

React and adjust to the patient's style of communication.

Generate and convey empathy.

Explore surface issues.

Develop and individualize goals.

Correct early problems

Generate an expectation of realistic gains.

duration? Will the therapist be available by phone? How much will the therapy cost the patient? There are useful guidelines for all these issues but no hard-and-fast rules.

Cost and frequency of sessions.   Cost may be a factor, as well as the acute or chronic nature of the problem. Supportive work with patients with schizophrenia can be maintained in meetings that are as infrequent as once every 2 months, whereas meeting more than once a week may create too intense a transference. On the other hand, acutely ill, hospitalized patients may need to be seen briefly more than once a day.

Trial versus fixed plan.   It is usually best to start with a trial of therapy rather than a specific commitment. Some therapists term this an *extended evaluation* and suggest that the therapist meet with the patient once or twice before responding to the patient's concerns with any specific suggestions. At the end of the trial period, therapist and patient make specific arrangements to continue.

Fixed versus variable duration.   In many medical settings—for example, internal medicine or surgery clinics—the physician generally controls the duration of the sessions, which end when the necessary procedures or assessments have been performed. Similarly, in many psychiatric clinic and hospital settings, the length of the session *must* be varied. For example, a psychiatrist in a medication clinic may wish to meet with a particular patient for as little as 5 minutes, if the patient is stable and simply requires medication renewal, or for as long as several hours (e.g., to speak to family and/or outside case managers, to conduct a treatment conference, or to arrange hospital admission).

Case Vignette

A 33-year-old surgical nurse with a 2-year history of inertia, sadness, pessimism, insomnia, apathy, ideas of reference, and an unwillingness to see her friends and relatives was fired from her job. Her condition failed to respond to combinations of antipsychotic medications, trials of two different antidepressants, 8 months of weekly psychodynamically oriented psychotherapy from a very experienced private-practicing psychiatrist, and 6 months of weekly psychodynamically oriented psychotherapy from a very experienced clinic psychiatric resident. Finally, she was seen by a first-year resident, who was asked to provide her with supportive psychotherapy. To obtain a detailed history, in the third session he spent 95 minutes with her rather than the usual 30–50 minutes that had been allotted her by other clinicians. From that point on there was a substantial improvement in her energy level and outlook, and a lessening of her insomnia and ideas of reference. She became eager to see her relatives and to return to work.

By seeing her for 95 minutes, the psychiatric resident apparently gave her a sense of caring and support that she had not experienced in 2 years of treatment.

Such arrangements are not feasible if the patient pays for a specific length of session. However, when the session length will vary, it should be explained at the outset. If the therapist is planning to vary the duration, the patient will often wish to exercise similar control. For example, sometimes when the patient arrives late, the therapist may extend the time of the session, but not always. Not knowing when the session will end can create anxiety for a patient who cannot terminate it herself. If it ends earlier than expected, the patient may think that she has angered the therapist and is being rejected. On the other hand, if the patient finds that time is always extended when there are pressing problems, she may invent some. The rules regarding length of session must therefore depend on the therapist's assessment of the patient's realistic ability to countenance the variations.

Treatment Contracts and Contingent Agreements

Some outpatient clinics present the patient with a written treatment contract that spells out the mutual expectations of therapist and patient. Individual therapists, recognizing that certain behaviors (especially substance abuse) are very difficult to treat in individual therapy, may also wish to make treatment contingent on the patient avoiding such behavior—that is, the patient must be free of such behavior to enter into and continue with therapy. However, such contingent contracts are usually undesirable in supportive psychotherapy. Although the patient's failure to progress in therapy *because of* the undesirable behavior may eventually prove a reason for termination, the use of the treatment contract as a threat or motivator is usually ineffective.

Key Therapist Functions

Developing your own impression.   You want to avoid locking into a diagnosis and formulation and ceasing to really listen to the patient. Change of diagnosis and formulation is common in psychiatry as you get to know the patient's experience in greater detail. You should compare her diagnosis with the previous record, but should not let the record prevail, because you may be the first person to *really* know the patient. Another interesting possibility is that you may find some secondary diagnosis—often a personality disorder—toward which much of the therapeutic work can be directed.

Reacting and adjusting to the patient's style of communication.   As you begin to respond to the patient (in the initial and subsequent sessions), you should develop a style that the patient finds receptive. This entails matching some aspects of your expressive style to the patient's established ways of perceiving and categorizing the world. For example, with the overly intellectual patient, you may need to offer intellectual explanations at first because these are the only ones to which the patient gives credence (Dewald 1971, p. 105). This therapist-patient matching occurs intuitively in many successful therapists; others must learn it. Matching also includes the use of metaphors that utilize the patient's preferred sensory modality (e.g., visual, auditory, tactile); again, this usually occurs without reflection in experienced therapists.

The patient also sees you and hears the most subtle intonations of your voice. Your nonverbal behavior, including facial expressions, gestures, and body language, often betrays the most fastidiously voiced words. A warning: Psychotic patients are often quite adept at appreciating nonverbal cues because they neglect or discount the verbal accompaniment.

Generating and conveying empathy.   Why must therapists, on stage as they are, be so attentive to their roles? *Empathy*, the combined emotional and cognitive experience in the therapist of what the patient's experience is like, must be developed in the therapist and conveyed to the patient. Havens (1978), for example, has written of the importance of simple statements such as "How awful," "It must have hurt," and "You wanted to be loved," which often extrapolate slightly from the patient's own statements to show that the therapist recognizes the former's state of mind. Sharing an "affective baseline" with the patient, the therapist learns to pursue actively the patient's less obvious feelings (Havens 1978). More complex empathic statements can begin with the recognition of the patient's isolation ("No one understands you") and the validation of the patient's responses to experience ("No wonder you were frightened"). These statements of recognition can be built into "bridging statements" that acknowledge conflict without presuming that the patient is at fault (Havens 1979).

Learning genuine empathy rather than contriving it is a difficult art. Effective, highly empathic therapists still retain the ability to modulate their feelings and adapt to a succession of different patients. To learn this art, the beginner should think about the persons in his or her own life who have struck him or her as sincere versus insincere and consider their differences in empathy. Havens' concept of "self-effacing empathy" is reminiscent of Hawthorne's description of the physician who cautiously seeks a patient's secrets:

> A man burdened with a secret should especially avoid the intimacy of his physician. If the latter possess native sagacity and a nameless something more—let us call it intuition; if he shows no intrusive egotism, nor disagreeably prominent characteristics of his own; if he has the power, which must be born with him, to bring his mind into such affinity with his patient's, that this last shall unawares have spoken what he imagines himself only to have thought; if such revelations be received without tumult, and acknowledged not so often by an uttered sympathy as by silence, an inarticulate breath, and here and there a word, to indicate that all is understood; if to these qualifications of a confidant be joined the advantages afforded by his recognized character as a physician—then, at some inevitable moment, will the soul of the sufferer be dissolved, and

flow forth in a dark, but transparent stream, bringing all its mysteries into the daylight. (Hawthorne 1850/1937, p. 157)

Exploring surface issues. Explorations in initial meetings must be mostly patient-directed and superficial. You begin, in a matter-of-fact but empathic way, to explore surface issues ("You have been coming to this clinic for a long time." "This has been a difficult time of your life."). The explorations become deeper as they turn to the patient's feelings about events in his life ("You seem to be worried about the financial burdens your illness is putting on your family." "You've told me that the voices you hear have been bothering you less since you started taking medicine."). Summaries can be made, which are an extension of the patient's chief complaint ("It seems that the most important problem in your life is getting your own place to live.").

Developing and individualizing the goals. From these initial explorations come the patient-specific issues of the therapy such as compliance with medication and reduction of family stress. You will often see immediately that a patient is invested in one set of goals but denies or neglects what you perceive as the real set of goals. This dichotomy is not the result of limited education or intelligence and may be seen in either a research biologist or a maintenance worker. The former may deny the seriousness of his myocardial infarction. The latter may act out her paranoid delusions. Or vice versa.

Often a patient's goals include getting a job and finding friends, whereas you see more internal obstacles, such as noncompliance with medication, basic personality defects, or educational/vocational deficits, that the patient is not willing to admit to or remedy. You must be willing to accept some initial goals that may later become less important. For example, an unemployed, depressed man's initial expectations of therapy may be that it will lead to a job; this may be part or none of the "real" solution to his problem, but it is *his* goal and should be acknowledged until he can be convinced of another.

A goal that may be slow to develop, but can be most important, is the patient's investment in the therapy itself. The relationship with the therapist, at first just a means to an end, may eventually become an end in itself as the therapist develops in the patient's mind into a trusted, accepting individual to whom the patient can bring her problems.

Correcting early problems. The patient dropout rate is high in all forms of treatment, including supportive psychotherapy. Because a positive therapeutic alliance, as described earlier, may have predictive value for the success of therapy, it is important early to assess the state of that alliance. Following our earlier guidelines, a positive alliance need not be interpreted, but studies indicate that good therapeutic outcome correlates with a therapist's early attention to a patient's problematic feelings about the therapist (Foreman and Marmar 1985).

Generating an expectation of realistic gains.   As we indicated at the start of this chapter, psychotherapies may be effective because they generate an expectation of success. For example, a patient will often talk in a second session of getting his "first good night's sleep" after the first session. But it serves little purpose to *tell* patients, whether research biologists or maintenance workers, that you will be a warm, supportive force in their lives who will lighten their burdens and lift their spirits. Although treatment documents in your clinic or practice may say that there is no guarantee of success and that there is a small but distinct possibility that therapy may make them worse, we urge you to try to foster positive expectations and minimize negative ones by the encounter itself, its emotional subtleties and understatements, and maturation of trust.

The Middle Course of Therapy

The middle course of therapy has no consistent pattern in supportive psychotherapy, although this phase can be quite specific when a given psychiatric disorder or symptom is narrowly being discussed. A common question in this phase is, "Are we making progress?" In supportive psychotherapy, progress is measured by the patients' statements as to whether they are subjectively less distressed, whether their behavior is less disturbing, and whether they are less disabled by their illness. You should not become concerned if patients' "understanding" of or "insight" into their disorder is not improving if they are improving in the area of distresses, disturbances, and disabilities. What patients learn in supportive psychotherapy is often not expressed in words but is shown in behavior. For example, the therapist may observe a realistic accommodation of personality to loss or deficit even as the patient continues to complain about problems. Resistance to progress may occur because the patient continues to be inhibited from speaking freely to the therapist. For example, a patient who wants to impress her therapist may withhold negative information and relate a catalog of her successes. You need to work with such a patient to develop more unconditional trust. Repetition, the mainstay of nearly all therapies, may take the form of helping her to arrange her life so that new reinforcers (e.g., income, job satisfaction, interpersonal rewards, internalized self-approval) come to replace old ones (e.g., satisfaction from substance abuse, self-esteem replenishment from delusional fantasy or projection) and so that she gradually achieves competence in more demanding settings.

If you conclude that progress is less than expected, you may wish to explore the suggested causes of therapeutic stalemate or failure of the therapy to thrive that are listed in Table 5–6. You should not be terribly upset to find that several of these are present in a given therapy—most of us experience several of these "causes" in the typical course of therapy with a patient.

Termination and Transfer to Future Care

Therapy may be terminated unilaterally by the patient or therapist, or by mutual agreement. At the time of termination, you may consider the therapy to be successfully complete, successfully progressing, or stalemated with either a positive or negative relationship.

A successfully completed therapy ought, in theory, to be terminated by mutual consent, as often happens when brief supportive therapy for bereavement or other crisis is ended. However, unresolved dependency by the patient or a continuing wish for nurturing on your part may prolong the therapy. If the problem is the patient's, the continuing dependency should be taken as a sign that the treatment is not yet successful. Tapering sessions in either length or frequency is desirable. Scheduling infrequent appointments or allowing the patient to ask for a follow-up is another strategy. In supportive therapy, the door must often be left open permanently. Many patients face a lifetime of chronic illness with exacerbations and remissions. It is most important for you to consider: What attitude should the patient have toward future treatment? The attitude you want to foster is that patients come to feel deeply that if early signs of a psychiatric illness emerge, they will turn to the clinic/therapist for help. Thus, termination ideally only takes place when the patient has that knowledge and that attitude.

A successfully proceeding therapy is frequently terminated by the therapist for reasons beyond his control, as often happens in postgraduate training programs. Both parties to the therapy will feel the loss, but if a useful institutional transference has developed, the patient will usually be able to continue with a new therapist. July is not a common time for suicides in most epidemiological studies (which show a springtime peak), but the highest rate of suicide in train-

Table 5–6.   Causes of therapeutic slowdown

Causes primarily in the therapeutic relationship

Disturbed transference (either addressed or unaddressed)

- Erotic

- Hostile

- Parental

Lack of relationship or therapeutic alliance (patient is not meaningfully engaged in the supportive relationship with the therapist)

Absence of transference

Causes primarily in the patient

Absence from therapy (unless caused by therapist's poor technique)

Deflation of initially high expectations

- From the therapy

- From the therapist

- From the mental health system

Anxiety too high from therapist's interpretations

Weakening of patient's defenses (e.g., inability to externalize cause of his or her failures)

Patient's feeling of being manipulated

Worsening of patient's underlying biological condition (progression or exacerbation of disease)

Change in patient's circumstances (e.g., relationships, financial, job, educational)

Negative therapeutic reactions

Causes primarily in the therapist

Countertransference reactions

Difficulty in relating to patient with empathy (when patient is accessible)

Interpretations incorrect or too deep

ing centers may occur in July because of the termination of therapy in June. Inadequate preparation for therapist change can be lethal.

Terminations can also provide transitions to a new therapist who can start a stalemated therapy moving again. Transitions must be approached from the standpoint of the new therapist who "inherits" someone else's caseload. Idealization or devaluations of the previous therapist commonly occur. The former is often an attempt to adjust defensively to the fait accompli of a therapist's change and the patient's perceived helplessness. The latter is expressive of the fear that the new therapist will not be as good as the old. Therapists may find the following guidelines useful:

1. Devaluation and idealization are usually transitory. They can initially be left alone.
2. If it is necessary to explore them, this should be done in the context of the patient's thoughts about the new therapist. In this way, the new therapist does not have to challenge the patient's previous judgment.

All too often, a new therapist must deal with a patient's surprise and rage at discovering that his previous therapist has left. Failure to tell a patient that you are leaving is undesirable from an ethical and countertransference point of view. Even from a self-serving perspective, you may wish to consider that you are likely to meet the patient again in some other setting and need to deal with the termination inevitably. You should also consider that in matters of transition, the patient may be more of an expert than you are, because in most mental health settings, patients are already familiar with the frequent changes of treatment teams as the patients move between inpatient and outpatient settings.

When should a patient be told? To tell the patient too early may prevent the development of the therapeutic alliance. The following guideline may help: When starting the therapy, tell the patient the minimum time that she will be seen. Whether or not the patient raises the issue again, she should be warned that the therapy will be ending as that date nears.

Changing Modes of Therapy

It is easier to change modes of therapy than one might imagine. Most psychodynamic therapists have had occasion to switch to a supportive mode at the time of an intercurrent medical crisis. The flexibility of transition can be appreciated by reports of complete role reversals in which the therapist became ill and the patient temporarily became supportive to the therapist. In the supportive therapy of patients with psychosomatic disorders, for example, Karasu (1986) states that insight-oriented treatment can be established 6–12 months into the therapy, once the patient can acknowledge dependency and has developed a strong positive transference. Phrased in this way, one can see that the transition involves loss as well as gain.

Directing the Content

So far, we have described the elements and structural components of supportive psychotherapy. Now let's "drill down" as we describe the actual work (both interactional and in the therapist's mind) during face-to-face sessions.

Inexperienced therapists may initially think that general interest or sociability is all that is required in order to get the patient to "fill the hour" with conversation. However, they soon learn that they must be more directive of content, especially in settings in which they are meeting with the patient as infrequently as once a month. In insight-oriented therapy, a therapist often listens to a variety of topics and finds a central theme running through them all. In supportive therapy, the therapist does more than locate or comment on these veins of thought; she must do the actual mining by taking a more directive stance. The more important aspects of this task are discussed below.

Updating Outside Activities

It is helpful to ask, at some point during each session, for an update on the patient's activities since the last session, starting, if possible, with a problem that was left unsolved the last time. Similarly, goals set in a previous session can be reviewed. Such techniques establish session-to-session continuity and indicate to patients that you have found the sessions important and memorable.

Focusing on Specific Issues

Practitioners of brief psychotherapy use a focus, or central issue (e.g., interpersonal relationships, educational problems), for the course of therapy. A similar concept has been used in long-term therapy under the name of *sectoring* (Deutsch and Murphy 1955). The desirability of a focus in supportive therapy depends on the patient. Some patients can be trusted to identify and address their most pressing problems without assistance; others will need frequent refocusing when they forget the treatment goals or avoid confronting them.

With either limited time or a high level of resistance, it is often necessary for the therapist to move around to cover different topics and update his knowledge of the patient's situation. This is especially important when a patient is known to be reticent on important issues such as conflict with family or suicidal intent. This method, which contrasts with sectoring, has been called *distributive psychotherapy* (Holmes 1988). For some, this may require a fairly complete psychosocial assessment and mental status review in each session.

Simple techniques, such as echoing and tracking, can be used to differentially reinforce areas of the conversation that the therapist wishes to explore. You may sometimes need to be more explicit, as in the case of a patient who spends the first half of the session mulling about his inability to get a job: "I see that you are concerned about getting a job, but I don't think we'll get anywhere if we continue to talk about that problem now. Let's see what else we can help you with."

Repetition without resolution, as illustrated in this patient, probably serves defensive functions, but you must decide whether to point this out to the patient. If left to his own devices to structure his therapy sessions, he may effectively avoid contact with any issues that draw attention to his current problems in functioning. Confrontation with the fact that he is doing so may be useful at times, or it may just be a restatement of the obvious. You must consider that time is limited, and it is often more important simply to address the issues rather than the patient's defensive avoidance of them.

Some questions you might try to answer for each session are as follows:

- Do I know what has happened in my patient's life since the last session?
- Is the patient relating material that is relevant to the treatment plan? (Or does the treatment plan need to be changed?)
- What is the current status of the transference and countertransference?
- What is the patient's current level of functioning?
- What is the patient's symptomatology?
- Have I forgotten the patient's history (because it has been so long since I asked him about it or read the chart)?

Kernberg (1984, p. 161) has additional suggestions:

- Find out early on what environmental interventions or limit setting will be needed for the patient's safe treatment.
- Set up a way to monitor the patient's outside activities.
- Determine if pharmacological treatments will be needed early on.
- Evaluate the patient's personality and dominant character patterns in his external life.

The timing, selection, and meaning of interventions will depend on the answers to these questions. For example, if the patient is decompensating, more exploratory interventions must be held in abeyance and the session directed toward maintenance. Also, if the patient has, say, just lost her apartment and is living on the street, it is more important to talk about her housing than her substance abuse. Effective supportive psychotherapy requires the adept and economical use of time to do the most good for the patient.

In addition to what may be called "macroscopic" questions, pertaining to the psychotherapy session as a whole, moment-to-moment "microscopic" decisions are part and parcel of any therapy. Whenever a patient says *anything*, you have the choice of being abstinent (e.g., saying nothing), neutral, empathic, exploratory, interpretive, directive, or even strongly limit-setting. The correct choice at any point depends on your knowledge of the patient. As a supportive therapist you should at least (by now!) be able to sort out *supportive* from *nonsupportive* interventions and choose how supportive to be at a given moment. In addition (and this is by no means a minor point), the *emotional tone* with which a comment is delivered can make the difference between the comment being supportive and it being literally vicious. Some therapists can virtually "get away with anything" in terms of critical comments because of their warm, empathic, or considerate style. Others, often because of unexamined personality or countertransference problems, manage to impart a sadistic tone to the most matter-of-fact remark.

Curveballs

We define a *curveball* as an unexpected, unusual, or unanticipated setting or behavior that the therapist must deal with immediately—or "strike out." Of course, just as a batter prepares to hit curveballs, and hence expects to deal with the unexpected, you can develop some general strategies for returning curveballs. Practice with such situations always helps.

Special Settings and Situations

Therapists who work with patients in an office setting are familiar with the often striking differences in behavior between the "official" part of the session and the unofficial greetings, leave-takings, or chance meetings in the hallway. The supportive therapist often has the appropriate opportunity to observe the patient on the ward and many other places in the hospital and clinic. Unobserved, a taciturn or mute patient may start chattering to her friends, or a polite patient may be heard to mutter curses at his doctor. Often there is the chance to conduct "casual therapy" while escorting a patient to the medical clinic or emergency room.

Chance observations in unusual settings are an opportunity to gather information that is unavailable in other types of therapy. Conducting therapy in unusual settings is a challenge that may lead to significant improvement that is not possible with "standard" therapy. For example, settings outside the office may be helpful to some patients by creating less anxiety. If it is appropriate and safe, you may consider visits to the patient's home or workplace along with the patient's case manager or job counselor. At the extreme, there is the patient who talks to you regularly by phone and picks up prescriptions punctually but always avoids seeing you in person. With these "absent but therapeutically engaged" patients, one can try to find ways of meeting in person that are less threatening than the standard parameters. For example, you might deliberately tell the patient that only a few minutes are available to see her between sessions with other patients, thus ensuring that the meeting will be brief. However, there are indeed some patients who can tolerate only very brief sessions, and if so, why not make that part of the treatment plan? Of course, the proliferation of online therapy services has created a whole new realm of video therapy services, many of which are selected by patients who have logistical issues as well as therapeutic issues in avoiding face-to-face therapy.

Extra sources of information are commonplace in the mental health clinic. The same psychiatrist may treat several members of a family or at least hear about their psychiatric histories. The challenge, then, becomes one of preserving confidentiality yet still making use of the information in some way.

Gifts to and From the Therapist

In the 1950s and 1960s, psychiatrists were usually taught the following guidelines about gifts: "If a neurotic, they should not accept the gift but interpret it; if a sicker patient, they should first accept the gift and then attempt to interpret it; and, for the sickest patient, they should simply accept the gift and thank the patient" (Hurst 1989, p. 14). However, times have changed, and the determining factors are applicable laws, ethical standards, and clinical judgment based on therapeutic purpose. How valuable is the gift? Is it personal, or is it an item that can be shared with the clinic? What is the occasion of the gift (holiday or personal event)? What is the apparent meaning of the gift for the patient? Can that meaning be discussed with the patient? Is the gift returnable? What will be the anticipated impact on therapy if you reject the gift? Can this occasion be used to establish or change future policy?

A gift may be a substitute for payment, a token of friendship, or (as with business gifts) a way of rewarding and cementing a business relationship. If the meaning is personal, it may express a wish to have a personal relationship with the therapist. For some patients, it is wrong to deny such a wish outright; it may even be unnecessary to interpret the wish.

In developing a therapeutic relationship with patients who have schizophrenia, we generally approve of the acceptance of small gifts (see Chapters 6 and 17). However, we believe that personal gifts of significant value must be returned. To acquiesce in accepting them may signal to the patient that you need to be "bought" or are corrupted, and that you do not appreciate the patient as a human being and the patient must buy the relationship. This will confirm the patient's view that you are not interested in the relationship for its own sake.

Because many supportive therapy patients do not pay for treatment, the gift may represent an opportunity to pay or gratify you, expressing the fear that you need such gratification to want to see them. Therefore, whether or not you accept the gift, this aspect needs to be explored. However, the patient's wish to pay for or express gratitude for treatment may be deflected into some minor service to the clinic or a gift that can be shared among patients and staff.

Gifts from therapist to patient are similarly problematic. When the gift is an item of therapy, such as a book of cognitive therapy exercises, it may be entirely appropriate. Related items, such as a blank pad to list problems for the next therapy session, are also appropriate links to the therapy and may even be encouraged. After this somewhat innocuous category of gifts comes the "loan," often permanent, of more general reading material, money, and personal apparel. We again suggest that this be made into an institutional practice if the patient really needs such things. For example, the therapist might say: "Mr. Jones, I've noticed that your shoes are really worn out and you've just come in from the snow. The staff here at the clinic have put together a supply of shoes and winter clothing for our patients. Would you like to take a look at what we have and see if something suits your needs?" With a more highly functional patient, the therapist should consider that the heartfelt sympathy behind a gift may be interpreted as pity instead.

Unusual behaviors require a similar empathy with the patient's motivations. The patient may be smoking, reading a book, hallucinating during the session, or reporting unusual body images. He may give you a Life Savers candy or begin to eat a pastrami sandwich. Psychodynamic interpretations of these behaviors (such as the Life Savers!) are possible, but are they always desirable? The offering of candy is a gift and an attempt to "sweeten" the session symbolically. Smoking and reading could mean that the patient expects unpleasantness during the session and is trying to soothe himself and guard against it. In each case, you should appreciate the meaning of the behavior before deciding what to do about it.

Excavating "Hidden Issues"

Much of psychotherapy involves the bringing into awareness of issues that are hidden to the patient. However, issues may remain forever hidden unless the therapist "excavates" them. A brief suggestive outline of some hidden issues is given in Table 5–7. Although the last category—patient's wishes, needs, and psychological defenses—might suggest that some hidden issues will be difficult to uncover, it is likely that you can discover them through a reasonably diligent effort.

For example, histories of sexual assault and abuse are common, and studies have shown that failure to elicit such information is usually a result of not the patient's defenses but the therapist's *failure to ask*. Thus, Jacobson and Richardson (1987) provide a set of routine questions for eliciting a detailed sexual and physical assault history. Traumatic material can be approached gradually by inquir-

Table 5–7.   Hidden issues

A.   **Recent experiences or activities patient may not be reporting**

  1.   Substance use

  2.   Side effects from medicines, especially sexual dysfunction

  3.   Abuse by others (e.g., by spouse)

  4.   Significant life change that patient does not wish to talk about (e.g., failed a college course, laid off from work)

  5.   Symptoms

    a.   Concealing symptoms (e.g., not telling the therapist about hallucinations)

      1)   To please the therapist

      2)   To discontinue the therapy

    b.   Exaggerating symptoms

      1)   To continue the therapy

      2)   To defeat the therapist's efforts

      3)   To gain sympathy

  6.   Noncompliance with treatment programs, especially with medication

B.   **Past history**

  1.   Abuse

    a.   Physical abuse (by others or of others)

    b.   Sexual abuse (by others or of others)

  2.   Previous losses that have not been grieved or mourned

C.   **Ongoing educational needs that patient is ashamed to reveal**

  1.   Family planning

  2.   Sex education

  3.   Literacy

Table 5–7. Hidden issues *(continued)*

D. Wishes, needs, and psychological defenses that the patient is expressing in the therapeutic relationship

   1. Needs

      a. To be sick or to play the sick role

      b. To remain dependent on the therapist

   2. Defenses

      a. Avoiding issues that might offend the therapist

      b. Lying to the therapist

ing about the way the patient was punished as a child or the results of marital disputes, but you must be comfortable questioning the patient about the details, circumstances, and effects of assaults when the patient begins to talk about it.

The untruthful patient presents particular problems. In a broad sense, the failure to be truthful represents *resistance*, but the therapist may choose either to confront it directly or to interpret it psychodynamically. Lying that relates to the transference needs to be explored. Other occasional lies of a defensive nature (e.g., about reasons for absences, denials of drug use) can be confronted. A pattern of chronic lying, typical in patients with antisocial personalities, may make therapy impossible.

Case Vignette

A morbidly obese 57-year-old woman with a paranoid psychotic disorder had recently entered a psychosocial rehabilitation program, which she enjoyed very much. Part of her treatment involved receiving prescriptions for an antipsychotic medication. The psychiatrist had great difficulty in finding a medication and dosage that would relieve her symptoms but at the same time cause a minimum of tremor and dizziness. Eventually, he found a medication that created a significant amount of tremor but no dizziness. He asked the patient if the tremor was acceptable, and she assured him that she did not mind it.

The patient received prescriptions for a few months until the psychiatrist found out from the patient's caseworker that the patient had been throwing her morning dose of medicine in the trash. Rather than confront this patient directly, the psychiatrist apologized to her. He said he was sorry that he had scared her so much that she could not tell him the truth about her nonadherence. This strategy worked well, because the patient readily admitted to her nonadherence and the fact that her discomfort from the tremor had been too uncomfortable to bear. With the psychiatrist's help, she recalled the times when she was paranoid a few months earlier and agreed that she would like to avoid being paranoid in the future. Her adherence even improved while the psychiatrist continued to look for a better medication regimen.

The outwardly well or adherent patient presents another problem. Weiner (1982) describes how many patients, especially in involuntary hospital treatment, learn to exhibit *institutional insight*: they play by the rules in order to be released from a treatment situation that they perceive as captivity. This phenomenon, in which a patient denies illness or minimizes symptoms in order to receive freedom from treatment or medication, has been observed in voluntary patients as well. Institutional insight may evolve into genuine insight—that is, suppression of symptoms to appear well may result in a sense of self-control and social praise that improve the patient's functioning. However, feigned wellness may also be deceptive, leading to premature discontinuation of medication and precipitous relapse.

You can often discover inconsistencies in the patient's adherence and symptoms from discussion with other staff. The combined therapist/medicator is especially apt to be deceived by a patient who wants to appear to be well and to be taken off medication. Outward adherence or wellness has many causes, including unconscious ambivalence. However, when the therapist detects it, there are ways to confront it. For example, one might observe: "You've been telling me you're not hallucinating, but when I saw you in the hallway, you were talking to yourself. Is there something going on?"

Judging the Effectiveness of Interventions

How do you know when an intervention has been effective? When an interpretation is effective in supportive psychotherapy, you will see behavioral changes and verbal material resulting from that interpretation. Often, the patient incorporates new defenses and coping strategies in stages, as follows:

1. *Remembers and echoes back advice or knowledge that was given.* The patient may remark: "I just wasted my paycheck on cocaine. That was really stu-

pid." Sometimes the patient seems to have understood your interpretation but throws it back at you because it has failed: "You said I was just fooling myself about the reasons for taking drugs. Well, I went out this weekend and got high anyway." (These retellings of your statements are also tests of your patient's memory.)

2. *Begins to internalize the therapist's reasoning* in statements of the form, "I remember you said *X*, so I did *Y* [something that follows from *X*]." For example, a patient who was confronted about spending money that was to be used for clothing on drugs (see Chapter 3, "Principles of Supportive Technique: Explanatory Techniques") might (ideally!) come back the following week and report: "My friend asked me to smoke some crack on Friday night, but I thought about what you said, and I went out and finally bought that winter coat."

3. *Begins to use more mature defenses and coping strategies.* For example, in Chapter 4, we spoke of providing the defense substitution of having to work to refuse an invitation to use drugs, because the patient otherwise "felt like a wimp" to turn down her friends. One will hope that the patient reports back at some later time: "My friend offered me some crack, but I told him I had to work."

You must capitalize on such moments. Whereas interpretation may be delayed until, in Pine's (1984) phrase, the "iron is cold," reinforcement should be offered when the iron is hot to establish a connection between the patient's positive affect and the action. So, you might tag on the following: "You felt good about turning down the crack. You knew that was the right thing to do." And one hopes the patient will agree: "Yes, I said to myself that I needed the money for a new coat, and I wasn't going to waste it like I did the last paycheck."

Management and Feedback: A Session Dialogue

Session management is dynamic; it requires adjustment within each session and strategy development between sessions. In the following extended case vignette, we look at how the therapist adjusts to the patient's remarks and controls the depth of interpretation.

Case Vignette

Mr. Buchanan, a 25-year-old man with dependent traits, relates that he met a "former girlfriend" who had once asked him to spend the night with her. The therapist knows that Mr. Buchanan has had some heterosexual relationships in the past but has not expressed much recent interest in women and does not have a current relationship.

THERAPIST: Are you still interested in Rachel?

PATIENT: No. She's got a new boyfriend now and he's (*patient flexes his muscles*) a real macho type.

THERAPIST: You don't want to tangle with him?

PATIENT: No, it's not worth it.

THERAPIST: But you were interested in Rachel. Wasn't it last year she made you that offer?

PATIENT: Yes.

THERAPIST: A lot of men wouldn't turn down an offer like that. [Note: This is a potentially vicious remark. The patient appears to agree, however.]

PATIENT: Yeah…and Rachel is a real knockout, but you know, I was scared, it just wasn't my night. People will talk, and I didn't want her talking to the other girls and saying things about me.

THERAPIST: If you didn't perform?

PATIENT: Yeah.

THERAPIST: If you were impotent.

PATIENT: No, I'm not worried about being impotent. Well, they say that the mind controls the body, so what happens up here can affect what's down there. And I just wasn't in the mood.

THERAPIST: Have you ever had a problem before?

PATIENT: No. Well, when [a past girlfriend] was interested in me [2 years ago], it turned out she told me she was a virgin and I didn't know what you did with a virgin, so I left her alone, and I think she told her friends about it and I didn't like that.

THERAPIST: They said some insulting things about you, and it hurt.

PATIENT: Yes, I didn't like that.

THERAPIST: But you know, it's significant that you haven't been interested in women lately—we haven't heard much in the therapy about them.

PATIENT: No, I haven't mentioned a woman in months.

THERAPIST: Maybe it would help to talk about that some more now. [This is a tentative offer to allow patient control.] That's something I might be able to help you with.

PATIENT: Well, I've been so busy getting started at work. [He has been in his new job a month, is doing well, and has gotten an excellent evaluation.] I thought I'd better concentrate on work.

THERAPIST: I'll bet you're meeting some new women at work.

PATIENT: Yes. [He related in a previous session that there was a woman who kept talking to him at work, kind of bothering him.] But I…well…I need another paycheck to get a new pair of glasses. I hate these glasses sometimes—I'd like to smash them.

THERAPIST: They don't look too bad to me! What's wrong with them?

PATIENT: Well, it's not the glasses, it's me. My hair is too long. I've got to get some of these waves cut back, have them take half of it off. I haven't been to the barber in 2 months. I really need to go twice a month….I don't know what those women want from me.

THERAPIST: But you don't think you're attractive to women?

PATIENT: I don't know what to think.

THERAPIST: Maybe it would help to kind of review things. Were there any other bad experiences that have made you feel that you were rejected or unattractive?

PATIENT: Remember Nicki?

THERAPIST: Yes, she was your girlfriend when you were 16.

PATIENT: And she was 23! But she was… [describes how he attempted intercourse but was unsuccessful].

THERAPIST (*perhaps getting a bit discouraged and letting it show*): Maybe I should have asked you which experiences have been *good*.

PATIENT: Well, except for Janet—I was real comfortable with her—nobody! And I've had to pay for street women.

THERAPIST: Have you done that recently?

PATIENT: No, the last time was 2 years ago. I got off the bus at [a well-known corner for prostitution] and…$100 for 20 minutes. I was trying to save money. She was so dirty…I had to wash myself when I got home.

THERAPIST: You found it disgusting.

PATIENT: Besides, I want a long-term relationship. I tend to fall in love with women.

THERAPIST: Who were you last in love with?

PATIENT: You know—Joan really wanted to get to know me better and I f—ed it up. That was one of the reasons I even went back [to her town], and then I was real cold to her. Last year I even went back there, but she had moved, and I went to the post office to get her new address, and of course they wouldn't give it to me. She must've moved far away, anyhow. But sometimes I wonder if I'll ever meet her again. Some of the girls here remind me of her.… Well, anyway, I'm going to get my paycheck tomorrow. I think I'll spend it on a few beers. I like playing pool. There's a bar where they have pool tables that I really like. It's hard to drink beer alone. I took Janet there once, and I forgot they had go-go girls. She didn't like it.

THERAPIST: You're not interested in the go-go girls.

PATIENT: No, not really. I used to talk to them sometimes, but I didn't know what to say.

THERAPIST: It's hard for you to talk to your male friends about this.

PATIENT: Yes, I wanted some advice from Larry, but he thinks I'm a real stud and he just laughed. He thought I was kidding him or something, and I expected some sympathy.

Even without going into the details of the intentions of this therapy, we can tell that this session is quite productive. The therapist draws out connected recollections of good and bad experiences (mostly the latter). The patient is often defensive and hesitant but readily gives way to true and painful recollections of humiliation and embarrassment in sexual experiences. The therapist avoids imposing his values, although some therapists might use this occasion to point out that casual sex involves the risk of HIV infection. Perhaps that would be therapeutic, because it would give the patient a defense against the sexual encounters that he finds so embarrassing and fails at anyway. Nor does the therapist necessarily second the patient's expressed wish for a long-term love relationship, which in this context appears to be a defense against his fear about sexual performance rather than a closely held value.

In more minor matters, such as the patient's appearance, the therapist expresses a direct opinion. Sometimes the therapist is too formal and literate in speech, and in at least one instance he is sarcastic, but the patient is not put off by it. Usually, however, the therapist does a good job of echoing, restating, and leading the session, using empathic statements in the format preferred by Havens (1978). Sometimes the therapist may appear to be putting words in the patient's mouth, but this particular patient is willing and able to hold his own.

As a result of the therapist's directive pressure, a lot of ground is covered in the session, yet the therapist does not relate it to possible homosexual or incestual fears. In fact, this patient was homosexually raped as a child, and his one satisfactory sexual relationship was with a much older, motherly woman. In addition, the therapist does not (in this session) interpret why Mr. Buchanan "forgot" that the bar he went to with Janet had go-go girls, or why Mr. Buchanan did not know that this would offend her.

How far to go into such issues depends on the patient's responses. You must not assume that the patient will eventually bring up important topics when he is ready. The therapist here must be active, for this patient is seen only weekly (if that frequently). He has missed many sessions but has been coming to therapy for 2 years and has never expressed a desire to stop.

This is not a regressed, hallucinating patient for whom such a session would be far too intrusive. But Mr. Buchanan has had multiple suicide attempts in the past and has been called a "borderline personality." Indeed, his diagnosis (including those dependent traits) would seem to be of a personality disorder, and the therapy promises to be a long-term process.

This is a supportive therapy case, and the session is a good example of empathic, directive, supportive work. Some therapists, however, might consider this patient suitable for long-term psychodynamic therapy. Indeed, many insight-oriented processes are bound to occur, even in this primarily supportive mode.

Key Points

- Supportive psychotherapy should not be chosen automatically and without forethought. It is effective and suitable for a wide variety of patients, but it should not be chosen when a more effective therapy is readily available (e.g., an exposure therapy for a phobic patient) or for a patient with dementia who cannot benefit.

- Treatment planning is an important component of all therapies, but its importance in supportive psychotherapy is enhanced by the need for more advanced planning of the patient's goals and activities. Treatment plans should change dynamically, and a good rule for chronically mentally ill patients is to make only one change at a time.

- Therapy can be divided into phases of initiation, middle therapy, and termination.

- The therapist has many tasks in initiating therapy, not just covering the mechanics of the therapy, but conveying empathy and exploring surface issues.

- In the middle course of therapy, key tasks will be development of trust between therapist and patient and repetition and timing of interventions to ensure progress.

- In managing therapy, skill is needed to direct the content to make progress toward the treatment goals. However, there will always be a need to unearth hidden issues and be prepared for unexpected events, or "curveballs," which require a willingness to change the parameters of the session to prevent therapeutic slowdown, stalemate, or abject disruption of the treatment.

- In the termination of therapy, the therapist wants to arrange for a safe transition to independent function, other agencies, or a return to therapy if needed.

References

Adams N, Grieder DM: Treatment Planning for Person-Centered Care: Shared Decision Making for Whole Health. Waltham, MA, Academic Press, 2014

Bandura A: Social Learning Theory. Englewood Cliffs, NJ, Prentice Hall, 1977

Conte HR, Plutchik R: Controlled research in supportive psychotherapy. Psychiatr Ann 16:530–533, 1986

Deutsch F, Murphy WF: The Clinical Interview, Vol 2: Therapy: A Method of Teaching Sector Psychotherapy. New York, International Universities Press, 1955

Dewald PA: Psychotherapy: A Dynamic Approach, 2nd Edition. New York, Basic Books, 1971

Eisenthal S, Emery R, Lazare A, Udin H: "Adherence" and the negotiated approach to patienthood. Arch Gen Psychiatry 36(4):393–398, 1979 426605

Fauzia R, Sholihah Q: Reassurance supportive therapy for reducing depression in paraplegic patients due to Bantul earthquake. The European Journal of Social & Behavioural Sciences (eISSN: 2301-2218):1410–1416, 2013

Fluent TE, Kuebler J, Deneke DE, et al: How best to engage patients in their psychiatric care. Curr Psychiatr 12(9):22–25, 35–36, 2013

Foreman SA, Marmar CR: Therapist actions that address initially poor therapeutic alliances in psychotherapy. Am J Psychiatry 142(8):922–926, 1985 4025587

Frances A, Clarkin JF: No treatment as the prescription of choice. Arch Gen Psychiatry 38(5):542–545, 1981 7235855

Havens L: Explorations in the uses of language in psychotherapy: simple empathic statements. Psychiatry 41(4):336–345, 1978 715094

Havens L: Explorations in the uses of language in psychotherapy: complex empathic statements. Psychiatry 42(1):40–48, 1979 760133

Hawthorne N: The Scarlet Letter (1850), in The Complete Novels and Selected Tales of Nathaniel Hawthorne. New York, Modern Library, 1937

Holmes J: Supportive analytical psychotherapy: an account of two cases. Br J Psychiatry 152:824–829, 1988 3167469

Hurst DM: Freud's principle of abstinence in therapeutic relationship reexamined. Psychiatr Times 6(12):1, 14–15, 1989

Jacobson A, Richardson B: Assault experiences of 100 psychiatric inpatients: evidence of the need for routine inquiry. Am J Psychiatry 144(7):908–913, 1987 3605402

Karasu TB: Psychosomatic medicine and psychotherapy. Psychiatr Ann 16:522–525, 1986

Kennedy JA: Fundamentals of Psychiatric Treatment Planning. Washington, DC, American Psychiatric Press, 1992

Kernberg OF: Severe Personality Disorders: Psychotherapeutic Strategies. New Haven, CT, Yale University Press, 1984

Makover RB: Treatment Planning for Psychotherapists: A Practical Guide to Better Outcomes, 3rd Edition. Arlington, VA, American Psychiatric Association Publishing, 2016

Maruish ME: Essentials of Treatment Planning. New York, Wiley, 2002

Pine F: The interpretive moment: variations on classical themes. Bull Menninger Clin 48(1):54–71, 1984 6692050

Ryback RS, Longabaugh R, Fowler DR: The Problem Oriented Record in Psychiatry and Mental Health Care, Revised Edition. New York, Grune & Stratton, 1981

Taylor CB, Liberman RP, Agras WS, et al: Treatment evaluation and behavior therapy, in Treatment Planning in Psychiatry. Edited by Lewis JM, Usdin G. Washington, DC, American Psychiatric Association, 1982, pp 151–224

Weed LL: Medical Records, Medical Education and Patient Care. Cleveland, OH, Case-Western Reserve University Press, 1969

Weiner MF: The Psychotherapeutic Impasse. New York, Free Press, 1982

Werman DS: Technical aspects of supportive psychotherapy. Psychiatr J Univ Ott 6:153–160, 1988

Yee WK: Psychiatric aspects of psychoeducational family therapy. Psychiatr Ann 19:27–34, 1989

PART II

Diagnostic Applications

6

Schizophrenia and Hallucinations

Diagnostic Considerations

According to DSM-5 (American Psychiatric Association 2013), a person diagnosed with schizophrenia will display at least two of the following symptoms:

1. Delusions
2. Hallucinations
3. Disorganized speech
4. Grossly disorganized or catatonic behavior
5. Negative symptoms

These five symptoms can be presented in 26 different symptom combinations. Focusing on the symptoms, not the syndrome, will help you develop a patient-specific treatment plan. If only the syndrome by itself is addressed, then some specificity is lost. Moreover, rapport with the patient can often be easier to achieve if you stress a complaint, such as voices, or other people disagreeing with the patient's ideas, than by asking the patient to accept that he has "schizophrenia."

But although many people still associate schizophrenia with the occurrence or predominance of hallucinations, more recent research has shown that hallucinations can be a prominent symptom in other illnesses, including mood disorders and posttraumatic stress disorder. Many therapists (especially in Europe) have changed direction so as to normalize rather than demonize the presence of hallucinations in many conditions, including schizophrenia, claiming that "[s]ome experts think the problem is how doctors and society treat people who hear things, not the voices themselves" (Morin 2014). In defense of this view may be cited the classic experiment reported in "On Being Sane in Insane Places" in which fake patients presented themselves at 12 hospitals complaining of voices that said "empty," "hollow," and "thud" (Rosenhan 1973). All of the fake patients were treated with antipsychotics and held for 7–52 days even after ceasing to complain of their voices. In today's realm of managed care, there is little likelihood of that happening (not to mention the ethics of running such an experiment). However, it is also unlikely that a therapist would or should treat an isolated or single-word hallucination. If you should hear of such a thing, you need to consider what is going on. It is not likely to be schizophrenia, in which the hallucinations have a content or contain commands or create dangerous delusions. Is there a danger created by occasionally hearing the word *thud*? Could there be some kind of temporal lobe seizure?

We should not overreact to the complaint of hallucinations—a good point to avoid misdiagnosis in the case of persons malingering the symptom for secondary gain. Therapists working on the content of hallucinations now try to direct scrutiny on negative or insulting voices that seem to be the interrogations of other figures who rejected the patient. Specific methods include rescripting imagery (Ison et al. 2014), in which the person lessens his distress from the voices. There is also benefit to be found in having patients interact with their voices (Shaikh-Lesko 2014, summarizing the work of Marius Romme). Some of these patients have schizophrenia, and some do not. Another resource is a manualized therapy for auditory hallucinations (Jenner 2016).

Supportive Psychotherapy in Schizophrenia

Throughout this book, we have urged readers to pay attention to the evidence basis for psychotherapy in specific conditions. In the case of schizophrenia (and, later in this chapter, for delusional disorder), there has been a major meta-review by the Cochrane Group of relevant studies (Buckley et al. 2015). Citing and reiterating many of the issues we described earlier in this book, such as the varying definition of supportive psychotherapy and its frequent use as a control treatment rather than the study treatment, the review authors concluded that "there does not seem to be much difference between supportive therapy, standard care and other therapies. Future research would benefit from larger studies where supportive therapy is the main treatment."

Surprisingly, therefore, we find ourselves in much the same position as we were in when we advocated the methods and treatments that we had developed in the first edition of our book. To quote some of the major researchers in the field: "[M]any researchers believe that aspects of ST (Supportive Therapy), such as the therapeutic alliance, the provision of support and advice, and efforts to minimize stress, may be beneficial in their own right...and incorporating lessons learned from ST may strengthen the effect of cognitive behavioral therapy [CBT] on schizophrenia" (Penn et al. 2004, p. 101). This is because, in the past few decades, there has accumulated evidence that CBT for the syndrome is effective (Opoka and Lincoln 2017; Smits and van der Gaag 2010). However, one can also find a major study that showed that cognitive therapy was ineffective (Lynch et al. 2010; University of Hertfordshire 2009). Finally, we note that in a study comparing supportive psychotherapy with treatment as usual in first-episode psychosis (which one does not normally find), the intervention was found to be superior (Rosenbaum et al. 2012).

We conclude that supportive psychotherapy should still be a fundamental treatment in the repertoire of a therapist for schizophrenia, but we urge readers to keep up to date with evidence-based methods as they are developed. In addition to the obvious centrality of one-on-one psychotherapy, these include the wide-ranging and standard "arsenal," if you want to call it that, of treatment, including the following, all of which are described in Chapter 4 of the text by Spaulding et al. (2017):

- Rehabilitation counseling and related modalities
- Neurocognitive therapy
- Contingency management
- Social skills training
- Problem-solving skills training
- Independent living skills training
- Specialized integrated treatment for co-occurring substance abuse
- Supported employment and occupational skills training
- Family therapy
- Peer support and self-help groups

- Acute treatment and crisis intervention and related services
- Specialized models for service integration and provision (e.g., clubhouse model; social learning programs; assertive community treatment; high-risk, first-episode, and early intervention programs; supported housing)

Patients should participate with the treatment team in the development of the treatment plan to the degree they are able, including lifestyle recommendations, medications, and referrals. To varying degrees, each session of supportive psychotherapy with a patient who has schizophrenia requires the treatment team to work with the patient to identify the present signs of illness and the signs of impending exacerbation that need to be addressed. Outside of the sessions with the patient, the therapist may also need to take on some advocacy tasks such as maintaining contact with those agencies to whom the patient has been referred.

The therapist performing supportive psychotherapy is often the command center for the treatment. Even with the most competent of case managers, the therapist will still want to maintain an "omniscience" as to the patient's treatment, such as directly receiving the art therapist's findings or keeping fully aware of developments in treatment groups. Treatment plans can then be altered, as long-term responses to the current treatment plan may require changes. For example, a patient may experience the therapist as overly controlling and react negatively to direction (Meaden and Van Marle 2008).

In addition, the therapist may be in the best position to monitor the patient's physical health. Recent estimates are that 50%–60% of people with schizophrenia have comorbid medical illnesses (El-Mallakh et al. 2010). Many patients will not complain of, or even notice, certain physical difficulties. In one study of chronic outpatients, 53% had undiagnosed medical problems (Farmer 1987). In a study of the California public health system, 14% of the patients had significant medical conditions but had not so informed the mental health staff (Koran et al. 1989). Health risks are increased because of the illness itself, unhealthy lifestyle behaviors, and side effects of the medications. Relative to the side effects of medications, psychoeducation or cognitive-behavioral interventions may help prevent weight gain that is common with antipsychotic medications (Alvarez-Jiménez et al. 2006; Evans et al. 2005).

People with schizophrenia often have other mental illnesses. Concomitant substance use disorders are common in people with schizophrenia, enhancing the therapeutic challenges. Fifty percent or more of patients have significant drug or alcohol abuse (Winklbaur et al. 2006). Treatment of the patient with a substance use disorder(s) and schizophrenia is discussed in Chapter 9. Signs of depression and anxiety are common, and in Chapters 7 and 8 we address their management.

Natural Course of Schizophrenia

A knowledge of the natural course of schizophrenia underlies successful psychotherapy. Schizophrenia is a chronic illness with a course of partial remissions and exacerbations. The need for supportive psychotherapy occurs throughout the illness—at the onset, during exacerbations, and especially during periods of remission. The exact nature of the techniques and interventions will vary with the stage of the illness, the specific symptoms, previous history of response, and so forth.

The exacerbation of symptoms is basic to the disease process and will not usually be totally eliminated by treatment, whether it be pharmacotherapy, supportive psychotherapy, or any combination of treatments. Supportive psychotherapy has a major role, usually not in banishing exacerbations, but in preventing them from turning into chaos and disorganization of the patient's life (Mendel 1989). Supportive psychotherapy accomplishes this through diminution of symptoms, lifestyle changes, enhancement of coping skills, recognition of the value of the therapeutic relationship, and provision of a long-term perspective, which includes elements of insight, reality testing, and trust.

Important characteristics of supportive psychotherapy in schizophrenia include

- The value of the real relationship between the patient and the therapist.
- Specific emphases in technique during therapeutic sessions.
- Emphasis on family and significant others.
- Emphasis on outside activities.
- Modeling and identification with the therapist (in many cases).

The Real Relationship

The therapist, to provide supportive therapy for a patient with schizophrenia, must be more than a distant figure given to silence, analytic interpretations, and total frustration of transference gratification. Indeed, the relationship between the therapist and the patient is crucial. Studies have shown that patients with schizophrenia who have formed good alliances with their therapists, in comparison to patients who have not, demonstrate greater acceptance of treatment, better medication adherence, less total medication use, and better long-term outcome. The better overall outcome occurs in a variety of measures of psychopathology, cognitive functioning, ego functions, social functioning, and work performance (Frank and Gunderson 1990).

Patients with schizophrenia can help adjust and modify their social deficits by interacting in real ways with the therapist and by discussing their social perceptions and achieving consensual validation of their perceptions or modifying their views based on the therapist's input. Patients may also adjust their social deficits by learning from the therapist and by modeling their behavior on the therapist's behavior. Social functioning is rarely improved by medication alone, yet it is "one of the strongest predictors of current functioning and long-term outcome in schizophrenia" (Penn et al. 2004, p. 101).

Case Vignette

One patient made a very serious suicide attempt. Months later, the telephone rang during a session; the therapist reached to answer the phone but then said, "I don't have to do that." A year or so later, the patient was again in a suicidal crisis and was about to make another serious attempt, when she remembered the therapist's behavior; repeated to herself, "I don't have to do that"; and did not attempt suicide. (The patient later related the incident to the therapist.)

The therapeutic advantages of the real relationship between patient and therapist are outlined in Table 6–1. As we indicated in Chapter 5, gifts and personal relationships must always be handled diplomatically. In general, however, therapists working with patients with schizophrenia can legitimately accept small or symbolic gifts, interact as real human beings, and attend special events such as graduation exercises or weddings.

Emphases in Individual Sessions

In this section we delineate some of the techniques and parameters for individual supportive sessions. However, this discussion is not meant to be all-inclusive.

Table 6–1.   Therapeutic advantages of the real relationship

Growth of interpersonal and social skills

Improved reality testing

Consensual validation

Promotion of identification with therapist

Enhanced patient self-esteem

Greater calmness in crisis

Frequency and Duration of Sessions

For individual sessions, flexibility should be maintained for frequency, duration, and even mode of contact. A patient experiencing exacerbation of symptoms, strong suicidal urges, command hallucinations, or another crisis may have to be seen more frequently than is usually planned. Some system of availability—whether through an answering device, a rotation of coverage among clinicians, or provision of emergency services at an accessible clinic—is mandatory when treating extremely ill patients.

For many patients, a 50-minute session may be too long, increasing anxiety or interfering with attention span. Although a 20-minute session is ideal for some patients, the exact duration should depend on each patient's characteristics and needs and should be as flexible as possible. Some patients may need to be seen in 50-minute sessions every 2 weeks when they are stable but may require 20-minute sessions once or twice a week during periods of exacerbation.

Availability may be more important than mode of contact. Telephone calls can be crucial during crisis, and contact by letter, postcard, or social media can be helpful at times. It is vital, of course, to document the content of the communication.

Giving Advice

In Chapter 4 we discussed many ways of giving suggestions, advice, and guidance. Here we shall simply add that the judicious giving of advice is natural during supportive psychotherapy with patients with schizophrenia. While not imposing your own ideology or values, you can certainly assist the patient in examining decisions, represent external reality for the patient, and at times strongly advise the patient—for example, "That sounds crazy" or "Illegal drugs and medication don't mix" or "Splendid! Going shopping by yourself is a real accomplishment."

Repetition

You may achieve a major piece of work with the patient, clarifying a situation (e.g., the interpersonal relation with Person A) and helping the patient acknowledge the emotions involved, which may even lead to more adaptive behavior. In the next session, you may become flabbergasted when an almost identical situation occurs and the patient appears to have learned nothing but is repeating the same self-defeating attitudes and behavior.

Concreteness of thinking, a failure to generalize, and a difficulty in switching psychological sets are among the deficits in schizophrenia. Insight into Situation A does not translate into insight into Situation A1, even if the differences between A and A1 appear minuscule to you. You may have to explain the same basic thing over and over. In addition to teaching patience, this process is a form of working-through, enabling the patient to apply the insight or recommendation to situations with slightly different variables, and each time with a new angle or a new cast of characters.

Emphases Outside the Sessions

Families are enlisted for support, information gathering, and crisis intervention; they are not seen as pathogenic agents and not ignored (Siegler and Osmond 1974). Chapter 15 discusses interactions with families in more detail.

Your initial contact with the family may come during a hospitalization or crisis and consists principally of information gathering. Later, with the patient's permission, you can give an explanation to the family of the illness's symptoms, course, treatment, side effects of medications, and so forth. This explanation serves many purposes. It can alleviate the family's unfounded guilt or anxiety, as they see that you do not blame them for the illness. Knowing facts about the course of the disorder can dispel irrational beliefs and unrealistic expectations of doom or keep the seriousness of the condition from being minimized.

Explanation and education will also help to correct misperceptions or fears on the family's part arising from improvement in the patient. For example, the family or caregivers of the poorly functioning patient may have become accustomed to her apathetic behavior and blunted affect. Treatment, however, may lead to an increase in the patient's level of activity, autonomy, or assertiveness. This change may be misperceived by the family or caregivers, or even interpreted as hostility (Mason et al. 1990). Appropriate educational efforts, especially in the context of regular ongoing contact, can help dispel these misperceptions. Family members and significant others are usually the first persons to notice the small symptoms or changes that herald an exacerbation and can thus alert the therapist in time to prevent a major disorganization. In addition to giving support, the family members, with coaching from the therapist, can provide reality testing and appropriate limit setting in the midst of the patient's severe anxiety. All these elements can decrease the patient's anxiety, improve her interpersonal skills, and contribute to enhance self-esteem. And finally: don't neglect the abundance of competent Internet resources for family members (e.g., Smith 2018).

Flexibility in your dealings with family members may allow them to function as facilitators of the treatment, and even co-therapists in a certain sense. There are many benefits of judicious contacts with family members (see Table 6–2). We will elaborate on these benefits and introduce some important caveats in Chapter 15.

Emphasis on Outside Activities

A great deal of the patient's progress will depend on increased social and interpersonal skills, ability to function in work environments, and ability to handle environment stress. Emphasis on rehabilitation and outside activities must be considered an intrinsic part of your role as therapist. In addition to discussing these issues and emphasizing their therapeutic value, you may need to communicate with rehabilitation workers, visit sheltered workshops and other sites, attend concerts in which the patient performs, and so forth.

Modeling and Identification With the Therapist

As we mentioned in Chapter 4, supportive psychotherapy allows for modeling and identification with the therapist. Patients can learn from the therapist's behavior without specific direction. It can also be used in group therapy for social skills training. The original concept for modeling was introduced by Bandura (1969) and elaborated by Decker and Nathan (1985). For example, in learning how to prepare for a job interview, you can teach patients to rehearse

Table 6–2.   Benefits of therapist-family cooperation

Information gathering

Reinforcement of the therapist's supportive relationship to the patient

Calming of overemotional family atmosphere

Dispelling of myths, guilt, and unrealistic expectations

Appropriate limit setting

Detection of early symptoms of exacerbations

their interview behavior. Modeling is often used as pat of a cognitive-behavioral treatment for schizophrenia. For an easily accessible review of techniques, see the article by Gaudiano (2006).

Response to Special Symptoms

The effective response to such special symptoms as hallucinations, delusions, and ideas of reference is a major part of the art of supportive psychotherapy. Although we have found reason to modify many of our recommendations on the basis of the discussion earlier of normalizing hallucinations, we still think it is generally contraindicated for the therapist to agree in total with the content of the patient's delusions. Such a false agreement can increase the patient's anxiety, further confuse his reality-testing skills, and reinforce the psychotic content.

Rather, the change in the newer therapies is to engage in mutual investigation with the patient of the predecessors, triggers, and meaning of hallucinations and other psychotic thought content. Instead of saying, "The CIA is not targeting you, that is a delusion," you can start with "Why would you think the CIA has targeted you?" Or more personally, "Why is that voice criticizing your looks? Do you have concerns about your looks?" You should develop an informed judgment on when and how to respond, when to note and store away for future response, and when to be silent in the presence of such symptoms. A basic strategy is to convince the patient that who she "really is" is more worthwhile and important to you than the identity provided by the hallucinations, delusions, or ideas of reference. Often a satisfactory goal is to reach an understanding by the patient that her belief is not accepted by others and that it is a mistake to talk about it in general conversation with others because they would not understand her.

Hallucinations

As we mentioned already, hallucinations are such a major symptom of schizophrenia that the disorder is sometimes defined in the lay community and by patients as one of "hearing voices." However, the degree of distress and disability generated by hallucinations varies greatly. Some patients enjoy or derive satisfaction from their hallucinations (Modell 1960), as was the case with a 50-year-old man who was comforted by auditory hallucinations of a kind nurse who had cared for him many years previously. When you are inquiring about hallucinations, it is always important to determine the patient's feelings, both individual and in general, in response to the hallucinations. If the hallucinations are pleasant, it is less important to focus on them and more important to turn your attention to the disabling psychopathology. We explain to patients at the outset that we have a particular concern about hallucinations that are hurtful or unpleasant or that command them to do dangerous things. When you are addressing hallucinations, the basic therapeutic attitude is to communicate that you do not hear the voices or see the visions, but to continue to maintain cordiality and relatedness. At times, this is accomplished by a simple statement such as "Tell me more about that experience, because I have not had that myself and I don't hear that voice," or "I realize that this is an important experience, but maybe there's another way to make sense of it." If you have the time, you can utilize a multiplicity of forms for the patient to describe his psychotic thoughts in detail and consider alternative explanations for their occurrence at this time in his life (Wright et al. 2014).

Therapeutic intervention starts with establishing the circumstances under which the hallucinations occurred. A calm investigation of the setting helps place the experience in context for the patient, emphasizing not just the abnormal experience itself but the total context. In many cases, it is more important to interpret the occurrence of the hallucination than its content. For example, investigation may show that the hallucinations occurred at a time of loneliness or of interpersonal disappointment, leading to decreased self-esteem. It is quite common for hallucinations to occur when the patient is alone (e.g., going to the bathroom). Making this connection for the patient will place the experience in context and diminish its frightening nature.

The hallucination may take the form of voices belittling the patient. It is more important to interpret the occurrence ("This disappointment causes you to experience this symptom") than to interpret the content ("A classic expression of castration anxiety"). Silvano Arieti contended that a very careful examination of all hallucinations in schizophrenia will show them to be a reaction to some perceived assault on the patient's self-esteem, and that establishing this will eventually result in the disappearance of this symptom (Arieti 1974). Obviously, if you continue this examination thoroughly and the hallucinations persist, you should go in another direction.

Case Vignette

A woman in a sheltered workshop had a combination of auditory and visual hallucinations, combining the word of God with religious and sexual symbols. The therapist examined the context of these hallucinations and concluded that an unrequited crush on an authority figure led to the experience. Instead of interpreting the oedipal content of the hallucination, the therapist commented on the patient's sense of disappointment in relation to the authority figure. The patient continued to believe in the reality of the hallucination for some time, but there were no further examples of this hallucination.

Keep in mind that a successful interpretation of the conditions giving rise to hallucinations is not a one-shot deal. The mechanisms may have to be explored numerous times and may have to be explained to the patient over and over.

At times, hallucinations are so disturbing to the patient that therapeutic accessories may be required. There are reports, for example, of elimination of auditory hallucinations by increasing external stimulation through the use of a radio with stereo headphones (Feder 1982). In some patients, humming or singing will also help reduce or eliminate auditory hallucinations. As Torous and Keshaven (2016, p. 190) point out, "Social media tools have the potential to offer new services to patients, although the clinical evidence base for such is still nascent." However, there are now applications to help (Firth and Torous 2015; Nott 2013).

There are other occasions when therapeutic wisdom consists not in directly addressing the hallucinations, but rather in de-emphasizing them, or in maintaining a temporary strategic silence, while focusing on positive matters such as gains in daily living abilities or work skills.

Command hallucinations necessitate very careful evaluation, including attention to the content of the command, the occurrence of previous acting out of the commands, the presence of other symptoms such as delusions, and the determination of whether the patient can identify the voices. Command hallucinations alone may not create greater risk for dangerous behavior (Hellerstein et al. 1987). However, in one study it was found that if the patient could identify hallucination-related delusions and hallucinatory voices, then it was more likely that he or she would act out on the command; the degree of dangerousness of the command did not appear to be a factor in compliance with the command (Junginger 1990).

Increased medication and even hospitalization may be indicated. At times, however, the patient may gain greater control and be able to differentiate between the psychotic thinking and more rational behavior if the therapist points out to the patient that she has been able to resist the commands in the past and asks what has contributed to that ability (Sarti and Cournos 1990).

When the hallucination is disabling, antipsychotic medication is always indicated. The integration of medication with supportive psychotherapy is discussed below and in Chapter 16. Therapeutic ways of responding to hallucinations are given in Table 6–3.

Delusions and Lack of Self-Awareness

Delusions in schizophrenia, although initially more disabling, are less difficult to treat than delusions not related to a specific psychiatric disorder. This view is consistent with a Cochrane Report that concluded: "Despite international recognition of this disorder in psychiatric classification systems such as ICD-10 and DSM-5, there is a paucity of *high quality* randomized trials on delusional disorder" (Skelton et al. 2015). The authors found only one relevant study comparing supportive psychotherapy with CBT but concluded that there is insufficient evidence to make evidence-based recommendations for treatments of any type for people with delusional disorder.

The therapist's acceptance or acquiescence in the delusional belief is usually countertherapeutic. Patients will react to the therapist's agreement with the delusions by exhibiting increased agitation, seeing it as confirmation of their worst fears, or concluding that the therapist himself or herself no longer has a grip on reality!

Table 6–3.   Therapeutic responses to hallucinations

Do not agree with the reality basis for the hallucination.

Examine the circumstances of the hallucination.

Interpret the occurrence (e.g., as a reaction to a blow to self-esteem).

Explain the mechanism again and again.

Try to treat the patient's condition with an increase in external stimuli (e.g., radio headphones).

Ask patient to drown out hallucinations with humming or singing.

Deemphasize the hallucinations and focus on positive matters.

Write out "coping cards" with specific strategies of thinking or doing to counteract the psychosis,[a] such as "I'm a good person. I don't need to believe what the voices say."

[a]Wright et al. 2014; see also http://www.treatingpsychosis.com.

Many delusions are firmly held. It is not unheard of for delusional beliefs to persist unchanged for decades as a circumscribed delusional system, even in the absence of other overt psychotic material. In the case of an absolutely held delusion, it is best to make a mild questioning, such as "I wonder if there is another way to explain that" or "I find that hard to believe," rather than to confront the delusion bluntly.

In many instances, a delusional patient goes through three specific phases while recovering from an acute psychotic episode:

1. A delusional phase, with full belief in the delusions
2. A double-awareness phase, in which the delusions coexist with more accurate reality testing (i.e., the patient may question the delusions, may simultaneously accept and reject them, or may conceal or try to suppress them)
3. A nondelusional phase, in which no delusions or only residuals of the delusion exist (Sacks et al. 1974)

This sequence of stages determines the timing for therapeutic challenging of delusions.

If the patient has no doubt whatsoever of the reality of the delusion, confrontation of the delusion should consist of only very mild questioning. A lack of sense of self may be tied to the delusion or may itself be a separate sign of illness.

Metacognition

People with schizophrenia often lack metacognition, and this contributes to their poor quality of life and adversely affects their recovery (Lysaker and Dimaggio 2014; Pesek 2009). Metacognitive treatment approaches that have supportive qualities include the following:

- Metacognition reflection and insight therapy (Vohs et al. 2018)
- Group-based metacognition-oriented social skills training (Inchausti et al. 2017, 2018)
- Metacognition using a focus on narratives (Schweitzer et al. 2017)
- Metacognition as a way of helping adolescents seeking treatment (Koren 2014)
- Mentalization-based psychodynamic psychotherapy (Brent 2009)

Some advice about timing: If the patient displays any doubt at all about the reality of the delusions, you should begin to confront the delusions (Rudden et al. 1982). This can be done by reinforcing the "observing ego" of the patient, by questioning the reality of the delusion more forcefully, and by beginning to investigate the circumstances around the formation of delusion. If the patient has recovered sufficiently so that he no longer believes the delusions, or if he has achieved sufficient psychological distance from the delusions, you should explore more thoroughly the process of formation of the delusions and may at times interpret the content of the delusions.

Therapeutic ways of responding to delusional material are summarized in Table 6–4. Even the most bizarre delusions often contain kernels of truth. As Golda Meir said to Henry Kissinger during the 1973 Sinai peace talks, "Even paranoids have enemies." (While this remark seems to have happened, it is a common refrain in popular culture, dating back at least as far as Freud and is a useful concept in understanding patients [Pierides 1998].) Indeed, the suspiciousness, poor interpersonal skills, and emotional withdrawal of delusional patients may create the very reactions and emotional conspiracies the patient fears (Cameron 1959). The therapist should provide consensual validation for those elements of reality in a delusion, the better to have credibility when eventually confronting the elements of unreality. For example, the therapist may agree that the patient's boss is bothering her, while questioning whether the CIA and FBI are involved.

Some delusions, even with a patient who has a firm, unquestioning belief, can be interpreted in such a way that the interpretation does not challenge the patient, yet sets the stage for a double awareness of the delusion and for future integration of the insight.

Case Vignette

A middle-aged man complained vigorously that his parents were wild Martian monsters. The therapist doubted the reality of this genealogy but commented that there was a poetic truth in what the patient was saying. Some months later, the patient could talk about the delusion, still believing it in part, but emphasizing that maybe it was just a poetic way of expressing his feelings about his parents.

Even when a direct interpretation or an introduction of a seed of doubt cannot be made, the therapist may gain major insight into the patient by understanding the delusion in a symbolic manner.

Case Vignette

A patient had the delusion that he was Darth Vader, the villain of the Star Wars movies. He dressed up as Darth Vader, attempted to frighten children in his neighborhood in that costume, and kept repeating emotion-laden sentences from the movie series. The therapist understood this delusion to reflect the patient's ambivalent relationship to his father (similar to the hero Luke Skywalker's relationship to Darth Vader). Although the therapist did not directly interpret this, awareness of this meaning resulted in the therapist's directing attention to the relationship with the father, and especially to a pathological identification with the aggressor (Rojcewicz 1987). The eventual changes in the family dynamics did lead to improvement in the patient.

At times, a delusion can have its intensity reduced if put into a context that emphasizes the human nature and the delusion. Providing such a context can serve to decrease the anxiety and the sense of bizarreness that the delusion elicits in the patient. For example, you may respond as follows to a patient with the delusional belief that he is entitled to huge amounts of money: "We all have wishes we know are not true but we act as though they are true. I some-

Table 6–4. Therapeutic responses to delusions

Express mild questioning or skepticism.

If patient has any doubts whatsoever, begin to confront the delusion and to explore its formation.

If patient becomes nondelusional, further explore the process of delusional formation and possibly interpret the content.

Offer consensual validation for elements of reality in the delusion.

Interpret the delusion as "poetic truth."

times think that I will win the lottery, and I sometimes assume that I will live forever; but there's also a side of my mind that says it is not true. Your wish that the army owes you a million dollars because of a dishonorable discharge is understandable."

Patients may be inclined to give up a delusion or to consider it with a double awareness when convinced that they are accepted as they "really are" by the therapist. The delusion, as Freud pointed out in the Schreber case (Freud 1911/ 1958), is often a secondary symptom. It is a reaction—a compensation or an attempt at restitution because of a more primary fear (such as in the Schreber study, as Freud hypothesized, a fear of homosexuals) or a sense of low self-esteem. For some patients, acceptance by the therapist, even in areas that the patient feels are shameful or guilt-ridden (e.g., sexual preference, marginal work performance, sordid family background), is a major factor that allows the delusion to fade.

Of course, when a delusion is disabling or dangerous, you should consider antipsychotic medication or changes in the medication regimen.

Ideas of Reference

Ideas of reference can be addressed in ways like those of addressing hallucinations and delusions. Furthermore, ideas of reference often form in the very early stages of a psychotic decompensation, as the patient struggles to make sense of intense anxiety and confusion. You may do well to make an empathic statement, commenting on how frightening this time is for the patient. As rapport is established, you can combine the empathic statement with a comment that perhaps the patient experienced the ideas of reference as some way of making sense of things when everything was confusing and nothing seemed to make sense.

Ideas of reference also develop in more chronic stages. The patient may obtain a sense of importance, not elsewhere realized, from this symptom. If the television is talking about her, she must be important. A therapeutic technique here would be an empathic statement about perceived assaults on her self-esteem or about her need for increased self-esteem, perhaps to be followed later by further interpretations.

As with hallucinations and delusions, if the ideas of reference become dangerous or disabling, you should consider changes or additions to the antipsychotic medication.

A supportive psychotherapy approach to ideas of reference based on levels of awareness and corresponding therapeutic response is given in Table 6–5. The basic strategy is the creation of the impression in the patient that who he "really is" is more interesting and worthy than the "who" implied by the ideas of reference. Over time, the therapist hopes to reach the stage at which the patient is predominantly able to think realistically (i.e., Level G), but may often have to be satisfied with the patient being able to have a double awareness (i.e., Level F). With many schizophrenia patients, development of social awareness (i.e., Level E) is all that can be achieved, yet this does not preclude the patient's working, marrying, or having a fulfilling life.

Denial of Psychotic Episodes

Recovery from an acute psychotic decompensation takes many forms, on a continuum ranging from denial of or amnesia for the psychotic episode (i.e., "sealing over"), through some awareness of the psychotic symptoms, to partial insight into why certain symptoms may have occurred, and, at times, to a fuller understanding and integration of the entire episode (McGlashan et al. 1975). All too often, the patient experiences denial for the most significant acute symptoms, thus decreasing the chances of learning from experiences and of preventing similar recurrences.

Early in supportive psychotherapy, you may not be able to address this denial or amnesia directly. As the therapeutic alliance develops, you should not ignore this phenomenon, but instead start to make some mild comments that can help your patient integrate the experience. For example, you can comment

Table 6–5.   Levels of therapeutic response to ideas of reference

Patient's level of awareness	Level of therapeutic response
Fixed ideas of reference (not safe to challenge cognitively; rapport with therapist uncertain)	A. Address the fears and concerns the patient is feeling as a result of such thoughts, without agreeing with the content.
Fixed ideas of reference (some rapport with therapist)	B. Acknowledge that the beliefs help make sense of the experience or observations without agreeing to the validity of the patient's conclusions.
Weakening ("dissolving") ideas of reference (subject to discussion)	C. Discuss and suggest other "possible" explanations for the experience or observations.
Some self-observation occurring (and patient begins to express)	D. Encourage the patient's ability to observe himself (i.e., fertilize any hints that the patient has doubts).
Development of social awareness	E. Encourage the patient's realization that others will not agree and that it serves the patient poorly if he talks about the ideas of reference (to persons other than the therapist).
Double-awareness stage (i.e., patient has a sense of reality coexisting with the ideas of reference)	F. When the patient has reached the double-awareness stage, encourage doubts as to the validity of the ideas.
Predominantly realistic thinking (sometimes with residue of ideas of reference)	G. At this stage, help the patient to understand the situations during which these ideas develop. Be as current and concrete as possible (e.g., use phrases like "feel threatened" rather than "in an oedipal situation").

that the decompensation occurred when the patient was "experiencing anxiety from rejection" or that "stopping medication played a role" in what happened. The patient can then have some cognitive, cause-and-effect explanation of the psychotic episode, allowing him to make some sense out of what previously made no sense whatsoever.

With even an inexact explanation of the episode, your patient may be able to tolerate further exploration. As he finds acceptance rather than feared condemnation or ridicule, he can remember more and more of the episode. The aim is not to compile an exhaustive catalog of the symptoms, but to gain a basic awareness of what occurred and some understanding of the process leading up to the decompensation.

Negative Symptoms

Of the patient's symptoms, amotivation, alogia, blunted affect, and apathy are often the most challenging to change. Various cognitive approaches have been tried with limited results.

Lifestyle Issues

Smoking, diet, physical exercise, and other lifestyle issues, as with the rest of us, need to be addressed to achieve the maximum possible health for people with schizophrenia. The clinician providing supportive psychotherapy may be the person most likely to influence the patient's lifestyle. The best hope for a person with schizophrenia and diabetes, a common comorbidity, is to learn to eat correctly. The supportive psychotherapist may be the person most likely to help the patient's healthy eating.

Supportive psychotherapy includes asking people about their diet. It may help to ask, "What is your favorite food?" People with schizophrenia often make poor dietary choices, choosing high-fat and low-fiber foods, contributing to an obesity independent of that caused by their medications. While medications and a lack of opportunity can contribute to little exercise, the illness itself is associated with anergy. Additionally, poor diet can contribute to medications not working, as some essential nutrients are needed for an adequate medication response. Furthermore, should a patient actually do an admirable amount of physical exercise, a poor diet may restrict the potential benefit. Lack of zinc in the diet, for example, can prevent the benefit of physical exercise.

Depression in Schizophrenia

A frequent therapeutic obstacle is the presence of significant depression, especially while the patient is recovering from an acute psychotic episode. Opinion is divided over whether such episodes of depression in schizophrenia patients represent bona fide new episodes of depression, the revelation of already existing depression previously masked by florid psychotic symptoms, or a basic aspect of schizophrenia per se (McGlashan and Carpenter 1976; Taylor 1992).

Published surveys of the occurrence of depressive symptoms in schizophrenia range from 7% to 75% (Siris 2000). The reason for such a wide range is partly due to the need for accurate instruments to measure depression in psychotic people (Chemerinski et al. 2008). It appears that in the majority of patients, the psychotic and the depressive symptoms run the same course over time, suggesting that in these patients the depressive symptoms are an integral part of the schizophrenia. However, in approximately 15% of patients (9%–22% in various studies), the course of the depressive symptoms is not the same as that for the psychotic symptoms. The term *postpsychotic depression* applies to this group, which itself comprises three different subgroups (Leff 1990):

1. A group in which the depressive symptoms remit more slowly than the psychotic symptoms
2. A group in which the depression starts after the acute psychosis has almost resolved
3. A group in which the depression starts as much as 1 year after the psychosis has remitted

In any case, the occurrence of depressive symptoms presents a therapeutic challenge. In addition to considering appropriate antidepressant medication, you must carefully address the depressive phenomena. Getting a clear picture of the symptomatology is often the first step; this requires a judicious balance of exploratory questions and empathic, supportive statements. A patient who has been relatively verbal may now become very quiet and less likely to participate in conversational give-and-take. Explanatory statements about the common occurrence and the nature of postpsychotic depression often give the patient a cognitive interpretation of the experience and help the patient to tolerate the dysphoric affect. At times, especially when fatigue is very prominent, it helps to point out that such feelings are common with many medical situations, such as pneumonia or recovery from surgery. The analogy with a nonpsychotic illness may be an easier explanation for the patient than one that uses psychological terms.

Extra efforts to reinforce rapport may be needed, if the rapport has seemed to be well established. Missed sessions by the patient could represent the lethargy, lack of motivation, or other symptoms of depression, rather than an acting out against the therapy.

As the psychodynamics become clearer, you may choose to address certain issues. Common themes are those of grieving and mourning, ambivalence toward the psychic episode, and real-life issues that could cause depressive symptoms in anyone. It may very well be that the patient suffered a loss some time previously but was unable to mourn the loss thoroughly, possibly because of undergoing a psychotic decompensation (Roth 1970). You should now encourage the work of mourning, prompting verbalization, expression of affect, and recall of memories of the lost object, with frequent use of empathic statements.

At other times, the patient has been experiencing, without full conscious awareness, profound ambivalence toward having a psychotic episode—for example, on the one hand shame and embarrassment and on the other hand some gratification of wishes and needs (such as for dependence or grandiosity). If the patient is unaware of or is minimizing this ambivalence, he is likely to become depressed and/or to express the ambivalence in an extremely concrete way. A task of supportive psychotherapy is to make the patient aware of this ambivalence, including awareness of the gratifying or self-reinforcing aspects of the illness. This must be done with diplomacy. (Patients may add humor and creativity on their own.)

Case Vignettes

A young patient had become more depressed following a psychotic exacerbation. He had been staying at home, not getting involved in any activities, but receiving special attention from his distinguished parents. He experienced a hallucination in which he was told that he had the condition "Lu-ke-me-a," pronounced both "leukemia" and "lucky me." Therapy then focused on his ambivalence toward his situation giving him extra attention, the absence of certain expectations and responsibilities, and so forth. This therapeutic concentration allowed him to acknowledge his ambivalence; he became less depressed about his unfortunate situation and started a rehabilitation program shortly thereafter.

Another young man was discouraged after a recurrence of a psychotic decompensation. He wondered if there were advantages at all to having schizophrenic episodes. He concluded that there were no advantages and that he had to "grin and bear it," resulting in police custody because of his nudity.

Any situation or conflict that can lead to depression in a nonschizophrenic patient can also lead to depression in a patient with schizophrenia. Full attention should be given to these underlying conflicts and losses, similar to the therapeutic attention given identical phenomena in any depressive syndrome. However, several important concerns and modifications may apply.

You should keep in mind the danger of suicide in schizophrenia. Suicide remains a high risk, even if the patient is not overtly psychotic. Suicidal ideation and intentions must be evaluated in the patient with schizophrenia as thoroughly and as delicately as in the patient with primary affective disorder. Establishing an excellent rapport with the patient with schizophrenia can itself increase the patient's risk for suicide when she feels that the therapist is going to be lost. This may be especially true for patients who have had few close relationships in their lives. The loss of that one close relationship with the therapist may be more than they can handle. You must pay very close attention to this danger at times of transitioning from another therapist, preparing for termination, or undergoing July turnover in residency training programs (Ravenscroft 1975).

Sometimes the patient may seem more demoralized by the depressive symptoms than by the florid psychotic symptoms. One possible comment about the issues leading to depression, serving both to reassure and to promote the therapeutic process, might be: "What previously made you crazy is now making you depressed. This may be very painful, but it is a step higher, a process in your recovery." A repertoire of therapeutic responses to depression in schizophrenia is provided in Table 6–6.

Integration of Medications With Therapy

The relationship of medication and psychotherapy is so significant that it will be examined in depth in Chapter 16, but we shall introduce some of the issues here.

Working with patients with a diagnosis of schizophrenia, you must be comfortable, if not a master, in several fields (i.e., individual therapy, family and group dynamics). Even if you are not a prescriber, you need to know a lot about psychopharmacology. It is impossible to treat schizophrenia in most instances without

Table 6–6.   Therapeutic responses to depression in schizophrenia

Look for and ask about symptoms of depression.

Respond emphatically to the patient's depressive feelings.

Pay attention to suicidal ideation.

Encourage appropriate mourning for earlier losses and for losses due to the illness.

Help the patient to acknowledge ambivalence toward psychotic episodes.

Address conflicts that lead to depression.

Use reassurance with explanation—for example, "What previously made you crazy is now making you depressed."

concomitant use of psychotropic medication. Nonphysician therapists and ortho-dox psychoanalysts may adjust to this issue by referring the patient elsewhere for medication. For many patients, this may not be a problem; for a few patients, this may even represent a decided advantage. However, for many patients, there is a therapeutic benefit to having the same professional manage both the psychother-apy and the medication prescription. This emphasizes to an often fragmented pa-tient his unity as a person, allows the therapist to observe subtle changes following moderate or minor medication adjustments, and keeps the therapist aware of un-comfortable side effects. The objective or subjective restlessness of akathisia, for example, may be easily misunderstood and misdiagnosed as anxiety or depression, and thus mishandled, by a therapist not attuned to psychopharmacology.

Meaning of Changes in Medication

Starting, making changes in, and stopping medication are meaningful to all patients. The therapist should not begin making changes in medication at the first visit but should first develop a baseline impression of the patient over several visits (Siris 1990). In addition, the concreteness and the inability to integrate fully one's own lived history (i.e., failure of historicity), which are character-istic of patients with schizophrenia, complicate the use of medication.

Case Vignettes

A patient had been doing well taking 10 mg of trifluoperazine at night. The pharmacy suddenly substituted two 5-mg tablets for the one 10-mg tablet;

there was no switch to a generic medication, and the total dosage was identical. The patient was convinced she was taking something different and began decompensating, only to reconstitute when the 10-mg dose was resumed.

A patient was being treated in psychotherapy by a nonphysician, with medication prescribed by Dr. Jackson, whose name appeared on the pharmacy label. One day, Dr. Jackson was absent, and Dr. Taylor prescribed the identical medication. Over the next week the patient began experiencing increased symptoms, and he told his therapist that the medicine prescribed by the doctor, a medicine whose name the patient identified as "Taylor," was not as effective as the medicine named "Jackson" that had been prescribed by the previous doctor.

The supportive psychotherapist must be highly alert to the meaning to the patient of changes in medication or changes in the act of prescribing the medications. In work with schizophrenia patients, as has been pointed out in work with borderline patients, focusing on medication does not obstruct the therapy or obscure its goals, but instead provides essential information and is fundamental to the therapy itself (Waldinger and Frank 1989).

Guidelines for Medication

Flexibility

When medicating, you must be flexible, increasing or decreasing the medication as required by circumstances, changing or adding medication to respond to various symptoms, and enlisting the patient's participation in this flexibility. If a good therapeutic rapport has been established, the patient can be instructed to make certain changes within a specified range under defined circumstances (Hansell and Willis 1977). The range of changes can include increasing the medication twofold and decreasing it by 25% or even 50%; the defined circumstances can include sudden crises or exacerbations of symptoms on the one hand, and excessive drowsiness on the other hand.

Case Vignette

A middle-aged man working in an office had established an agreement with the therapist whereby the patient was free to double the medication on his own if he developed paranoid delusions, severe anxiety, or prominent insomnia. The same patient could decrease the medication by 25% if he experienced excessive drowsiness that interfered with work. The patient would discuss these changes with the therapist at their next session, or by telephone if the symptoms persisted. This arrangement allowed the patient to modify his medication regimen rapidly, allowing better work adjustment and a greater sense of control.

However, such an agreement is not for every patient; a fair amount of responsibility and an adequate power of self-observation are required.

Premonitory Symptoms

Presence of prodromal or premonitory symptoms may be one of the strongest indicators for medication change. Exacerbations of psychosis are almost always preceded by early symptoms, and in a particular patient the same symptoms may precede all exacerbations. However, these prodromal symptoms may not be the most prominent symptoms of the acute exacerbation once it becomes full-blown. The most common prodromal symptoms are nervousness, difficulty in concentration, insomnia, depression, and social withdrawal; many of these symptoms may seem to be affective symptoms at first glance (Herz 1985). Increased psychotropic medication may help prevent the exacerbation from turning into disorganization or chaos. It is the antipsychotic medication that should be increased in these circumstances; this is true even if the prodromal symptoms appear to be primarily affective in nature. This guideline, of course, assumes that one has made a proper differential diagnosis of schizophrenia from bipolar disorder and major depression.

Case Vignette

A graduate student had experienced two acute psychotic episodes characterized by paranoid delusions, auditory hallucinations, ideas of reference, and severe anxiety. Both episodes were preceded for several days by tactile hallucinations, but the tactile hallucinations were not prominent during the florid psychotic episodes. For 2 years the student had been keeping up well with her studies, although she had had major difficulties in interpersonal relationships. Most of the time, while she was taking psychotic medication, the patient experienced excessive drowsiness, interfering with her schoolwork. On several occasions, the patient developed tactile hallucinations that were interpreted in various ways (e.g., she thought that she had walked into a spiderweb, that some pollutant had gotten on her skirt). Several days later, the psychotic symptoms became more marked. Medication was started or increased after each episode of tactile hallucinations; although periods of psychosis sometimes followed, these episodes were time-limited and did not require hospitalization. On several occasions, no full-blown psychosis at all developed. The patient was able to pay attention to this prodromal symptom and thus minimize the medication requirements at other times.

Emphasis on Positive, Personal Benefits

Medications must be presented in ways that make sense for that particular patient (Diamond 1983). An explanation of medication usage as a way to decrease auditory hallucinations may not match the immediate goals of a particular patient; such an explanation may not mean anything for that patient and may neither enhance medication adherence nor contribute to the therapeutic alliance. A more effective presentation would be to emphasize positive benefits for the particular patient. For example, a patient may be told that medication can help eliminate distractions from his ability to concentrate so that he can enjoy reading the sports pages. Another patient may be told that medication will enable her to watch television without experiencing disturbing ideas of reference. The positive benefits should 1) be presented in as concrete a manner as possible, 2) be relevant to the activities of the patient's daily life, and 3) involve some pleasure, satisfaction, or improvement in the quality of life.

Attention must be given to issues of medication nonadherence, both voluntary and inadvertent. One method is to ask the patient regularly what medication is being taken. This method emphasizes the importance of the patient's knowledge and identification of the medications and enables the therapist to keep abreast of attitudes toward medication and toward changes in adherence. At times, it will prove useful to have the patient bring in all the medications for a pill count. This can be a powerful nonverbal action about the importance of adherence (Siris 1990).

On many occasions, you may have to enlist the aid of family members, caregivers, group home landlords, and so forth to monitor and encourage medication adherence. In such cases, major changes in medication may have to be communicated to the significant other.

Guidelines for discussing medication in supportive psychotherapy are given in Table 6–7.

Difficulties in Supportive Psychotherapy With Patients With Schizophrenia

Risks for the Patient

Supportive psychotherapy, like all medical treatments, has its indications and its benefits and risks. Indeed, the very success of supportive psychotherapy in

Table 6–7.   Approaches to talking about medications in supportive psychotherapy

Determine the meaning of medication to the patient.

Design a flexible medication plan.

Specify circumstances and a range for increase/decrease in medication.

Allow for flexibility in dosing schedule based on the patient's lifestyle.

Pay attention to prodromal symptoms.

Look to premonitory symptoms as an indicator for medication changes.

Consider an increase in antipsychotic medication even if prodromal symptoms appear to be affective.

Present the benefits of medication.

• Emphasize positive benefits, such as increase in pleasure.

• Be concrete.

Monitor adherence.

enhancing the lives of patients with schizophrenia carries with it the risk of inappropriate or excessive therapy. There will be times when the proper medical treatment is hospitalization, no matter how successful previous outpatient supportive psychotherapy has been. There may be times when the success of supportive psychotherapy tempts the therapist to engage the patient in a more intense insight-oriented psychotherapy. Although this may bring early positive results, there is a danger that the patient may not be able to handle the more intense transference. Inappropriate insight-oriented therapy may become overstimulating and intrusive, leading to severe decompensation and regression, premature termination, and alienation from family and caregivers (Drake and Sederer 1986).

Countertransference Issues

Working with patients with schizophrenia places you in close contact with intense anxiety, primary-process thinking, projective identification, and an atmosphere of loss of ego boundaries. It would not be unheard of for you to experience the fear of going crazy yourself (Searles 1966). You should not panic if this fear develops, but should instead look at it as a consequence of empathy with the patient. In many ways this fear is similar to the experience of many medical students in their initial exposure to patients: the students see in themselves the symptoms of cancer and other dread diseases.

At times you may develop unrealistic expectations in work with a particular patient, leading to disappointment in yourself, or subtle pressure on the patient to improve more than can be expected. At other times, you may have overly pessimistic expectations, settling for only minor changes in the patient or even giving messages that the patient should not strive for further progress.

Work with patients with schizophrenia can be very satisfying. One therapist expresses appreciation for the "moments of meeting" that can punctuate long-term therapy with a schizophrenia patient and writes that "[s]uch privileged moments in which the unspeakable becomes spoken can occur in a supportive process" (Rogan 2000, p. 166). However, because schizophrenia is inherently a disease characterized by remissions and exacerbation, many patients will experience regressions and crisis regardless of the quality, or even brilliance, of the treatment. The risks of supportive psychotherapy in schizophrenia and some suggestions for minimizing them are schematized in Table 6–8.

Do not let your professional satisfaction be replaced by discouragement and burnout. You must maintain your equilibrium, have a satisfying life apart from your profession, and place your work with patients with schizophrenia in the context of the natural history of the illness and a long-term perspective on the benefits of treatment.

Table 6–8. Risks of using supportive therapy in schizophrenia and strategies for minimizing these risks

Risks	Strategy for minimizing risk
For the patient	
Dangers of inappropriate intensive psychotherapy	Understand your individual patient's needs and abilities, and use limited or superficial interpretations at first.
Increased depression; change in suicide risk	Build in safety by seeking feedback from the patient about these issues, and be able to offer extra support when needed.
Premature termination	Maintain appropriate distance; avoid overstimulation and intrusion into patient's life before such issues can be handled.
Countertransference problems	
Fear of going crazy	Recognize the fear as an empathic understanding that you are on a continuum with the patient; seek mixed caseload that includes nonpsychotic patients.
Unrealistic expectations	Understand the course of prognosis of the illness, and, in particular, become knowledgeable about cognitive deficits in schizophrenia.
Overly pessimistic expectations	Consider that pessimism may be a way of protecting yourself from doubts about your own competency; however, *pessimism can become self-fulfilling*.
Therapist burnout	There is no easy answer to this, but avoid staking your reputation on curing any one patient, and balance the deadly seriousness of professional life with nonprofessional activities.

Key Points

- According to newer conceptualization of hallucinations, they are more frequent and less pathological than in previous conceptualizations, and these newer viewpoints are helpful to patients themselves in understanding their experiences.

- It is important to establish a connection (a professional yet still a real relationship) with patients who have schizophrenia.

- You can make your therapy more effective but Y the course of schizophrenic illness and how patients deal with the various stages of illness, such as recovering from a psychotic episode.

- The therapist's repertoire of skills should include asking about experiences outside the sessions, responding to special symptoms such as ideas of reference, responding to negative symptoms, and helping the patient with medical needs and lifestyle issues.

- You can improve your timing of interventions by recognizing the patient's ability to benefit from the interpretation at that time (e.g., when the patient is in a "double-awareness" phase of the illness and is amenable to challenging his delusions).

- As you learn about the illness of schizophrenia, you will be better able to handle your own countertransference reactions in therapy.

- Many patients with schizophrenia will benefit from a combination of medication and psychotherapy, but you must individualize your approach if you are to overcome objections to medications as well as mitigate the side effects of medications.

References

Alvarez-Jiménez M, González-Blanch C, Vázquez-Barquero JL, et al: Attenuation of antipsychotic-induced weight gain with early behavioral intervention in drug-naive first-episode psychosis patients: a randomized controlled trial. J Clin Psychiatry 67(8):1253–1260, 2006 16965204

American Psychiatric Association: Diagnostic and Statistical Manual of Mental Disorders, 5th Edition. Arlington, VA, American Psychiatric Association, 2013

Arieti S: Interpretation of Schizophrenia, 2nd Edition. New York, Basic Books, 1974

Bandura A: Principles of Behavior Modification. New York, Holt, Rinehart & Winston, 1969

Brent B: Mentalization-based psychodynamic psychotherapy for psychosis. J Clin Psychol 65(8):803–814, 2009 19572277

Buckley LA, Maayan N, Soares-Weiser K, et al: Supportive therapy for schizophrenia. Cochrane Database Syst Rev (4):CD004716, 2015 25871462

Cameron N: The paranoid pseudo-community revisited. Am J Sociol 65:52–58, 1959

Chemerinski E, Bowie C, Anderson H, Harvey PD: Depression in schizophrenia: methodological artifact or distinct feature of the illness? J Neuropsychiatry Clin Neurosci 20(4):431–440, 2008

Decker PS, Nathan BR: Behavior Modeling Training: Principles and Applications. New York, Praeger, 1985

Diamond RJ: Enhancing medication use in schizophrenic patients. J Clin Psychiatry 44(6 Pt 2):7–14, 1983 6133855

Drake RE, Sederer LI: The adverse effects of intensive treatment of chronic schizophrenia. Compr Psychiatry 27(4):313–326, 1986 2873959

El-Mallakh P, Howard PB, Evans BN: Medical illness in people with schizophrenia. Nurs Clin North Am 45(4):591–611, 2010 20971339

Evans S, Newton R, Higgins S: Nutritional intervention to prevent weight gain in patients commenced on olanzapine: a randomized controlled trial. Aust N Z J Psychiatry 39(6):479–486, 2005 15943650

Farmer S: Medical problems of chronic patients in a community support program. Hosp Community Psychiatry 38(7):745–749, 1987 3610070

Feder R: Auditory hallucinations treated by radio headphones. Am J Psychiatry 139(9):1188–1190, 1982 7114315

Firth J, Torous J: Smartphone apps for schizophrenia: a systematic review. JMIR Mhealth Uhealth 3(4):e102, 2015 26546039

Frank AF, Gunderson AG: The role of the therapeutic alliance in the treatment of schizophrenia: relationship to course and outcome. Arch Gen Psychiatry 47(3):228–236, 1990 1968329

Freud S: Psycho-analytic notes on an autobiographical account of a case of paranoia (dementia paranoides) (1911), in The Standard Edition of the Complete Psychological Works of Sigmund Freud, Vol 12. Translate and edited by Strachey J. London, Hogarth Press, 1958, pp 1–82

Gaudiano BA: The cognitive-behavioral treatment of schizophrenia: the state of the art and the evidence. International Journal of Behavioral Consultation and Therapy 20(1):1–11, 2006

Hansell N, Willis GL: Outpatient treatment of schizophrenia. Am J Psychiatry 134(10):1082–1086, 1977 900258

Hellerstein D, Frosch W, Koenigsberg HW: The clinical significance of command hallucinations. Am J Psychiatry 144(2):219–221, 1987 3812793

Herz M: Prodromal symptoms and prevention of relapse in schizophrenia. J Clin Psychiatry 46(11 Pt 2):22–25, 1985 2865253

Inchausti F, García-Poveda NV, Prado-Abril J, et al: Metacognition-oriented social skills training (MOSST): theoretical framework, working methodology and treatment descriptions for patients with schizophrenia. Psychologist Papers 38(1):204–215, 2017

Inchausti F, García-Poveda N, Ballesteros A, et al: The effects of metacognition-oriented social skills training on psychosocial outcomes in schizophrenia-spectrum disorders: a randomized controlled trial. Schizophr Bull 44(6):1235–1244, 2018 29267940

Ison R, Medoro L, Keen N, et al: The use of rescripting imagery for people with psychosis who hear voices. Behav Cogn Psychother 42(2):129–142, 2014 23920004

Jenner JA: Hallucination-Focused Integrative Therapy: A Specific Treatment That Hits Auditory Verbal Hallucinations. London, Routledge, 2016

Junginger J: Predicting compliance with command hallucinations. Am J Psychiatry 147(2):245–247, 1990 2301669

Koran LM, Sox HC Jr, Marton KI, et al: Medical evaluation of psychiatric patients, I: results in a state mental health system. Arch Gen Psychiatry 46(8):733–740, 1989 2787623

Koren D: Metacognition in non-psychotic help-seeking adolescents: associations with prodromal symptoms, distress and psychosocial deterioration. Isr J Psychiatry Relat Sci 51(1):34–43, 2014 24858633

Leff J: Depressive symptoms in the course of schizophrenia, in Depression in Schizophrenia. Edited by DeLisi LE. Washington, DC, American Psychiatric Press, 1990, pp 1–23

Lynch D, Laws KR, McKenna PJ: Cognitive behavioural therapy for major psychiatric disorder: does it really work? A meta-analytical review of well-controlled trials. Psychol Med 40(1):9–24, 2010 19476688

Lysaker PH, Dimaggio G: Metacognitive capacities for reflection in schizophrenia: implications for developing treatments. Schizophr Bull 40(3):487–491, 2014 24636965

Mason SE, Gingerich S, Siris SG: Patients' and caregivers' adaptation to improvement in schizophrenia. Hosp Community Psychiatry 41(5):541–544, 1990 2347571

McGlashan TH, Carpenter WT Jr: An investigation of the postpsychotic depressive syndrome. Am J Psychiatry 133(1):14–19, 1976 1247119

McGlashan TH, Levy ST, Carpenter WT Jr: Integration and sealing over: clinically distinct recovery styles from schizophrenia. Arch Gen Psychiatry 32(10):1269–1272, 1975 1180660

Meaden A, Van Marle S: When the going gets tougher: the importance of long-term supportive psychotherapy in psychosis. Adv Psychiatr Treat 14:42–49, 2008

Mendel WM: Treating Schizophrenia. San Francisco, CA, Jossey-Bass, 1989

Modell AH: An approach to the nature of auditory hallucinations in schizophrenia. Arch Gen Psychiatry 3:259–266, 1960

Morin R: Learning to live with the voices in your head. The Atlantic, November 5, 2014. Available at: https://www.theatlantic.com/health/archive/2014/11/learning-to-live-with-the-voices-in-your-head/382096. Accessed February 20, 2019.

Nott L: iPhone app helps schizophrenics block voices. Mental Health, August 7, 2013. Available at: https://www.elementsbehavioralhealth.com/mental-health/iphone-app-helps-schizophrenics-block-voices/. Accessed February 20, 2019.

Opoka SM, Lincoln TM: The effect of cognitive behavioral interventions on depression and anxiety symptoms in patients with schizophrenia spectrum disorders: a systemic review. Psychiatr Clin North Am 34(1):25–31, 2017 29080591

Penn DL, Mueser KT, Tarrier N, et al: Supportive therapy for schizophrenia: possible mechanisms and implications for adjunctive psychosocial treatments. Schizophr Bull 30(1):101–112, 2004 15176765

Pesek MB: Therapy and quality of life of patients with psychosis. Psychiatr Danub 21 (suppl 1):146–148, 2009 19789502

Pierides S: Even Paranoids Have Enemies: New Perspectives in Paranoia and Persecution. London, Routledge, 1998

Ravenscroft K Jr: Milieu process during the residency turnover: the human cost of psychiatric education. Am J Psychiatry 132(5):506–512, 1975 1119610

Rogan A: "Moving along" in psychotherapy with schizophrenia patients. J Psychother Pract Res 9(3):157–166, 2000 10896741

Rojcewicz S: Darth Vader: masks, power and meaning. Journal of Poetry Therapy 1(1):23–30, 1987

Rosenbaum B, Harder S, Knudsen P, et al: Supportive psychodynamic psychotherapy versus treatment as usual for first-episode psychosis: two-year outcome. Psychiatry 75(4):331–341, 2012 23244011

Rosenhan DL: On being sane in insane places. Science 179(4070):250–258, 1973 4683124

Roth S: The seemingly ubiquitous depression following acute schizophrenic episodes, a neglected area of clinical discussion. Am J Psychiatry 127(1):51–58, 1970 5426245

Rudden M, Gilmore M, Frances A: Delusions: when to confront the facts of life. Am J Psychiatry 139(7):929–932, 1982 6979944

Sacks MH, Carpenter WT Jr, Strauss JS: Recovery from delusions: three phases documented by patient's interpretation of research procedures. Arch Gen Psychiatry 30(1):117–120, 1974 4808730

Sarti P, Cournos F: Medication and psychotherapy in the treatment of chronic schizophrenia. Psychiatr Clin North Am 13(2):215–228, 1990 1972273

Schweitzer RD, Greben M, Bargenquast R: Long-term outcomes of metacognitive narrative psychotherapy for people diagnosed with schizophrenia. Psychol Psychother 90(4):668–685, 2017 28544223

Searles H: Collected Papers on Schizophrenia and Related Subjects. Madison, CT, International Universities Press, 1966

Shaikh-Lesko R: Imagining voices: a look at an alternative approach to treating auditory hallucinations. Stanford Medicine Scope, November 13, 2014

Siegler M, Osmond H: Models of Madness, Models of Medicine. New York, Macmillan, 1974

Siris SG: Pharmacological treatment of depression in schizophrenia, in Depression in Schizophrenia. Edited by DeLisi LE. Washington, DC, American Psychiatric Press, 1990, pp 141–162

Siris SG: Depression in schizophrenia: perspective in the era of "atypical" antipsychotic agents. Am J Psychiatry 157:1379–1389, 2000

Skelton M, Khokhar WA, Thacker SP: Treatments for delusional disorder. Cochrane Database Syst Rev (5):CD009785, 2015 25997589

Smith B: Helpful hints about schizophrenia for family members & others. October 8, 2018. Available at: https://psychcentral.com/lib/helpful-hints-about-schizophrenia-for-family-members-and-others/. Accessed February 20, 2019.

Smits CT, van der Gaag M: Cognitive behavioural therapy for schizophrenia [in Dutch]. Tijdschr Psychiatr 52(2):99–109, 2010 20146181

Spaulding WD, Silverstein SM, Menditto AA: The Schizophrenia Spectrum, 2nd Edition. Boston, MA, Hogrefe, 2017

Taylor MA: Are schizophrenia and affective disorder related? A selective literature review. Am J Psychiatry 149(1):22–32, 1992 1728181

Torous J, Keshavan M: The role of social media in schizophrenia: evaluating risks, benefits, and potential. Curr Opin Psychiatry 29(3):190–195, 2016 26967314

University of Hertfordshire: Cognitive therapy is of no value in schizophrenia, analysis of studies suggests. ScienceDaily, June 26, 2009

Vohs JL, Leonhardt BL, James AV, et al: Metacognitive reflection and insight therapy for early psychosis: a preliminary study of a novel integrative psychotherapy. Schizophr Res 195:428–433, 2018 29108671

Waldinger RJ, Frank AF: Transference and the vicissitudes of medication use by borderline patients. Psychiatry 52(4):416–427, 1989 2685859

Winklbaur B, Ebner N, Sachs G, et al: Substance abuse in patients with schizophrenia. Dialogues Clin Neurosci 8(1):37–43, 2006 16640112

Wright NP, Turkington D, Kelly OP, et al: Treating Psychosis: A Clinician's Guide to Integrating Acceptance and Commitment Therapy, Compassion-Focused Therapy and Mindfulness Approaches Within the Cognitive Behavior Therapy Tradition. Oakland, CA, New Harbinger Publications, 2014

7

Mood Disorders

T he supportive interventions in the previous chapter were primarily addressed to patients with serious thought disorders. Here we turn our attention
from cognitive to affective disturbances. Consistent with our emphasis on evidence-based treatments, we continue to find evidence supporting the use of
supportive psychotherapy in depressive disorders, but also a need for further
research (see, e.g., Jacobs and Reupert 2014, also cited in Chapter 1). However, there is no recent Cochrane review of psychological therapies for adult
depression. A review of somatic and psychological therapies (not including supportive psychotherapy) for adolescents was inconclusive: "There is very limited evidence upon which to base conclusions about the relative effectiveness
of psychological interventions, antidepressant medication and a combination of
these interventions" (Cox et al. 2014). Another Cochrane study on treatment-
resistant depression did not specifically examine supportive psychotherapy,
but it certainly did find that the psychotherapies studied were equally effective
(Ijaz et al. 2018).

However, various forms of short-term psychodynamic psychotherapy
(STPP), which included both supportive and expressive elements, were eval-

uated in a meta-analysis and found to be effective in the treatment of depression, and perhaps most importantly for our purposes, "[s]upportive and expressive STPP modes were found to be equally efficacious" (Driessen et al. 2010, p. 25). This provides a rather strong mandate for continuing to teach and urge the use of supportive psychotherapy for depressed adults. For adolescents, there is also a positive study of STPP as defined above (Dil et al. 2016). There are also positive studies for specific subcategories of depressed persons. Although mildly to moderately depressed patients do not necessarily need somatic therapies, we do remind therapists that depression requires consideration of somatic treatments, including pharmacotherapy and/or electroconvulsive therapy, supplemented by psychotherapy.

Some therapists, of course, may want to adopt programs from cognitive-behavioral therapy (CBT), interpersonal psychotherapy, or many of the other psychotherapy types available in various teaching programs. However, therapists should be guided by evidence and not just the historical dominance of one particular therapeutic school. We mention again the studies referenced in Chapter 6 about cognitive therapy being ineffective in schizophrenia, and these also showed that it was of minimal effectiveness in depression (Lynch et al. 2010; University of Hertfordshire 2009). Therefore, we are confident that the supportive techniques described here will form a good initial training for therapists who move on to use other methods. And of course, these techniques may be used to provide psychotherapy when coming from providers who are primarily medicators but who do want to maximize the effectiveness of all their interventions, both somatic and psychological.

Supportive psychotherapy approaches to several disorders with affective components are summarized in Table 7–1. More will be said about each of them here or in subsequent chapters, although there will not be a complete discussion of diagnostic issues.

Depressed States

It is likely that psychotherapy improves a different set of symptoms than does pharmacotherapy. Therapies that embrace some supportive measures include social learning (Lewinsohn et al. 1980), social skills (Hersen et al. 1984), self-control and reward programs (Rehm 1984), positive psychology (Seligman

Table 7–1. Supportive psychotherapy approaches to disorders with affective components

Disorder	Major defense mechanisms	Immediate source of disturbance	Effect on self-esteem	Supportive approach to treatment
Grief	Normal defenses typical for the individual (at times exaggerated); denial	Extrinsic	Traditionally said to be intact	Environmental supports, providing time perspective for self-healing and development of new social relationships
Depression of adjustment disorder with depressed mood	Introjection of ambivalently regarded love object; regression or fixation at oral stage of development	Sometimes extrinsic (i.e., exogenous depression or adjustment disorder), but usually involves endogenous biological and genetic factors, especially if patient has bipolar disorder	Acutely decreased	Improvement of self-esteem; improvement of cognitive and interpersonal processes to prevent depressive reactions to life events; displacement of aggression into reinforcing activities, often as adjunct to biological treatments
Dysthymic disorder	Defective defenses and coping capacity in a stable self	Mostly intrinsic (i.e., life history and genetic factors)	Chronically low	Restructuring dysfunctional defenses and counteracting chronically learned helplessness with improved coping strategies

Table 7–1.   Supportive psychotherapy approaches to disorders with affective components *(continued)*

Disorder	Major defense mechanisms	Immediate source of disturbance	Effect on self-esteem	Supportive approach to treatment
Borderline personality disorder	Splitting and other primitive defenses in an inadequately matured self	Mostly intrinsic (i.e., poor parenting, early trauma, some genetic association to mood disorders)	Defectively and unrealistically regulated; dependent on external supports	Limit setting; controlled provision of a gratifying primary object relationship; confrontations of dysfunctional behavior; improvement of skills in controlling impulsive behavior
Mania	Denial and grandiosity, possibly as defenses against underlying depression and low self-esteem	Intrinsic (i.e., strong genetic factors)	Increased, but may oscillate dramatically in mixed states	In acute manic state, limit setting and protection from destructive acts; as manic state subsides, compliance issues, defense mechanisms, and personality dysfunction can be addressed

Table 7–2. Supportive strategies for depression

At the start, take the patient's distress at face value.

While acknowledging the distress, always provide hope that the depression will get better rather than last "forever" as many patients feel it will.

Counter feelings of self-blame and responsibility for the depression.

When appropriate, introduce the biological theory of the illness.

Improve the patient's cognitive and interpersonal skills.

Improve the patient's self-image.

Counter reductions of self-esteem associated with chronic illness.

Improve compliance with medication and help patient to tolerate side effects.

Educate patient and family about biological course of illness.

To the extent possible, provide or refer to adjunctive sources of education such as brochures, books, Internet sites, and apps.

Provide monitoring charts for mood management (see section "Bipolar Disorder").

Offer crisis support and diminish probability of suicide.

2002), and behavioral activation (Tull 2018). Interpersonal psychotherapy employs elucidation of psychic conflicts only when necessary, preferentially using education, antidemoralizing measures, social manipulations, and problem-solving techniques. Therapists are specifically trained to be supportive and active but not overly active or directive (Klerman et al. 1984; Rousanville et al. 1984). In a major meta-analysis that compared several psychotherapies, including CBT, nondirective supportive treatment, and interpersonal psychotherapy, the latter was found somewhat more efficacious, but we emphasize that the nondirective therapy would naturally be thought less efficacious than the directive therapies we advocate in this book (Cuijpers et al. 2008).

Major supportive interventions useful with depressed patients are listed in Table 7–2. It should also be noted that pharmacological treatments can take weeks and that a substantial number of depressions are medication resistant; psychotherapy may be required in relapse or while appropriate medication dosage is being titrated. The therapist interested in supportive techniques may therefore wish to be conversant with one or more particular programs and to try them with appropriate patients. Brief summaries are available elsewhere (Hirschfeld and Goodwin 1988; Jarrett and Rush 1987).

Karasu (1990a, 1990b) has developed a detailed comparison of three major treatments—psychodynamic, cognitive, and interpersonal—with the goal of providing a selective treatment model that does not lock the therapist into any one modality. None of the three, however, has the broad applicability of supportive therapy. For example, cognitive therapy is not effective with many unmotivated, nonlogical patients and has decreased effectiveness in depressed patients with low social dysfunction (Sotsky et al. 1991). Psychodynamic treatment is too time-consuming and stressful for depressed medically ill patients.

Supportive psychotherapy also has an important role in treating depressed patients with other psychiatric problems or those who deny or somatize their illness. Given the show of effectiveness (as the minimalist placebo–clinical management treatment condition) in the National Institute of Mental Health (NIMH) study discussed in Chapter 1, it is important to *not* neglect supportive therapy when treating depression. With indebtedness to Karasu's work, we have reorganized his analysis of the other three therapies in comparing them with supportive psychotherapy (see Table 7–3). We redistributed Karasu's patient selection characteristics from his original table to accommodate the additional group of patients who can be treated most effectively with supportive psychotherapy (see Table 7–4).

An instructive early version of supportive therapy for depression was developed by Hollon (1962), who described a short-term psychotherapy that utilized a "maximum activity program" with a log of daily activities, a displaced attention to the patient's oral needs (including feeding), and a detailed recollection of the patient's life history that was used to enhance the patient's reality testing. The express aim was to create gratifying work that would displace the patient's attention from his or her depression. Modern versions of these techniques can be recognized in cognitive therapy, in logs for behavioral activation (Schuldt 2019), and in several of the supportive techniques mentioned below.

Depressed patients present in many ways. They may be anxiously seeking relief and pinning all their hopes on the therapist, or, being brought in reluctantly by family, they may parade their irritability and defensiveness. Supportive interventions are especially indicated for patients who passively express helplessness and do not volunteer information. A variable length for sessions is especially suitable for

Table 7–3. Comparison of supportive therapy with other therapies for depression

Type of therapy	Concepts of pathology and etiology	Major goals and mechanisms of change	Primary techniques and practices	Therapist role/ Therapeutic relationship	Some advantages	Some limitations
Psychodynamic	Ego regression: damaged self-esteem and unresolved conflict due to childhood object loss and disappointment	Promote personality change through understanding of past conflicts Achieve insight into defenses, ego distortions, and superego defects Provide a role model Permit cathartic release of aggression	Expressive/ empathic: fully or partially analyzing transference and resistance; confronting defenses; clarifying ego and superego distortions	Interpreter/ reflector: establishment and exploration of transference; therapeutic alliance for benign dependency and empathic understanding	Individual depth approach encourages patient to look inward for solutions rather than depending on external sources	Focus on intrapsychic phenomena may obscure other (e.g., interpersonal, environmental) factors; aggression = depression theory can be overgeneralized and lead to overreliance on catharsis

Table 7–3.   Comparison of supportive therapy with other therapies for depression *(continued)*

Type of therapy	Concepts of pathology and etiology	Major goals and mechanisms of change	Primary techniques and practices	Therapist role/ Therapeutic relationship	Some advantages	Some limitations
Cognitive	Distorted thinking; dysphoria due to learned negative views of self, others, and the world	Provide symptomatic relief through alteration of target thoughts Identify self-destructive cognitions Modify specific erroneous assumptions Promote self-control over thinking patterns	Cognitive/ behavioral: recording and monitoring cognitions; correcting distorted themes with logic and experimental testing; providing alternative thought content; assigning homework	Educator/shaper: positive relationship instead of transference; collaborative empiricism as basis for joint scientific (logical) task	Cognitive/ behavioral orientation is tangible and objective	Cognitive/ behavioral emphasis may neglect whole person, especially his or her affective component; symptom-oriented perspective overlooks past history, complex problem areas, and hidden conflicts

Table 7–3. Comparison of supportive therapy with other therapies for depression *(continued)*

Type of therapy	Concepts of pathology and etiology	Major goals and mechanisms of change	Primary techniques and practices	Therapist role/ Therapeutic relationship	Some advantages	Some limitations
Interpersonal	Impaired interpersonal relations; absent or unsatisfactory significant social bonds	Provide symptomatic relief through solution of current interpersonal problems Reduce stress involving family or work Improve interpersonal communication skills	Communicative/ environmental: clarifying and managing maladaptive relationships and learning new ones by communication and social skills training providing info on illness	Explorer/ prescriber: positive relationship, transference without interpretation; active therapist role for influence and advocacy	Interpersonal orientation addresses broader (e.g., social, family) context, useful in focusing on man-woman relations	Emphasis on four designated interpersonal problems can bias oneself toward preconceived themes; interpersonal orientation may stress marital/family factors while underplaying intrapsychic forces

Table 7–3. Comparison of supportive therapy with other therapies for depression *(continued)*

Type of therapy	Concepts of pathology and etiology	Major goals and mechanisms of change	Primary techniques and practices	Therapist role/ Therapeutic relationship	Some advantages	Some limitations
Supportive	Biopsychosocial, with significant contributions of genetic predisposition and neuroendocrine factors	Maximize patient function during crisis or if patient cannot perform tasks for himself or herself Support the patient's judgment with therapist's reasoning and decision-making skills Engender hope for recovery	Reality testing: is relatively accepting of existing defenses but attempts to restructure them; self-esteem-enhancing measures; enlistment of social supports	Warm, empathic, taking patient's side; offers some direct gratifications and secure "holding environment"	Tendency to present a unified understanding of grief; loss, depression under a common theoretical basis involving coping deficiencies that must be improved by supportive relationship and interventions	May underestimate the role of conscious, willful factors and character pathology that requires anxiety-provoking confrontations to ameliorate

Source.   First three categories adapted from Karasu 1990b.

Table 7–4.   Patient selection for four therapies: psychodynamic, cognitive, interpersonal, and supportive

Type of therapy	Selective patient variables
Psychodynamic	Chronic sense of emptiness and underestimation of self-worth
	Loss or long separation in childhood
	Conflicts in past relationships (e.g., with parent, with sexual partner)
	Capacity for insight
	Ability to modulate regression
	Access to dreams and fantasy
	Little need for direction and guidance
	Stable environment
Cognitive	Obvious distorted thoughts about self, world, and future
	Pragmatic (logical) thinking
	Real inadequacies (including poor responses to other psychotherapies)
	Moderate to high need for direction and guidance
	Responsiveness to behavioral training and self-help (high degree of self-control)
Interpersonal	Recent, focused dispute with spouse or significant other
	Social or communication problems
	Recent role transition or life change
	Abnormal grief reaction
	Modest to moderate need for direction and guidance
	Responsiveness to environmental manipulation (available support network)

Table 7–4.   Patient selection for four therapies: psychodynamic, cognitive, interpersonal, and supportive *(continued)*

Type of therapy	Selective patient variables
Supportive	Failure to progress in other types of therapy
	Suicidal ideation or behavior (supportive psychotherapy is both suitable and necessary for such patients)
	Cognitive impairment and illogical thinking
	Acute or chronic medical illness
	Presence of somatization or denial of illness
	Like cognitive therapy, suitable for patients with real inadequacies, who require high levels of guidance or who are responsive to behavioral methods; however, the behavioral methods need not be verbal

Source.   First three categories adapted from Karasu 1990b.

taciturn patients because it does not force them to fill the time anxiously. Psychotic features (e.g., delusions of worthlessness or persecution), as in schizophrenia, are generally not worth challenging directly but can be worked with in the ways we have described in the preceding chapter. Anxiety, present in the majority of depressed patients, can be addressed by the techniques discussed in Chapter 8.

It should be remembered that *somatic complaints* are fundamental to the DSM-5 (American Psychiatric Association 2013) definition of depression and must be addressed directly and not approached merely as psychological defenses. Somatic complaints should be taken seriously; their discussion can be useful as a displacement from more painful psychological issues.

Primary Techniques and Emphases in Treatment of Depressed States

Giving Reassurance

A starting point for many patients, cooperative or not, is the giving of appropriate hope and reassurance. They can be told that there is light at the end of the tunnel and that their depression will probably be of finite duration. Often this reassurance will be rejected but will be remembered by the patient when the recovery process begins. To bypass the conscious rejection of reassurance, some therapists have effectively used metaphorical reassurance, as by reminding the patient of the wandering of the Israelites in the Sinai desert (Barker 1985, p. 125). Another analogy is the comparison of depression to the loss of energy in physical illness. The patient is reminded: "When you don't have energy, as when you are knocked out by the flu, you are unable to do the ordinary activities of living, but it's remarkable how soon you feel better. So you shouldn't worry about your limitations now. When your depression improves, you will have your energy back again." This analogy can be used as a rationale for delaying precipitous decisions as well as warding off suicidal actions. Also well known are the memory complaints found in depression, and the decisions you can make to work up, delay workup, or provide reassurances that problems will improve as the depression resolves. A good resource for patients that might save them an expensive workup is the overview by Scaccia (2016).

Giving reassurance can be dangerous if it is not believable, as in the following case.

Case Vignette

A depressed man had the delusion that his bank account was too deficient to provide a cushion for the future national economic woes that he was sure were just over the horizon. A psychiatrist assured him that his bank account was sufficient and that the economic forecasts were rosy. The patient became even more despondent, perhaps because he felt his concerns were not being recognized, and hanged himself.

Reassurances should, therefore, never be too far removed from the patient's beliefs and feelings and may need to be softened with statements like "You will find this hard to believe, but…[give the reassurance here]." Reassurance should not be given automatically but must be based on assessment of its compatibility with the patient's needs.

Facilitating Medication

When medication is offered, achieving compliance and developing tolerance of minor side effects become goals of the therapy; this may require discussing the patient's guilt and dependency at having to take medication. We do not advise giving unduly optimistic reassurances about medication. Discussions of medication often reflect a displacement of discussions of the therapist-patient relationship into the medication-patient sphere, just as Hollon's focus on food (see above) provided ways to talk about gratification and oral needs without mentioning the therapist directly. If you wish to apply psychoanalytic theory to this supportive situation, you can conceptualize depression as involving a resurgence of oral needs with reluctance in admitting them, and therefore use the topic of medications to address these needs vicariously.

Addressing Guilt

You should attempt to restore self-esteem and dispel self-accusatory modes of thought. You should not actively encourage morbid or guilty ruminations, nor encourage these ruminations by long silences (which, in the depressed patient's viewpoint, imply tacit agreement). In addition, the patient who does not feel like conversing may feel additional guilt in not holding up her side of the conversation. Depression is bad in itself, but it is the additional dimension of hopelessness and failure that is especially malignant. Therefore, the patient's "depression about depression" needs to be addressed, and the patient needs to be counseled to disconnect the pessimistic meanings attached to depressed feelings. Depression frequently involves a masochistic component, and, without attempting to interpret this component, it is supportive and consistent with that defensive style to tell patients that they are too harsh with themselves just because their standards are so idealistic.

Managing Dependency

A supportive therapist may need to allow some dependency but must also set limits to it. Some patients evoke a strong countertransference irritation because of their obsessive ruminations or clinging behaviors. Others stir up a profound sadness and an inclination to offer more support than is realistic. As in offering reassurance, there is no absolute rule about the degree of dependency to allow. It depends on the patient's need.

Addressing Loss

As in grief (to be discussed in Chapter 11), depression involves a loss that must be empathetically addressed. In this case, it is the loss, through devaluation, of the patient's evaluations of self, past, and future, and probably of imagined evaluations by others. However, you must be guarded in making attributions of responsibility for the loss. Or perhaps you may think that the patient is digging herself into the depression and refusing to climb out. A consequence may be to interpret the depression as a defense (such as avoidance of responsibility) or an attempt at oral gratification or secondary gains. Of course, this will only worsen the depression. Similarly, a well-meaning exhortation like "You can work yourself out of this" will not take root, and the patient may interpret the failure for it to do so as another sign of deficiency. If such an approach is pushed to the extreme with the attribution of personal responsibility to depression, suicide may even result. By contrast, Perry (1990) stresses the use of a medical model to both patient and family, telling the patient that the feelings she experiences are out of conscious control and are not like everyday ups and downs.

Noticing Improvement

Another characteristic of depressed patients is that their behavior often improves before they themselves realize it. Observer ratings of their depressions improve sooner and are "leading indicators" of response to therapy. To point out that the patient is spending more time in productive activities and is showing more enthusiasm is an effective reassurance once the patient has developed a trusting relationship with the therapist. It is during the recovery, however, that you should know the patient well enough to gauge if he is concealing a suicidal plan and gaining the energy to carry it out. The suicide risk can be increased for up to 8 months during the recovery phase.

Working With the Family

Educating patient and family about the biological course of the illness and preventing the family from sabotaging treatment are important goals. A depressed patient's ventilation of feelings, whether appropriate or not, generates reactive hostility and anxiety, which therapists may need to accept. Thus, Sederer (1986) points out the need to help the patient "limit to whom, when, and how much he shares his grief" (p. 28). He notes that direct expression of hostility (to the therapist or anyone else) is not necessarily therapeutic, but it is naturally to be expected toward a therapist who must frustrate some of the patient's dependency needs. Inevitably, therefore, there will be anger in the transference related to the patient's losses and disappointments. As a way of preserving the patient's social contacts, it is useful to channel a patient's anger into the therapy rather than at family or spouse. Conversely, families must also be prevented from casting the patient in an unnecessarily dependent role or creating the potential for secondary gain.

The Depressed Patient in Remission

Because about half of patients with major depression will have a recurrence, patients must be primed to seek additional treatment if symptoms recur. Issues in long-term therapy will include use of maintenance medications, the loss of self-esteem and delay of life goals from the chronicity of the illness, and adjustments of the family to the patient's loss of function. It is in the remission, or maintenance, phase that much effective work can be done, and current opinion favors the view that combined medication and psychotherapeutic treatments of several years' duration reduce the relapse rate (Klerman 1990). However, to the patient who does well and discontinues treatment, the therapist should still give the message: "You may never need me (or the clinic) again, but you should not view it as a failure if you do." The patient should be encouraged to contact you if there is occurrence of early or moderate symptoms, such as insomnia, change in activity, change in mood, difficulty in concentration, and so forth. Prodromal symptoms often precede the full affective syndrome by weeks or months, thus allowing for early and perhaps more effective treatment (Fava and Kellner 1991).

Dysthymic Conditions and Dysphoric States

The resolution of major depression, while leaving fears of recurrence, may result in relatively normal functioning. Often, however, the therapist discovers residual symptoms, personality problems, or cognitive dysfunctions that may predispose the patient to future depression. The patient may also have had a premorbid depressive neurosis, traditionally considered to represent chronically defective character traits such as a punitive superego. The closest representative to this disorder in DSM-5 is persistent depressive disorder (American Psychiatric Association 2013). Often such patients have a history of loss, trauma, or deprivation. A major review by Kocsis and Frances (1987) provided evidence for three subtypes of chronic or intermittently chronic depression:

- Depression with insidious onset that sometimes progresses to a major depression
- Depression that develops after an acute major depression
- Depression associated with other disorders, including possibly personality disorders; with chronic stress; or with medical disorder

Therapy of these chronic states may include antidepressants (see Kocsis and Frances 1987 and Akiskal 1983 for a discussion of responsive subtypes) and modifications of the previously discussed types of psychotherapy. In such cases, it is helpful to determine to what extent the patient's depressive tendencies reflect the traditional overly punitive superego and the failure to resolve internal conflicts that result in decreased self-esteem. Long-term psychoanalytic therapy or cognitive restructuring may be most useful in those cases.

Another group, including patients with depression secondary to medical illness, includes patients whose capacities and strengths fail to live up to usual cultural expectations. Such patients will benefit most from realistic support of self-esteem and a necessary decrease in expectations.

A third group of chronically depressed patients comprises those who tend to be masochistic and self-defeating, and who persistently support their depressions with existential, political, and personal arguments, inviting the therapist to join them in their despair. Such ploys may be sympathetically viewed as their adaptations to chronically depressed mood, and the existence of such cognitive features does not establish what caused what. For example, a study by Lewinsohn et al. (1981) showed that depression-related cognition concurred with episodes of depression but was not present in nondepressed control subjects or in persons who became depressed during the study.

Despite the effectiveness of cognitive therapy in treating depression, many such patients are basically irrational in clinging to depressive modes of thought, and they cannot be argued out of their depression even by sophisticated methods. Supportive psychotherapy, however, can be effective in providing a model therapist whose optimism is as contagious as the patient's pessimism. In other words, the nonverbal aspects of the relationship with an encouraging therapist are likely to be more effective than cognitive techniques. At the least, such patients will benefit from your assistance in acquiring better social skills and supports, vocational training, and increased self-control over contributing factors such as alcohol abuse.

Bipolar Disorder

Although bipolar disorder is much less common than unipolar depression, there has been much attention to the development of evidence-based treatments for the various phases of bipolar disorders. Supportive techniques such as establishing a therapeutic alliance are still going to be at the core of all therapies for bipolar disorder. Since the first edition of our book, we were pleased to find that both supportive and cognitive-behavioral therapies were demonstrated to be equally effective in the treatment of bipolar disorder (Meyer and Hautzinger 2012; Pedersen 2018). However, we do recognize that therapists of bipolar patients may want to practice other evidence-based therapies in addition to supportive psychotherapy by choosing one or more evidence-based well-known mainstream therapies for regular use with bipolar patients. The two that we have found most useful are interpersonal and social rhythm therapy (IPSRT; Frank 2007) and CBT (Basco and Rush 2007), and we have incorporated some of their techniques into our presentation. A fundamental tenet of IPSRT is that vulnerable individuals can change moods because of changes in their biological and social rhythms, such as sleep, activity and light exposure (the signals to the body known as zeitgebers or "timegivers").

Manic States

An understandable limitation of both IPSRT and CBT is the difficulty of treating acutely manic patients. Thus, it is suggested that "the best time to initiate IPSRT is when a patient is either acutely ill (for depressive episodes) or just beginning to recover (for manic or mixed episodes)" (Frank 2007, p. 41). Therefore, we think it remains important to discuss supportive techniques that begin at a time when the patient is acutely manic and that may then segue into an established or time-limited brief therapy for stabilization.

Acute mania usually requires hospitalization. However, supportive psychotherapy can contribute to the treatment of acute mania and to the continued treatment of the patient's bipolar illness. Although we have usually discussed outpatient treatments in this manual, we shall take this opportunity to show the continuity of supportive methods from inpatient to outpatient settings.

The maneuvers used by manic patients include the following (Janowsky et al. 1970):

1. Manipulation of others' self-esteem
2. Perceptiveness and ability to exploit vulnerability and conflict
3. Projection of responsibility onto others
4. Progressive limit testing
5. Alienation of family members (which is often the outcome of mania, as well as an interpersonal maneuver by the patient)

These tactics are aptly illustrated in the following example.

Case Vignette

Mr. Johnson, a self-ordained minister of his own church, was brought in as an emergency patient by police after he was found crawling on the floor in the supermarket. Loud and grandiose, he offered some explanation for his behavior and demanded to be released. The clinician performed the initial assessment and terminated it, but Mr. Johnson returned time after time to argue the same point. The clinician emphasized his concern for the patient's physical health and the need for sleep. He noted that Mr. Johnson could not carry out his ministerial work in his current condition and was therefore defeating his own interests. Nevertheless, the patient continued to interrupt the clinician, who was alone in his office at the end of the ward hallway. Finally, the clinician said, "I know that you are an expert on spiritual affairs, which I know very little about. But one thing I do know is that the spiritual world is not directly visible to us, but you can perceive many such things. Therefore, let us imagine that there is a line across the hallway. If you cross that line, I will order you into seclusion."

Mr. Johnson was familiar with seclusion and argued that it could not be legitimately used for that purpose. The clinician said that he would order it anyway and went back to his office. Mr. Johnson crossed the line and was immediately put in seclusion, where he complained loudly for about an hour. After an hour, the clinician came by and asked him if he remembered where the imaginary line was across the hallway. Mr. Johnson said that of course he did, since he remembered the whole incident and would use it as evidence in court. The clinician delegated to the other staff the power to draw imaginary lines anywhere else on the ward to set other limits for Mr. Johnson's activities. He then let Mr. Johnson out of seclusion. For the next two days, Mr. Johnson asked permission of staff whenever he wanted to cross one of the imaginary lines. He developed a warm relationship with the clinician, who continued to be his outpatient therapist, and frequently joked about how the therapist had won the battle of wits. He respected the therapist for that and was open to the therapist's other advice about managing his affairs.

What kind of (limited) agenda can be developed that will benefit the patient without destroying the therapist? First, you must be prepared to deal with the patient's uncanny ability to manipulate your self-esteem. After telling you "I'm so glad I met you because you're the first person who has ever understood me," the manic patient will demand more and more attention and try to get you to buy into his defensive scheme of justifications for irrational behavior. It is certain that any "mistake" you make (e.g., being late for an appointment, forgetting some jot from the patient's previous hospital record) will be used against you. Your own weaknesses (e.g., your residual need for flattery after years of your own therapy) and differing staff opinions about the patient's management will be exploited to the hilt. The patient may evoke sympathy or rage by saying, "You don't know what I've been through and you don't care." You will be enlisted in investigating claims of staff mistreatment. You must keep expectations reined in and avoid any personal investment in the patient's improvement, however likable the patient. Nevertheless, you can use the patient's own characteristics as tools of the therapy, as the therapist did with Mr. Johnson.

A second agenda item, based on the preceding discussion, is the need to set limits both inside and outside the therapy. Proper limit setting requires an authoritarian approach, yet, as Gunderson's (1974) survey of fire-setting manic individuals showed, patients who deny their problems and demand release "trigger the common guilt-evoking conflict that is found when the setting of limits is expected of people who want above all to be helpful" (p. 144). Premature accommodations or privileges, perhaps offered to buttress a shaky therapeutic alliance, will usually lead to patient infractions and staff crackdowns that fulfill the manic patient's prophecy of draconian treatment.

Invariably, the manic patient will violate some of the limits within psychotherapy sessions, such as verbal abuse of the therapist. In such cases you should warn the patient that this behavior is not productive, and the sessions should be terminated without an overt display of anger, with a comment such as "We need to talk further, but now isn't a good time. I'll plan to see you tomorrow at the regular time." Manic patients are at high risk for violence and assault, and it is difficult to give precise advice on how to manage verbal abuse. Verbalization may be ventilation, or it may be a prelude to a physical assault, but in either case patients should not be allowed to continue with you in a one-to-one setting.

A third agenda item concerns the patient's family. The patient will enlist family members to argue for her release. Some family members will present to you with a double agenda: on the surface (often with the patient present) they argue for discharge, while beneath the surface they hope the patient will remain hospitalized. You can, if necessary, address both issues in the same conversation, reframing the hospitalization as a chance for more intensive psychotherapy. The spouse of the manic patient may or may not be allied to you. In general, marriages of bipolar patients are reported to have a poor prognosis (see, e.g., Davenport et al. 1977; Janowsky et al. 1970). Spouses who express the desire to separate are likely to do so and are not merely asking for reassurance or reconciliation. Others will remain faithful to the end, using massive denial or rationalization at times to minimize the seriousness of the illness. This is not to imply that all marriages of bipolar patients are worthy of dissolution. As one husband remarked after being evicted from their apartment because of his wife's manic behavior, "I know she looks bad now, but she's the most loving person when she's well." However, you will also encounter spouses who have been physically and psychologically abused.

Destructive aspects of the patient's behavior must always be on the agenda of treatment as the patient returns to normal mood so that she can institute protective measures to maintain long-term social relationships. While the patient is still manic, the more limited agenda can put the patient's unimpaired faculties, such as memory and perception, to use. The patient who says, "You don't know what I've been through," can be asked to prepare a chronology of his past admissions and a problem list for the next therapy session. The patient who starts giving away all her money can be told, "You are managing a lot of projects, but I'd be interested in seeing a written financial plan." Each therapeutic tactic should be seen as a reality-enhancing countermove to the manic person's reality-denying defenses.

You must remain aware that the experience of mania and hypomania may provide considerable direct pleasure for the patient. This enjoyment can reinforce denial and interfere with the patient's compliance with medication and overall treatment. The issue has to be addressed whenever it becomes a major stumbling block to treatment. Your acknowledgment of the pleasure experienced by the patient may be a useful preliminary to any of the appropriate supportive techniques discussed in this chapter.

You should also remember that manic patients suffer from both thought and mood abnormalities. They are often totally irrational and cannot be argued out of their grandiosity. However, it is often possible to select some aspects of manic behaviors that are defensive (as opposed to biologically fueled) and interpret them to the patient. In addition, there has been increasing recognition of the occurrence of mixed manic states that consist of rapid alternations or simultaneous expressions of depressed and elevated moods (Himmelhoch and Garfinkel 1986). Such patients represent a more seriously ill group, but they are often better able to discuss the depressed aspects of their moods with therapists and to ask for help.

A summary agenda for treatment of the acutely manic patient is presented in Table 7–5. When an agenda such as this is put into operation, the restraining care established early will be remembered by the patient later when a more formalized therapy is useful.

The Manic Patient in Remission

Manic patients in remission may be as typical as anyone else and benefit from various forms of psychotherapies in addition to maintenance medications. However, they are especially suited for supportive psychotherapy, because bipolar illness is predominantly psychophysiologically caused, and it is often difficult to use therapies whose core concepts are psychological or social.

Education about the illness is one of the first items on the agenda. A useful start is the NIMH resource "Bipolar Disorder" (National Institute of Mental Health 2018).

A principal goal of therapy is obviously to prevent mood disturbances, but also specifically to arm the patient against the recurrence of mania or depression. By "arming" we mean giving them "weapons" to fight the recurrence of mood episodes. Knowledge about the disease is probably a weapon of sorts, but there are more active things patients can do on a daily basis to make them feel they have some control over the illness. Patients who are well enough to implement the techniques of IPSRT, for example, can learn to stabilize their social rhythms, starting with sleep and then behavioral patterns. All of these techniques involve the use of mood-monitoring charts or applications. Therefore, in our introduction to therapy for well patients, we begin with an introduction of social rhythms and provide a mood-monitoring chart. Many such charts are available from the relevant treatment manuals and internet sites. One

Table 7–5. Agenda for treatment of the acutely manic patient

Establish yourself as firm, caring, and supportively restraining.

Do not buy into the manic person's point of view.

Develop a consistent therapeutic and staff approach that counteracts the manic patient's tactics, utilizing the patient's own beliefs about self.

Use many frequent and short interventions when they work.

Ask for feedback from the patient to see if your interventions are remembered and accepted.

Do not continue talking when you realize that there is no more therapeutic benefit to be had in that particular psychotherapy session.

Maximize understanding of and compliance with treatment.

Set limits within therapy (including avoidance of fruitless interactions so as to reinforce fruitful ones).

While setting limits, do not take risks or "be a hero" by continuing sessions when there is ample evidence of violence risk.

Set protective limits outside therapy (including interactions with staff, family, and strangers).

Work closely with family to develop realistic options for them.

that we recommend is the NIMH Life Chart (National Institute of Mental Health 2019).

Addressing Comorbid Illnesses and Personality Issues

It is general knowledge that patients with bipolar illness may have other major mental illnesses, so it has to be routine to diagnose these comorbidities. One finding worth mentioning here, however, is that about half of bipolar patients report a history of impairing panic symptomatology (Frank et al. 2002).

MacVane et al. (1978) showed no significant differences between a group of 35 lithium-stabilized manic patients and a like number of control subjects. However, we do believe, as do most therapists, that many previously manic patients have inter-episodic personality traits, usually narcissistic in nature, that may be seen as reasonable adjustments to their illness. Frank (2007, p. 61) notes that it is difficult to diagnose personality disorders in persons who have had manic episodes. They may appear borderline, antisocial, narcissistic, or dramatic, but it may not be known whether they really have one disorder or two separate comorbid disorders.

In MacVane et al.'s study, a frequent finding in bipolar patients could not be addressed—namely, denial of the possibility of recurrence—because the control subjects in the study had no illness to deny. For example, a patient who remembers giving away his life savings or assaulting his spouse is likely, even when well, to construct some measure of justification for his actions. Such problems may reflect residues of chronic mania, partially treated mania, hypomania, or neurotic elations.

Regardless of etiology, the therapist should address these issues, as in the following example.

Case Vignette

A 37-year-old woman with three previous hospitalizations for mania and one for depression was anxious to discuss her writings and research with the therapist. The therapist learned that the patient was receiving disability payments as well as $300 a month from her parents and $500 a month from her former husband. Her plan was to become a historian, but so far, at the rate of one course per semester, she had completed only half the required credits for a degree. The patient adamantly defended her progress.

The therapist could have confronted this behavior through interpretive work, but he decided to agree at first with the patient's defenses. He reviewed her life and pointed out that she was undeniably talented and deserved recognition. However, he pointed out that her current plans were not working. Her progress was too slow, and she was depriving herself of social companionship by spending all her time alone. What she needed was better career planning to make use of her abilities. He convinced her to attend a career-planning seminar, at which she made new friends and developed a wider range of social activities. Eventually, she was able to accept a reduction of payments from outside sources and live more independently.

The outpatient agenda, for this or any other previously manic patient, will continue to focus on protective measures for recurrence of mania (or depression).

Patients with bipolar illness are usually interested in understanding their disease and its pharmacological maintenance. If so, they should contact their local and national support groups and obtain detailed information about their illness. Their fear of relapse and of the destructive loss it brings needs to be discussed. Because elevation of mood is associated with noncompliance, the patient needs to learn to associate elevation of mood with that loss and turn to the therapist or medicator for protection. In regard to adherence (also discussed in Chapter 16), you should not be misled by how well the patient seems to be doing. Often, the only pathology evident may be the denial of illness itself and hence the resulting nonadherence.

Although many previous psychodynamic approaches interpreted mania as a defense against depression or the expression of a wish to return to an omnipotent childhood state, some studies have emphasized that there are a substantial number of therapeutic issues deriving from the disease itself. Kahn (1990) emphasizes several:

- Interruption (by the illness) of developmental tasks, such as forming extrafamilial relationships and career progression
- Discrimination of normal from abnormal moods and the tendency to fear strong emotions
- Demoralization from fears of recurrence
- Guilt at destructive efforts
- Concern about genetic transmission
- Losses due to the treatment itself (e.g., symbolic loss of self-esteem and the use of treatment as an excuse for unrelated failures)

You can provide education, guidance, and reassurance in most of these areas. Perhaps the most difficult task for you, as it is for your patient, is to remain vigilant to changes in mood that might signify relapse without clamping down or overreacting to the daily excitements and depressions of normal life. In this regard, the therapist who works in a clinic setting will often be approached by other workers involved in the patient's care with "warnings" that the patient is getting worse and needs medication. Even extensive experience does not always allow one to discriminate between false and genuine alarms—but it helps.

Key Points

- Many types of therapy are available to treat patients with mood disorders. These include supportive, psychodynamic, interpersonal, and cognitive behavioral.

- Using patient characteristics and life circumstances, you can select patients with mood disorders who are best suited for supportive psychotherapy.

- Somatic complaints must be addressed directly and not approached merely as psychological defenses. Such complaints should be taken seriously; their discussion can be useful as a displacement from more painful psychological issues.

- The primary techniques and emphases in treating patients in depressed states with supportive psychotherapy are giving reassurance, facilitating medication, addressing guilt, managing dependency, addressing loss, noticing improvement, and working with the family.

- When working with chronically depressed patients, some may need cognitive restructuring or long term psychodynamic therapy, but others will benefit from improvement of self esteem and learning optimism from their therapist.

- Management of acute manic states involves recognition of the behaviors seen in manic patients and countering them therapeutically.

- Educational interventions are important for the manic patient in remission. This includes knowledge about their illness and control of their social rhythms such as sleeping and behavioral patterns.

- It is important to address comorbid illnesses and personality issues.

References

Akiskal HS: Dysthymic disorder: psychopathology of proposed chronic depressive subtypes. Am J Psychiatry 140(1):11–20, 1983 6336637

American Psychiatric Association: Diagnostic and Statistical Manual of Mental Disorders, 5th Edition. Arlington, VA, American Psychiatric Association, 2013

Barker P: Using Metaphors in Psychotherapy. New York, Brunner/Mazel, 1985

Basco MR, Rush AJ: Cognitive-Behavioral Therapy for Bipolar Disorder, 2nd Edition. New York, Guilford, 2007

Cox GR, Callahan P, Churchill R, et al: Psychological therapies versus antidepressant medication, alone and in combination for depression in children and adolescents. Cochrane Database Syst Rev (11):CD008324, 2014 25433518

Cuijpers P, van Straten A, Andersson G, et al: Psychotherapy for depression in adults: a meta-analysis of comparative outcome studies. J Consult Clin Psychol 76(6):909–922, 2008 19045960

Davenport YB, Ebert MH, Adland ML, et al: Couples group therapy as an adjunct to lithium maintenance of the manic patient. Am J Orthopsychiatry 47(3):495–502, 1977 196507

Dil L, Dekker J, Van R, et al: A short-term psychodynamic supportive psychotherapy for adolescents with depressive disorders: a new approach. J Infant Child Adolesc Psychother 15(2):84–94, 2016

Driessen E, Cuijpers P, de Maat SC, et al: The efficacy of short-term psychodynamic psychotherapy for depression: a meta-analysis. Clin Psychol Rev 30(1):25–36, 2010 19766369

Fava GA, Kellner R: Prodromal symptoms in affective disorders. Am J Psychiatry 148(7):823–830, 1991 2053620

Frank E: Treating Bipolar Disorder: A Clinician's Guide to Interpersonal and Social Rhythm Therapy. New York, Guilford, 2007

Frank E, Cyranowski JM, Rucci P, et al: Clinical significance of lifetime panic spectrum symptoms in the treatment of patients with bipolar I disorder. Arch Gen Psychiatry 59(10):905–911, 2002 12365877

Gunderson JG: Management of manic states: the problem of fire setting. Psychiatry 37(2):137–146, 1974 4828976

Hersen M, Bellack AS, Himmelhoch JM, et al: Effects of social skills training, amitriptyline, and psychotherapy in unipolar depressed women. Behav Ther 15:21–40, 1984

Himmelhoch JM, Garfinkel ME: Sources of lithium resistance in mixed mania. Psychopharmacol Bull 22(3):613–620, 1986 3797567

Hirschfeld RMA, Goodwin FK: Mood disorders, in The American Psychiatric Press Textbook of Psychiatry. Edited by Talbott JA, Hales RE, Yudofsky SC. Washington, DC, American Psychiatric Press, 1988, pp 403–441

Hollon TH: A rationale for supportive psychotherapy of depressed patients. Am J Psychother 16:655–664, 1962 13961369

Ijaz S, Davies P, Williams CJ, et al: Psychological therapies for treatment-resistant depression in adults. Cochrane Database Syst Rev 5(5):CD010558, 2018 29761488

Jacobs N, Reupert A: The effectiveness of supportive counselling, based on Rogerian principles: a systematic review of recent international and Australian research. Melbourne, PACFA, 2014. Available at: https://www.pacfa.org.au/wp-content/uploads/2012/10/PACFA-Supportive-Counselling-literature-review-May-2014-Final.pdf. Accessed February 20, 2019.

Janowsky DS, Leff M, Epstein RS: Playing the manic game: interpersonal maneuvers of the acutely manic patient. Arch Gen Psychiatry 22(3):252–261, 1970 5413274

Jarrett RA, Rush AJ: Psychotherapeutic approaches for depression (Chapter 65), in Psychiatry, Revised Edition, Vol 1. Edited by Michels R, Cavenar JO Jr, Cooper AM, et al (eds). Philadelphia, PA, JB Lippincott, 1987

Kahn D: The psychotherapy of mania. Psychiatr Clin North Am 13(2):229–240, 1990 2191279

Karasu TB: Toward a clinical model of psychotherapy for depression, I: systematic comparison of three psychotherapies. Am J Psychiatry 147(2):133–147, 1990a 2405718

Karasu TB: Toward a clinical model of psychotherapy for depression, II: an integrative and selective treatment approach. Am J Psychiatry 147(3):269–278, 1990b 2309942

Klerman GL: Treatment of recurrent unipolar major depressive disorder: commentary on the Pittsburgh Study. Arch Gen Psychiatry 47(12):1158–1162, 1990 2244800

Klerman GL, Weissman MM, Rousanville BJ, et al: Interpersonal Psychotherapy of Depression. New York, Basic Books, 1984

Kocsis JH, Frances AJ: A critical discussion of DSM-III dysthymic disorder. Am J Psychiatry 144(12):1534–1542, 1987 3318511

Lewinsohn PM, Sullivan JM, Grosscup SJ: Changing reinforcing events: an approach to the treatment of depression. Psychotherapy: Theory, Research, and Practice 17:322–334, 1980

Lewinsohn PM, Steinmetz JL, Larson DW, et al: Depression-related cognitions: antecedent or consequence? J Abnorm Psychol 90(3):213–219, 1981 7288016

Lynch D, Laws KR, McKenna PJ: Cognitive behavioural therapy for major psychiatric disorder: does it really work? A meta-analytical review of well-controlled trials. Psychol Med 40(1):9–24, 2010 19476688

MacVane JR, Lange JD, Brown WA, et al: Psychological functioning of bipolar manic-depressives in remission. Arch Gen Psychiatry 35(11):1351–1354, 1978 708196

Meyer TD, Hautzinger M: Cognitive behaviour therapy and supportive therapy for bipolar disorders: relapse rates for treatment period and 2-year follow-up. Psychol Med 42(7):1429–1439, 2012 22099722

National Institute of Mental Health: Bipolar disorder. NIH Publ No QF 18-3679. National Institutes of Health, 2018. Available at: https://infocenter.nimh.nih.gov/pubstatic/QF%2018-3679/QF%2018-3679.pdf. Accessed February 20, 2019.

National Institute of Mental Health: Life chart. Stable Resource Toolkit, 2019. Available at: http://www.cqaimh.org/pdf/tool_edu_moodchart.pdf. Accessed February 20, 2019.

Pedersen T: CBT, supportive therapy equally effective for bipolar. August 8, 2018. Available at: https://Psychcentral.com/news/2012/07/08/cbt-supportive-therapy-equally-effective-for-bipolar/41324.html. Accessed February 20, 2019.

Perry S: Combining antidepressants and psychotherapy: rationale and strategies. J Clin Psychiatry 51(suppl):16–20, 1990 2403999

Rehm LP: Self-management therapy for depression. Adv Behav Res Ther 6(2):83–98, 1984

Rousanville BJ, Chevron ES, Weissman MM: Specification of techniques in interpersonal psychotherapy, in Psychotherapy Research: Where Are We and Where Should We Go? Proceedings of the 73rd Annual Meeting of the American Psychopathological Association, New York City, March 3–5, 1983. Edited by Williams JBW, Spitzer RL. New York, Guilford, 1984, pp 160–172

Scaccia A: Can depression cause memory loss? Healthline, July 5, 2016. Available at: https://www.healthline.com/health/depression/depression-and-memory-loss. Accessed February 20, 2019.

Schuldt W: Behavioral attraction. Therapist Aid, 2019. Available at: https://www.therapistaid.com/therapy-worksheet/behavioral-activation. Accessed February 20, 2019.

Sederer LI: Depression, in Inpatient Psychiatry: Diagnosis and Treatment, 2nd Edition. Edited by Sederer LI. Baltimore, MD, Williams & Wilkins, 1986, pp 3–35

Seligman MEP: Authentic Happiness: Using the New Positive Psychology to Realize Your Potential for Lasting Fulfillment. New York, Free Press, 2002

Sotsky SM, Glass DR, Shea MT, et al: Patient predictors of response to psychotherapy and pharmacotherapy: findings in the NIMH Treatment of Depression Collaborative Research Program. Am J Psychiatry 148(8):997–1008, 1991 1853989

Tull M: 8 tips for using behavioral activation for treating depression. December 3, 2018. Available at: https://www.verywellmind.com/increasing-the-effectiveness-of-behavioral-activation-2797597. Accessed January 31, 2019.

University of Hertfordshire: Cognitive therapy is of no value in schizophrenia, analysis of studies suggests. ScienceDaily, June 26, 2009

8

Anxiety Disorders and Related Disorders

Victor Chavira, Ph.D.

Anxiety disorders make up the most common type of mental illness in the United States, affecting approximately 10% of the U.S. population in any given 12-month period and more than 30% over the life span (Bandelow and Michaelis 2015). These disorders not only cause significant distress and functional impairments but also play a role in the manifestation of other mental disorders such as depression (Cummings et al. 2014) and other public health problems, including alcohol and drug use (Kaplow et al. 2001; Smith and Book 2008). Before we discuss treatment of anxiety disorders, it is useful to frame anxiety in a broader context. As we noted in the first edition, the reduction of anxiety is, except under truly extraordinary circumstances, always indicated.

It is self-evident that experiencing too much anxiety overwhelms us; it can be extremely debilitating, preventing us from doing all sorts of necessary, healthy, and

---

Dr. Chavira is a psychologist in private practice.

Table 8–1.   Therapeutic strategies for anxiety disorders

Ascertaining the patient's level of anxiety

Conveying empathy and interest and understanding

Framing: naming the problem, teaching, reframing

Universalizing

Conveying realistic optimism

Building skills

Identifying and reinforcing strengths and available resources

Imparting praise

Medication: encouraging collaborative exploration and patient decision making

exciting things. However, there is also such a thing as too little anxiety, and this also is not healthy. In his seminal book on the psychology of optimal experience, Csikszentmihalyi (1990) emphasizes an optimal balance between the challenge of any given task and the individual's ability to meet that challenge. In this framework, anxiety is the result of the challenge (or perceived threat of the challenge) being significantly greater than that person's ability (or self-perceived ability) to meet that challenge. Conversely, boredom is the result of the challenge posed by the task being significantly lower than the person's ability to meet the task. In this chapter we illustrate how supportive therapy helps the patient achieve a healthy level of anxiety not by avoiding the sources of the anxiety but by helping him to deal with them head-on, through the use of effective coping skills. First, we outline the general supportive therapy principles and techniques that are useful across the full spectrum of anxiety disorders (see Table 8–1); the effective use of these principles and techniques establishes the foundation for more specific interventions in the treatment of each of the various anxiety disorders. Table 8–2 summarizes the use of supportive therapy for anxiety in general and for specific anxiety disorders.

General Principles and Techniques

Ascertaining the Patient's Level of Anxiety

It may seem intuitively obvious, but it is worth emphasizing that very early in the first therapy session, you should gauge the amount of anxiety the patient is

Table 8–2. Therapeutic techniques for specific disorders

Disorder	Specific techniques
Generalized anxiety disorder	Relaxation training
	Controlled breathing
	Progressive muscle relaxation
	Cognitive restructuring
	Encouragement of exposure
	Physical exercise
	Sleep hygiene
Specific phobias	Discussion and rating of fears
	Encouragement of exposure
Panic disorder	Medical evaluation
	Reduction of caffeine and other stimulants
	Medication (antidepressants)
	Encouragement of exposure
	Family involvement, family therapy
	Treatment of associated disorders
Obsessive-compulsive disorders[a]	Validation of feelings
	Exposure and response prevention
	Medication (antidepressants)

[a]Obsessive-compulsive disorder is not categorized as an anxiety disorder in DSM-5, but we included it in this chapter as explained in the main text.

experiencing. At one extreme is the example of the patient who does not exhibit immediate symptoms, other than perhaps some nervousness about meeting you for the first time and concern about getting the appropriate treatment for her condition. The patient walks into the room confidently and speaks appropriately, making regular eye contact and engaging easily and pleasantly in conversation. Then she tells you she is doing "fine," except for the fact that she won't get on a plane because of her extreme fear. She clarifies that this has never been a cause of major problems in her life, but now she has to travel for her job and she is embarrassed to let anyone know about her nervousness and fear. At the other extreme is the case of a patient with very severe anxiety that is evident within seconds of his arrival in the therapy office. In the waiting room he alternates between sitting and pacing back and forth, constantly rubbing his hands together and looking at the clock every couple of minutes; he hesitates before entering your therapy room, stutters as he speaks, says he cannot shake your hand because he is afraid of getting germs, does not make eye contact, appears very distracted, then begins to hyperventilate as he complains about his heart starting to beat very rapidly and says he thinks he is going to have a heart attack. There are both important differences and similarities in the approaches that are most effective for each of these patients.

Conveying Empathy, Interest, and Understanding

Your interactions should express empathy and a sincere sense of interest and appreciation for the patient and her situation. Reflective listening and aptly timed (albeit simple) empathic statements such as "The thought of people judging you if you tell them about your fears makes you feel even more anxious" or an acknowledgement like "I hear you telling me it was very difficult for you to come here today" convey that you understand the patient's experience and can immediately help reduce anxiety.

Framing: Naming the Problem, Teaching, Reframing

Within your first session it is very helpful to identify and label the patient's anxiety symptom(s) and/or disorder. The process of briefly educating the patient, providing a diagnosis and a pithy explanation using nontechnical jargon, is inherently therapeutic. This not only acknowledges an accurate understanding of the patient's presenting problem but also helps establish the appropriate framework for therapy, creation of the treatment plan, and use of more specific interventions, whether in the same session or later on. For example, in the case of a patient who is worried that she has "lost control" and is fearful of having another panic attack soon, framing her symptoms in terms of activation of the sympathetic nervous system (fight-or-flight response) sets the stage for implementing relaxation exercises that invoke the parasympathetic nervous system and help the patient gain a sense of control. Similarly, framing the disorder in terms of a (maladaptive) learned way of coping (in contrast to the patient's view that "this is just the way I was born") helps instill the message of improvement through learning and utilizing new coping skills.

Yet another example is that of a patient who declines to consider psychotropic medication because "that's for crazy people and I'm not crazy." Directly educating the patient about the biochemical basis of the disorder not only may help reframe the condition and improve his motivation to consider medication but also is likely to help modify his stigmatized view of mental illness. A less direct and more collaborative reframing technique involves suggesting and critiquing alternative perspectives. For example, you may encourage the patient to think about (other) medical conditions that involve "chemical imbalances," such as juvenile diabetes, in which necessary chemicals (i.e., insulin) are not automatically produced or sustained by the body and medication is necessary to provide those chemicals and create the right balance.

Universalizing

Early in treatment you may want to use the supportive technique of universalizing to help patients realize they are not alone in experiencing anxiety disorder and its many complications and manifestations. Although anxiety disorders and symptoms may be relatively common, the patient is not necessarily aware of this (and it is a good idea not to assume otherwise, even in the age of the internet and social media). And this may contribute to feelings of shame and of not being understood by others. You can address this directly by informing the patient about the prevalence of the disorder and of the symptoms she is experiencing. However, keep in mind that not all patients may benefit from this technique and that for a few it may be counterproductive. The extent to which the patient responds favorably depends not only on whether she feels alone or alienated and on the severity and prevalence of her symptoms, but also on her level of psychological defenses. While many patients may find relief and comfort in your conveying to them that they are not alone, others, such as people with underlying personality disorders, may perceive this as your minimizing or devaluing the severity or uniqueness of their condition.

Conveying Realistic Optimism

As you conceptualize your initial treatment approach, you convey this to the patient in a manner that is both optimistic and realistic. Also consider a process that moves from general to more specific statements, consistent with where you are in your conceptualization. For instance, in the first session you can make statements like "Fortunately, most phobias are very treatable," "There are very effective treatments for anxiety," or "Most people find that their anxiety symptoms have decreased or resolved as the result of treatment." You may also consider providing information about the specific type of therapy and techniques that will be utilized (e.g., relaxation skills training, problem solving, cognitive-behavioral therapy [CBT]). Of course, it is usually not a good idea to make more specific pronouncements or estimations within the first session or two, as you are not likely to have sufficient information about the patient and his condition.

Building Skills

A core function of supportive therapy is that of helping the patient develop and implement the skills necessary to decrease or prevent anxiety symptoms so that daily functioning is no longer impaired. Among the most essential skills for people with anxiety are open expression (verbalization) of feelings, self-monitoring, relaxation/calming techniques, effective problem solving, organization, time management, physical exercise, and sleep hygiene.

Identifying and Reinforcing Strengths and Available Resources

Supportive therapy at its core is a strength-based approach. Early in the course of treatment you should assess the patient's "internal and external" strengths (e.g., positive attributes, skills, abilities, areas where she is functioning well). During this phase you also help the patient identify and organize external sources of support, such as family, friends, broader social networks, and more formal systems, such as community resources and faith-based affiliations. In today's age of internet and social media, it is advisable to take advantage of the available resources and tools, such as educational media, online support groups and directories, and interactive therapeutic/educational platforms.

Imparting Praise

We strongly encourage the use of praise. In the context of supportive therapy, it is most effective to use praise not only as a way of reinforcing the patient's adaptive coping skills but also as a way of helping the patient develop his own effective use of self-praise, based on his accurate appraisals of the challenges he faces and the steps he is taking to effectively face these challenges. In order for praise to be effective, it must be accurate (empirically based), client centered (praising the patient's behavior as it relates to his own values or goals, and not those of the therapist), and relevant and meaningful (the same behavior may demonstrate a major breakthrough or accomplishment for one patient but not for another); should focus on process/effort rather than ability; and should be communicated in a manner that is sincere (Mueller and Dweck 1998; Willingham 2005–2006).

Medication: Encouraging Collaborative Exploration and Patient Decision Making

Combining psychotherapy with medication is often more effective than psychotherapy alone (Bandelow et al. 2007). However, this is not always the case, and there are many factors to consider, including not only the type and severity of anxiety but also the patient's attitudes about (and prior experience with) medication. An essential first step in combining medication with supportive therapy is to ensure full patient participation in the decision-making process. For a variety of reasons, the patient may not initially be willing to consider taking medication, notwithstanding the demonstrated efficacy. While you are educating the patient about the benefits and risks of medication, it is usually most appropriate to maintain a neutral stance that is accepting of the patient's decision.

Specific Disorders

In this section we describe more specific approaches to the various types of disorders, These approaches are meant to be incorporated with the more general supportive therapy techniques outlined in Part I. The common features of all anxiety-related disorders are prominent symptoms of distress—for example, arousal, nervousness, fear, and discomfort—and avoidant behaviors that the patient uses as a primary way of coping with these symptoms. It is important to note that although obsessive-compulsive disorder (OCD) is no longer characterized as an anxiety disorder in DSM-5 (American Psychiatric Association 2013), we have included it in this chapter. The primary reason is that anxious states—and more specifically, avoidance or other maladaptive anxiety-reducing behaviors—are important characteristics of the disorder and are the focus of treatment.

Generalized Anxiety Disorder

Generalized anxiety disorder (GAD) is characterized by excessive worry and also often includes symptoms of restlessness, poor concentration, sleep difficulties, irritability, and somatic complaints, including muscle tension or pain and fatigue. Perhaps because of the latter symptoms, GAD is among the most common mental health disorders identified in primary care visits (Davidson et al. 2010; Kroenke et al. 2007). It is also highly correlated with other anxiety disorders (e.g., panic disorder), other mental health disorders (especially depression), and other conditions such as endocrine disorders, medication side effects, and substance withdrawal symptoms (Kavan et al. 2009). Therefore, you should always rule out the possibility that any of these may coexist with or mimic the presence of GAD. As with all anxiety disorders, it is important to assess and reduce the amount of caffeine, nicotine, and other stimulants the patient may be using.

Research over the past 15 years suggests that GAD is a complex disorder that involves physiological, cognitive, behavioral, and interpersonal domains, and there is evidence that the most effective treatment approaches address all of these domains (Crits-Christoph et al. 2004; Gould et al. 2004). In addition to experiencing distressing levels of arousal, people with GAD tend to have difficulty understanding and tolerating negative emotions, use worry as an avoidance-based coping strategy, have distorted perceptions and beliefs about problems, use ineffective problem-solving skills, and often lack knowledge or skills, such as those related to self-monitoring, organization, time management, and sleep hygiene (Craske 2018; Heimberg et al. 2004; Stein and Sareen 2015). Below we describe how supportive therapy techniques can be applied and integrated with other interventions to help the patient overcome these difficulties.

One of the most effective and fastest ways of treating the arousal and somatic symptoms of GAD is through relaxation training. In everyday practice, relaxation techniques are often used very early in the course of treatment and then incorporated with other interventions, including education, CBT, and medication. Consider the example of a patient who upon attending her very first therapy session tells you she is feeling extremely nervous, appears restless and unable to concentrate, and complains of general body aches and pains.

After responding with empathic statements and educating her about the symptoms and rationale for your approach, you introduce and practice in the session the relaxation technique. Almost immediately, the patient begins to experience a sense of calm. She may be pleasantly surprised and respond with remarks such as "This works!" or "I feel much better." This is a very powerful intervention that not only decreases the feeling of distress but also begins to help instill in the patient a sense of self-efficacy. Furthermore, practicing the relaxation exercise in vivo in the session provides you with the opportunity to observe the patient's response directly, rather than rely on the patient's account. You can then share your observations with the patient, gently recommend any adjustments as appropriate, and instruct her to practice the technique in her natural environments (e.g., home, work, school), in response to potential triggers of anxiety.

Two common relaxation techniques are controlled breathing (sometimes also referred to as "deep or rhythmic breathing") and progressive muscle relaxation. *Controlled breathing* is based on the premise that the anxious patient is (unknowingly) experiencing an activated autonomic system response, which includes hyperventilation (more than about 15 breaths per minute), and the goal is to counter this response by introducing optimal breathing at a reduced rate (of about 6–10 breaths per minute). There are several well-established variations on this technique, such as the following: The patient places one hand on his stomach, slightly above his belly button; then breathes in slowly through his nose (e.g., to a count of about 4 seconds) as he observes his stomach expanding; then holds his breath briefly (about 2 seconds); then exhales through his mouth; and finally pauses for about 2 seconds before taking the next breath. The patient repeats this process about six to eight times to the point at which he feels sufficiently calm. *Progressive muscle relaxation* is a technique utilized to increase the patient's awareness of tension throughout his body and to reduce such tension. It involves a two-step process whereby the patient alternately tenses and relaxes isolated muscle groups in a systematic manner under your specific direction. The effectiveness of this technique is also well documented, and there are several effective variations of this approach (see Mackereth and Tomlinson 2010).

It is very useful to incorporate CBT interventions to address the cognitive and behavioral components of GAD. Stated briefly, the rationale for CBT is based on evidence that people with GAD engage in a consistent pattern of cognitive distortions and avoidance behaviors. Specifically, they have difficulty tolerating negative emotions, overly attend to potentially threatening stimuli, negatively interpret ambiguous situations, overestimate the impact of negative events ("catastrophize"), and avoid perceived anxiety-provoking situations through ritualistic thinking and behaviors such as worry, rumination, excessive checking, and procrastination (Craske 2018; Newman et al. 2013). The therapist helps the patient develop these new thinking and coping skills by implementing an integrated set of CBT techniques—namely, self-monitoring, cognitive restructuring, and exposure exercises. Through self-monitoring the patient learns to gather accurate and relevant information, especially the instances of anxiety (e.g., arousal, excessive worry, avoidance behaviors) and the specific thoughts associated with these instances. *Cognitive restructuring* refers to the process of helping the patient identify and modify the cognitive errors (misappraisals) that have contributed to the anxiety. This is accomplished by helping the patient examine the validity of her cognitions, through carefully examination of the evidence that supports or refutes her thoughts.

Exposure refers to the patient's direct experience with situations or activities that in the past he has avoided because they provoke anxiety. This is accomplished by having the patient develop a list of items and organizing them from the least feared (least anxiety-producing) to the most feared (most anxiety-producing). Common examples of activities patients fear include asking someone out on a date (fear of being rejected), turning in an assignment or task before checking it many times to ensure there are no errors (fear of being reprimanded or fired), arriving extremely early at appointments (for fear of being late), and trying something new (fear of uncertainty). Next you prescribe that the patient gradually engage in each of these activities. In most cases, such as when the patient is being seen one session per week, you will probably want to prescribe that he practice one activity per week.

Imagery exposure is a similar technique and is the process of helping the patient to tolerate feeling negative emotions and autonomic arousal, by exposing her to vivid anxiety-provoking images that in the past she has avoided through rumination or worry. This is accomplished by having the patient generate a hierarchy of fear images related to the areas of rumination or worry and then exposing her systematically to each of these images. When you see that the patient no longer experiences high levels of anxiety in response to the fear image, you progress to the next image on the hierarchy.

The techniques described above work together as part of an integrated CBT approach, and thus we encourage you to implement them in this manner. However, many of the CBT techniques, especially exposure exercises, could be perceived as quite grueling to the patients and thus cause them to want to drop out of treatment. Thus, we emphasize that a strong therapeutic alliance, based on supportive therapy, is a necessary precursor to CBT interventions.

Patients with anxiety, particularly those with GAD, stand to benefit from therapy that specifically targets improving sleep hygiene. Research suggests that poor sleep not only is a common symptom of GAD (Comer et al. 2012) but also may exacerbate it, along with other disorders such as depression (Goldstein et al. 2013; Morin and Ware 1996). Patients should be encouraged and taught to practice good sleep habits. This includes setting aside sufficient time for sleep, establishing a daily routine prior to sleep, having consistent sleep and wake times, using the bed only for sleep or sexual activity (e.g., refraining from using the bed for television, internet, texting, reading), and refraining from consuming caffeine late in the day.

Finally, we strongly encourage that you consider prescribing a regimen of regular physical exercise to your patients with GAD. The many benefits of exercise in terms of both physical and mental health are well documented; this includes an increasing body of literature demonstrating anxiolytic effects (Knapen and Vancampfort 2013; Strickland and Smith 2014; Wipfli et al. 2008). The mechanisms through which physical exercise can reduce anxiety are not clear, but it is hypothesized that they involve both physical fitness (and related physiological and biochemical factors) and psychological improvements, such as increased self-esteem, distraction from rumination and worry, and decreased negative appraisals (Knapen and Vancampfort 2013).

Specific Phobias

Specific phobias (also called "simple phobias") are the most common type of anxiety disorder, affecting up to 10% of the population in any given 12-month period (Bandelow and Michaelis 2015). A phobia is a severe and persistent fear of a very specific object or situation; exposure or anticipation of exposure to the feared stimulus results in an anxiety response that usually takes the form of a panic attack in adults or tantrums, crying, and clingy behavior in children. Because of this, the patient tends to avoid the phobic situation. He may realize that the fear is irrational and the avoidant behavior is excessive. However, he is not likely to seek treatment until the symptoms are so frequent or severe that they have a major negative impact in his daily life. A common scenario where the patient feels compelled to attend therapy is where outside circumstances (e.g., job requirements) make contact with the feared stimulus unavoidable.

Usually the most effective core treatment consists of exposure to the stimulus, through the systematic method commonly known as *exposure and response prevention* (ERP), which is a subtype of CBT. In ERP, the patient learns to change maladaptive thoughts and behaviors that have previously served to reinforce the phobia. Being in the presence of the phobic stimulus without the usual avoidance is the most active ingredient of the treatment. However, we consider supportive techniques to be indispensable adjuncts to this treatment approach. The mere thought of "facing their fears" can be reason enough for patients to not want to return to therapy after the first session, and the research indeed suggests that many patients drop out of this kind of behavior therapy or do not engage in the prescribed between-session tasks (Strauss et al. 2015). Thus, effective treatment begins with the supportive therapist providing a safe (e.g., accepting, nonjudgmental) atmosphere in which to discuss the patient's fears and effectively practicing supportive techniques that build a strong therapeutic alliance. And in cases in which pure behavioral techniques may not be indicated or effective, you will still achieve very satisfactory results by sticking with the purely supportive approaches (Raj and Sheehan 1987).

For many patients a relatively detailed explanation of the rationale for the exposure approach may be most effective; this includes talking with the patient about the evidence that this treatment approach is highly effective. Similarly, you are encouraged to practice considerable flexibility in terms of the length of the session and the frequency and length of exposure intervals. Research suggests that sessions of prolonged exposure are more effective than those of shorter duration and that multisession treatments are generally more effective than single-session treatments (Abramowitz 1996; Podină et al. 2013). The exposure phase of treatment begins with assessing the breadth and severity of the specific phobias; this is achieved by identifying and discussing the patient's various phobias (feared objects/situations) and asking the patient to rate the amount of fear that is aroused (e.g., on a scale from 1 to 10, where 1 means very little fear/anxiety and 10 is very much). In this manner a hierarchy of the fears is created (from a stimulus that causes only minimal anxiety to one that constirutes the most feared situation). The patient is then gradually exposed to each object/situation in the hierarchy. Often the first steps involve imaginal exposure (i.e., the patient visualizes confronting the feared stimulus) and are followed by gradual in vivo exposure. After repeated exposure to a feared item results in the fear being reduced by half (e.g., from a 10 to a 5 on the patient's fear scale), the next item in hierarchy is introduced (i.e., the patient is exposed to it). The exposure exercises continue until the patient has been exposed to all the items in the hierarchy and the patient rates her level of anxiety as very low on the fear scale. Although in vivo exposure is considered optimal in the final exposure phase, there is now sophisticated technology (virtual reality) that closely approximates in vivo exposure (e.g., a flight simulator program and gear) and has demonstrated effectiveness (Opriş et al. 2012).

Panic Disorder and Agoraphobia

Panic disorder is associated with major social and health consequences, including other psychiatric disorders, substance abuse, suicide attempts, and impaired social functioning (Mendlowicz and Stein 2000; Nepon et al. 2010; Tilli et al. 2012). It is among the most common mental health disorders for which patients receive health services (Wang et al. 2005), often in primary care settings (Davies et al. 2017). Thus, when approaching the treatment of patients with panic disorder, you should bear the serious psychiatric, medical, and social consequences in mind. It is necessary to conduct a thorough assessment that includes a medical evaluation, determination of other psychiatric disorders, phenomenology and history of the panic attacks, precipitating factors or events, and factors that exacerbate or maintain the panic disorder (Dattilio and Salas-Auvert 2000). In terms of treatment, an integrated approach is likely to be most effective. This includes combining supportive psychotherapy with medication, using CBT techniques, treating associated psychiatric conditions, addressing environmental stressors, and improving family and social supports (Busch et al. 2010; Carr 2009). Thorough medical evaluation is indicated because of the many organic conditions (e.g., hyperthyroidism, hypoglycemia, caffeinism) that give rise to panic and anxiety (Raj and Sheehan 1987). The evaluation should determine the quantity of stimulants and caffeine used. Many patients are unaware of the large amounts of caffeine ingested through soft drinks, pain medications, and so forth. Reduction of caffeine, nicotine, and other stimulants may have major therapeutic effects.

Many of the relevant aspects of supportive psychotherapy to panic disorder and agoraphobia have been discussed earlier in this chapter. Empathic statements, reassurance, provision of a diagnosis or explanation of symptoms, and communication of a realistic optimism all help to restore the patient's morale and prevent further morbidity. In addition, the establishment of a therapeutic alliance allows the therapist to use persuasive powers to encourage the patient to take difficult actions (such as exposure in vivo) to overcome agoraphobic avoidance. Pharmacotherapy plays a crucial role in the treatment of panic disorders. Antidepressants and selected benzodiazepines have both demonstrated efficacy (Mitte 2005) and are especially indicated early in the course of treatment if the panic episodes are severe and/or frequent. Given that both classes of drugs are effective, selection of the best option depends on additional factors, such as side effects and the presence of other disorders (e.g., depression). In light of the side-effect profiles, treatment guidelines recommend selective serotonin reuptake inhibitors as the first choice in the treatment of panic disorder (Marchesi 2008). However, if the panic symptoms are relatively mild or mainly associated with particular situations, use of medication may not be necessary, or you may wait to recommend medication until other aspects of supportive psychotherapy have been tried.

Through supportive psychotherapy, medication, and behavioral techniques, the patient will likely experience a significant decrease in spontaneous panic, with an attendant rise in morale and self-esteem. However, he may still experience significant anticipatory anxiety and severe restrictions and avoidance in his life. Thus, you must guide the patient to expose himself to the feared situations. The strategy for encouraging exposure must be individualized for each patient. For some patients, an intellectual explanation of the process may be helpful, outlining the goal of greater exposure with attendant extinction of the panic response. For others, a very detailed, stepwise progression, with support available at critical moments, may be indicated. For example, a patient with severe panic symptoms with agoraphobia will be given gradual goals, the first of which is to stay outside or go to a feared location for a total of 5 minutes only. The date and time of the excursion are decided in advance, and the patient is instructed to call the therapist, who is available and awaiting the telephone call. After the patient has mastered 5 minutes in the feared situation, the exposure technique will follow gradually increasing times of exposure or more complex goals, until the panic response has been extinguished.

Supportive assistance by family members or other loved ones, such as accompanying the patient to the feared location, may be very helpful and should be encouraged as a type of co-therapist approach, which can be gradually modified and withdrawn. The patient's natural support system (e.g., friends, relatives) can play an essential role in other ways—for example, by encouraging the desired (exposure) behavior and not reinforcing the avoidance behavior. A few patients will require the presence of the therapist. In these cases, it appears that prolonged sessions of exposure with the therapist present are more beneficial than multiple short sessions of exposure. Many patients benefit greatly from referral to support groups or self-help groups for people with panic symptoms, agoraphobia, or simple phobia. These groups, which are readily available in many urban locations, are often led by professionals who have recovered from these disorders and serve to restore self-esteem as well as provide practical coping techniques and emotional support. In addition, you can consider treating patients with panic disorders and/or agoraphobia with combined group and individual psychotherapy. In this instance, much individual preparation is often required, because the anticipation of the first group session can evoke intense panic sensations. By the same token, the patient's experience of the first group session is never as bad as feared, and some extinguishing of panic symptoms may occur during that session.

We emphasize that early in the treatment of the panic disorder, you should be alert to the presence of additional psychiatric disorders or sequelae. Depression is frequently found and should be fully addressed. Even after the panic symptoms have apparently resolved, the patient may display low self-esteem, excessive worry, or personality problems that can then serve as the focus of therapy. In addition, relapse can occur, especially under major stress. The patient should be made aware that relapse is possible but is usually milder and temporary and often self-limited. Termination with the patient should include discussion of "booster" sessions in the future to handle these temporary relapses.

Obsessive-Compulsive Disorder

As a reminder, although OCD is not included with the major anxiety disorders in DSM-5 (American Psychiatric Association 2013), for the purpose of this chapter we are including it because of the major role that anxiety plays. The disorder is characterized by dysfunctional patterns of obsession and/or compulsions. According to DSM-5, obsessions are recurrent and persistent thoughts, urges, or images, which in most individuals cause marked anxiety and distress. Compulsions are repetitive behaviors that the individual feels driven to perform and are aimed at preventing or reducing anxiety or distress or preventing some dreaded event or situation. Thus, compulsions are the actions the individual produces to decrease the anxious states elicited by the obsessions.

OCD remains the most difficult of the anxiety-related disorders to treat with supportive psychotherapy; the most effective approach combines CBT (including ERP, as described below) along with medication. However, supportive therapy is a very useful part of the overall treatment strategy. First, by utilizing supportive therapy techniques, you develop a strong therapeutic alliance with the patient, which increases the likelihood that she will continue to participate in therapy and follow through with your interventions and prescriptions. Similarly, some patients, particularly those with OCD of the predominantly obsessive type, may not feel "safe" talking about their very "dark and shameful thoughts," and a great source of their anxiety is that something very bad will happen if they talk about their thoughts. Thus, they have ignored or consciously suppressed their feelings. Any spontaneous expression of feelings should be reinforced, and supportive therapy techniques alone may suffice to help the patient feel safe and extinguish such fears. Furthermore, supportive therapy can be utilized to help the patient develop effective coping skills for overcoming some of the complex challenges that often accompany OCD—namely, co-occurring disorders and problems such as depression, generalized anxiety, interpersonal problems and conflicts, and self-harm tendencies.

The most empirically validated treatment approach for OCD is CBT, including ERP and cognitive restructuring. Although a detailed explanation is beyond the scope of this book, we describe the approach briefly and refer you to some of the expert literature (see, e.g., Wilhelm and Steketee 2006). The premise of this treatment is that the patient's ritualistic thoughts and behavior (obsessions and compulsions) decrease discomfort in the short term but reinforce anxiety in the long term. The goal of ERP is to reduce (ideally eliminate) anxiety symptoms by systematically exposing the patient to the situations or things that trigger her obsessions and compulsions. Over time, through this exposure, the patient begins (learns) to respond differently as the anxiety decreases and the patient no longer has the need to engage in the rituals. Consider the example of a patient who engages in compulsions such as repetitive hand washing or avoidant behaviors (e.g., refusal to touch common items such as knobs or handles, or to shake people's hands) because of his obsession (excessive, unrealistic fear) that he will become contaminated and get sick. The first step in this approach is to work with the patient to identify the specific compulsions and to organize (rank) them from least to most severe (i.e., most to least bothersome, intense, or frequent). The next step is to expose the patient to the thing or situation that triggers the compulsion (this is the exposure component). Then you help the patient refrain from engaging in the behavior (this is the prevention component).

Depending on the severity of the patient's compulsions, you initially conduct the exposure and prevention exercises for relatively brief intervals and steadily increase them over subsequent sessions. Through repeated trials of prolonged ERP, the patient learns that although her anxiety initially increases and actually peaks, it also subsides and then remains low or nonexistent. Once the patient has mastered this experience, she is ready to move on to tackle the next most difficult compulsion. Both the exposure and the response prevention components must be implemented together as one treatment approach. Thus, throughout the treatment it is essential that you emphasize the importance of refraining from the compulsive rituals and that you help the patient to accomplish this by providing her with encouragement and guidance to prevent her from engaging in the ritualistic behavior (or other "safety behaviors" that could turn into rituals). Although we encourage the use of use in vivo exposure whenever possible, imaginal exposure is also effective and should be used when in vivo exposure is not feasible. For example, it may not be possible to re-create the triggers of some compulsions in the therapy session. Or the patient may have primarily an obsessive type of OCD ("obsessions about obsessions"), such as a patient who is overwhelmed by an obsessive image of him hurting someone.

Key Points

- It is useful to view anxiety on a continuum, in which usually extremes of neither very low nor very high anxiety are considered healthy or optimal for most people.

- The major goals of supportive psychotherapy are to help the patient develop and utilize more effective strategies for thinking

230 Clinical Manual of Supportive Psychotherapy

about and coping with anxiety-producing situations and practice skills that help achieve healthy levels of anxiety.

- Although the various anxiety-related disorders have important characteristics in common, there are also significant differences that call for adjusting the specific supportive techniques to be utilized.

- Supportive psychotherapy is effective in the treatment of anxiety disorders, both in its own right and as an adjunct to other forms of treatment.

- We recommend supportive psychotherapy as a first-line approach that promotes strong patient engagement in therapy, directly reduces anxiety symptoms, and facilitates the use of other empirically validated approaches and techniques.

References

Abramowitz JS: Variants of exposure and response prevention in the treatment of obsessive-compulsive disorder: a meta-analysis. Behav Ther 27(4):583–600, 1996

American Psychiatric Association: Diagnostic and Statistical Manual of Mental Disorders, 5th Edition. Arlington, VA, American Psychiatric Association, 2013

Bandelow B, Michaelis S: Epidemiology of anxiety disorders in the 21st century. Dialogues Clin Neurosci 17(3):327–335, 2015 26487813

Bandelow B, Seidler-Brandler U, Becker A, et al: Meta-analysis of randomized controlled comparisons of psychopharmacological and psychological treatments for anxiety disorders. World J Biol Psychiatry 8(3):175–187, 2007 17654408

Busch F, Oquendo M, Sullivan G, et al: An integrated model of panic disorder. Neuropsychoanalysis 12(1):67–79, 2010

Carr A: The effectiveness of family therapy and systemic interventions for adult-focused problems. J Fam Ther 31:46–74, 2009

Comer JS, Pincus DB, Hofmann SG: Generalized anxiety disorder and the proposed associated symptoms criterion change for DSM-5 in a treatment-seeking sample of anxious youth. Depress Anxiety 29(12):994–1003, 2012 22952043

Craske M: Psychotherapy for generalized anxiety disorder in adults. UpToDate, March 1, 2018. Available at: https://www.uptodate.com/contents/psychotherapy-for-generalized-anxiety-disorder-in-adults. Accessed February 20, 2019.

Crits-Christoph P, Connolly Gibbons MB, Crits-Christoph K: Supportive-expressive psychodynamic therapy, in Generalized Anxiety Disorder: Advances in Research and Practice. Edited by Heimberg RG, Turk CL, Mennin DS. New York, Guilford, 2004, pp 293–316

Csikszentmihalyi M: Flow: The Psychology of Optimal Experience. New York, Harper & Row, 1990

Cummings CM, Caporino NE, Kendall PC: Comorbidity of anxiety and depression in children and adolescents: 20 years after. Psychol Bull 140(3):816–845, 2014 24219155

Dattilio FM, Salas-Auvert JA: Panic Disorder: Assessment and Treatment Through a Wide-Angle Lens. Phoenix, AZ, Zeig, Tucker, 2000

Davidson JR, Feltner DE, Dugar A: Management of generalized anxiety disorder in primary care: identifying the challenges and unmet needs. Prim Care Companion J Clin Psychiatry 12(2):PCC.09r00772, 2010 20694114

Davies SJ, Nash J, Nutt DJ: Management of panic disorder in primary care. Prescriber 28(1):19–26, 2017

Goldstein AN, Greer SM, Saletin JM, et al: Tired and apprehensive: anxiety amplifies the impact of sleep loss on aversive brain anticipation. J Neurosci 33(26):10607–10615, 2013 23804084

Gould RA, Safren SA, O'Neill Washington D, et al: A meta-analytic review of cognitive-behavioral treatments, in Generalized Anxiety Disorder: Advances in Research and Practice. Edited by Heimberg RG, Turk CL, Mennin DS. New York, Guilford, 2004, pp 248–264

Heimberg RG, Turk CL, Mennin DS (eds): Generalized Anxiety Disorder: Advances in Research and Practice. New York, Guilford, 2004

Kaplow JB, Curran PJ, Angold A, et al: The prospective relation between dimensions of anxiety and the initiation of adolescent alcohol use. J Clin Child Psychol 30(3):316–326, 2001 11501249

Kavan MG, Elsasser G, Barone EJ: Generalized anxiety disorder: practical assessment and management. Am Fam Physician 79(9):785–791, 2009 20141098

Knapen J, Vancampfort D: Evidence for exercise therapy in the treatment of depression and anxiety. The International Journal of Psychosocial Rehabilitation 17(2):75–87, 2013

Kroenke K, Spitzer RL, Williams JB, et al: Anxiety disorders in primary care: prevalence, impairment, comorbidity, and detection. Ann Intern Med 146(5):317–325, 2007 17339617

Mackereth P, Tomlinson L: Progressive muscle relaxation: a remarkable tool for therapists and patients, in Integrative Hypnotherapy: Complementary Approaches to Clinical Care. Edited by Cawthorn A, Mackereth P. New York, Elsevier, 2010, pp 82–96

Marchesi C: Pharmacological management of panic disorder. Neuropsychiatr Dis Treat 4(1):93–106, 2008 18728820

Mendlowicz MV, Stein MB: Quality of life in individuals with anxiety disorders. Am J Psychiatry 157(5):669–682, 2000 10784456

Mitte K: A meta-analysis of the efficacy of psycho- and pharmacotherapy in panic disorder with and without agoraphobia. J Affect Disord 88(1):27–45, 2005 16005982

Morin CM, Ware JC: Sleep and psychopathology. Appl Prev Psychol 5(4):211–224, 1996

Mueller CM, Dweck CS: Praise for intelligence can undermine children's motivation and performance. J Pers Soc Psychol 75(1):33–52, 1998 9686450

Nepon J, Belik S-L, Bolton J, et al: The relationship between anxiety disorders and suicide attempts: findings from the National Epidemiologic Survey on Alcohol and Related Conditions. Depress Anxiety 27(9):791–798, 2010 20217852

Newman MG, Llera SJ, Erickson TM, et al: Worry and generalized anxiety disorder: a review and theoretical synthesis of evidence on nature, etiology, mechanisms, and treatment. Annu Rev Clin Psychol 9:275–297, 2013 23537486

Opriş D, Pintea S, García-Palacio A, et al: Virtual reality exposure therapy in anxiety disorders: a quantitative meta-analysis. Depress Anxiety 29(2):85–93, 2012

Podină IR, Koster EH, Philippot P, et al: Optimal attentional focus during exposure in specific phobia: a meta-analysis. Clin Psychol Rev 33(8):1172–1183, 2013 24185091

Raj A, Sheehan DV: Medical evaluation of panic attacks. J Clin Psychiatry 48(8):309–313, 1987 3301823

Smith JP, Book SW: Anxiety and substance use disorders: a review. Psychiatr Times 25(10):19–23, 2008 20640182

Stein MB, Sareen J: Clinical Practice: Generalized anxiety disorder. N Engl J Med 373(21):2059–2068, 2015 26580998

Strauss C, Rosten C, Hayward M, et al: Mindfulness-based exposure and response prevention for obsessive compulsive disorder: study protocol for a pilot randomised controlled trial. Trials 16:167, 2015 25886875

Strickland JC, Smith MA: The anxiolytic effects of resistance exercise. Front Psychol 5:753, 2014 25071694

Tilli V, Suominen K, Karlsson H: Panic disorder in primary care: comorbid psychiatric disorders and their persistence. Scand J Prim Health Care 30(4):247–253, 2012 23113695

Wang PS, Lane M, Olfson M, et al: Twelve-month use of mental health services in the United States: results from the National Comorbidity Survey Replication. Arch Gen Psychiatry 62(6):629–640, 2005 15939840

Wilhelm S, Steketee G: Cognitive Therapy for Obsessive Compulsive Disorder: A Guide for Professionals. Oakland, CA, New Harbinger Publications, 2006

Willingham DT: Ask the cognitive scientist: how praise can motivate—or stifle. 2005–2006. Available at: https://www.aft.org/ae/winter2005-2006/willingham. Accessed February 20, 2019.

Wipfli BM, Rethorst CD, Landers DM: The anxiolytic effects of exercise: a meta-analysis of randomized trials and dose-response analysis. J Sport Exerc Psychol 30(4):392–410, 2008 18723899

9

Co-occurring Disorders

Previously known as "dual diagnoses," co-occurring disorders will often be an issue for you and your patients to address. *Co-occurring disorders* refers to the coexistence of both a mental health disorder and a substance use disorder or certain behavioral problems, such as gambling. Supportive psychotherapy, which is not limited to one binding theoretical framework, is similarly not wedded to any one diagnosis or not always applying the same fixed techniques for the same patient. For example, for a young man with a diagnosis of schizophrenia who smokes cannabis rather than taking his psychotropic medicines, those who work with him may not view his occasional drug use as a problem, even though it worsens his paranoia. A second example is a woman who has been diagnosed with bipolar disorder and skips her medications during a manic episode, drinks heavily, and becomes sexually promiscuous (Singer 2006).

It will not be possible to cover every behavioral issue or substance your patient may abuse or to cover every possible co-occurring disorder in this chapter. The substance-related disorders alone in DSM-5 include 10 separate classes. However, there are numerous resources available for further information.

These include texts by Cavacuiti (2011), Galanter et al. (2015), Miller et al. (2019), and Mack et al. (2010).

Supportive psychotherapy includes the art of paying full attention to all the pertinent interacting factors and of maintaining maximum flexibility to modify techniques or emphases to address the uniqueness and possible multiple diagnoses of the patient.

If the symptoms of a mental health disorder are not treated, the disorder itself will hinder the individual's ability to remain clean and sober or to abstain from behavioral problems such as gambling. Conversely, if the substance use or gambling disorder is left untreated, mental health treatment will be ineffective. The most frequent connection between substance use disorder and mental illness is the individual's attempt to alleviate his mental health symptoms that are disruptive to his everyday functioning in society by using substances.

Individuals with co-occurring disorders are among the most challenging to treat, and there is a high rate of relapse. A 2001 study comparing consumption patterns of individuals with and without schizophrenia found that the most frequently used substances were cocaine, alcohol, and cannabis (Lammertink et al. 2001). Drake and Mueser (2000) suggest that the most effective treatment programs for individuals with co-occurring disorders combine mental health and substance use disorder interventions. They conclude that the practice of using separate services for mental health and substance use disorders places the burden of integrating services on patients rather than on providers.

Many of the patients who are well suited for supportive psychotherapy will have co-occurring or multiple diagnoses. According to the Substance Abuse and Mental Health Services Administration (SAMHSA) National Survey on Drug Use and Health (Center for Behavioral Health Statistics and Quality 2015), approximately 7.9 million adults in the United States had co-occurring disorders in 2014. Additionally, SAMHSA has identified the scope of substance use disorders as follows: "In 2014, about 21.5 million Americans ages 12 and older (8.1%) were classified with a substance use disorder in the past year. Of those, 2.6 million had problems with both alcohol and drugs, 4.5 million had problems with drugs but not alcohol, and 14.4 million had problems with alcohol only."

There is undoubtedly a connection between mental health disorders and substance use disorders, as noted by the National Bureau of Economic Research: "Individuals with an existing mental illness consume roughly 38 percent of all alcohol, 44 percent of all cocaine, and 40 percent of all cigarettes. Furthermore, the people who have ever experienced mental illness consume about 69 percent of all the alcohol, 84 percent of all the cocaine, and 68 percent of all cigarettes" (National Bureau of Economic Research 2019).

Substance use must be addressed from the first session or the first knowledge of the issue; however, this should occur matter-of-factly, as part of history taking. All patients, even those not initially suspected of alcohol or drug abuse, should be asked about drinking habits, the abuse of drugs, and their family history of substance abuse. This can be done informally or in a structured manner using one of the many questionnaires concerning alcohol or drug use. In the beginning, your patients will not have to acknowledge the full extent of alcohol or drug abuse or its effects on their mental illness; merely bringing up the topic with the patient can function as a good start, to be built upon as the therapeutic alliance becomes more secure and as you directly observe more of the patient's life.

Abstinence is a long-term goal, not the prerequisite for psychotherapy. Educational elements can be added whenever appropriate. For example, whenever starting or changing a medication, you can mention the negative interactions of alcohol or illicit drugs with that medication. As these situations occur, you can also discuss the effects of an illicit drug in causing certain symptoms or contributing to insomnia or difficulties in concentration, or the role of substance use in precipitating a hospitalization. This educational approach also allows some patients to focus on these issues in an impersonal way when personal discussion would be too threatening.

As therapy progresses, your patient can develop confidence that he is not being criticized, rejected, or judged to be hopeless. An atmosphere of frank discussion of substance use will have been established. Increased trust and more open communication will ensue. Referrals to peer support groups or special treatment programs will now come more naturally, and the substance use disorder can be addressed more fully.

Once the therapeutic relationship is well established, additional opportunities for interpretations and interventions will often occur, and you may be able to modify your treatment plan to shift focus to the mental health diagnosis. Interpretations should further the course of therapy; the interpretations should not be made mainly to display your insight or expertise. Understanding where, when, and with whom the patient uses substances is also important.

An understanding of patients' substance use settings and socialization will enable you to guide those with limited social skills to find non-substance-using settings for socialization.

Confounding Effects of Substance Use on Making a Mental Health Diagnosis

The high prevalence rate of co-occurring disorders may be a result of overlapping symptoms. For example, substance use symptoms can resemble the symptoms of depression and mania. Additionally, the symptoms of alcohol and stimulant intoxication can cause symptoms of mania, and withdrawal symptoms can manifest as symptoms of dysphoria and depression. The use of stimulants such as cocaine and amphetamines can produce symptoms that are typically seen in bipolar disorders, such as euphoria, increased energy, decreased appetite, grandiosity, and paranoia. Conversely, withdrawal from stimulants, especially cocaine, can bring about symptoms of anhedonia, apathy, depressed mood, and suicidal ideation. The chronic use of substances causing central nervous system depression, such as alcohol, benzodiazepines, barbiturates, and opiates, can cause depressive symptoms such as concentration difficulties, anhedonia, and poor sleeping patterns. Withdrawal from central nervous system depressants can result in anxiety and agitation. Before you make a clear-cut diagnosis, it is best to delay this process until the individual has had a reasonable amount of time being clean and sober; doing so will give the symptoms of intoxication or withdrawal time to decrease (Quello et al. 2005). Clearly, you will need to develop an accurate understanding of co-occurring disorders to provide treatment and prevention methods. Too often, particularly when a patient has had multiple admissions for substance use disorder, medical problems can be interpreted as symptoms of intoxication or withdrawal as in the following vignette. It is imperative for you to recognize the differences.

Case Vignette

S.R., a 35-year-old man admitted to the detox unit, has had several admissions for alcohol use disorder, and is well known to the nursing staff. He presented with some symptoms of alcohol withdrawal (headache, vomiting, confusion, and slurred speech). However, his presentation was alarming to the nursing staff as he "was not himself." He was slouched over in the chair and very lethargic and had urinated on himself. His usual presentation was not one of confusion and isolating to self, and he had never been in withdrawal to the point of being unable to make it to the bathroom on his own. He was sent to the emergency room and rushed into surgery with a subdural hematoma.

Upon release from the medical center, S.R. followed up with his therapist. He revealed to his therapist he had no recollection of the injury that caused the subdural hematoma because "I was drunk out of my mind." S.R. also indicated he felt he was unable to control his use of alcohol, voiced feelings of guilt, and noted he felt "like I am just stupid to keep drinking or maybe I am just weak." S.R. reported he was often depressed and used alcohol to lift his mood. He also reported he felt the need for alcohol when socializing because of anxiety. Over the next three sessions the therapist provided S.R. with education on substance use disorders and explained to him his diagnosis of alcohol use disorder, severe (American Psychiatric Association 2013). His therapist assured him he was not "stupid," reminding S.R. he was capable of learning new tasks and worked with him on improving his self-esteem. He was referred to AA and to a long-term rehabilitation residential program.

Motivational interventions are widely used for substance use disorders and can be achieved within the framework of supportive treatment. Motivational interviewing is empathic and patient centered. Psychoeducation is based on a disease model of addiction and focuses on the psychological and physical effects of substances and the fact that substances may be used to self-medicate (Winston et al. 2012).

Addiction and Substance Abuse Terminology

You will hear frequently the terms "addiction" and "dependence." However, DSM-5 has eliminated these terms and uses the neutral terminology *substance use disorder* with modifiers ranging from *mild* to *severe* based on the presence of symptoms (American Psychiatric Association 2013). Refer to DSM-5 for the specific diagnostic criteria for the substance-related disorders.

Substance Use Disorders and the Practice of Confrontation

The role of confrontation in the treatment of substance use disorder is widely debated. For decades, the standard of treatment of substance use disorders emphasized and endorsed the use of confrontation, and it was routinely practiced in residential programs. Additionally, many residential programs prohibit the use of medications and criticize the applicability of a medical model. Despite its usefulness in primary alcoholism and primary drug abuse, this technique of confrontation has major limitations when applied to patients with additional psychiatric diagnoses, especially chronic schizophrenia and rejection-sensitive depressions and personality disorders. The use of confrontation in these cases has been found to be counterproductive and associated with poor outcomes. A seminal study by Miller et al. (1993) revealed that the more confrontational the therapist, the more an individual would abuse alcohol. Clearly, a more empathic and supportive style of therapy is required.

Alcoholics Anonymous (AA) and Narcotics Anonymous (NA) employ confrontation as a major therapeutic element. Founded in 1935, AA has long been thought of as the standard treatment for recovering alcoholics. The program is based on the 12 steps of recovery, first published in 1938 (Alcoholics Anonymous 2017). Because of AA's strong emphasis on anonymity, research to determine its success rate is impossible. Another negative of AA and NA, noted by Johnson (2010), is AA's doctrine that when there is a relapse, the individual is powerless to stop drinking. A patient who believes this tenet is likely to experience a relapse that is longer and more damaging. White and Miller (2007) report that research has failed to show any effective results with the use of confrontational methods and that for the more vulnerable individuals this practice can be harmful. They recommend that therapists instead practice in a supportive style.

Supportive Groups: Alternatives to 12-Steps

Undeniably, AA and NA have helped many individuals. However, just as there is no one medication for depression that works for everyone, there is no one peer support group that will be effective for everyone. Therefore, as a supportive psychotherapist you should be aware of groups other than AA or NA that may be more appropriate for the individual with whom you are working. There are several alternative groups that provide peer support and give individuals in recovery methods to reduce episodes of relapse. Two such groups are Women for Sobriety (https://womenforsobriety.org) and SOS (Secular Organizations for Sobriety) (www.sossobriety.org). Women for Sobriety consists of 13 acceptance programs and is supportive and does not hold to the doctrine of being powerless when one has substance use disorders (Women for Sobriety 2017). SOS does not focus on any one area of knowledge or theory of substance use disorders and encourages scientific research of substance use disorders (Secular Organizations for Sobriety 1985). As noted by Mercer (2001), participation in peer support groups is indeed a beneficial treatment for those with substance use disorder. The benefits include assisting individuals with the development of a social support network outside their treatment program, helping participants learn the skills needed to recover, and helping them to take responsibility for their own recovery. Buddie (2004) identifies other treatment programs as alternatives to programs based on the 12 steps.

Goals and Objectives of Supportive Psychotherapy for Individuals With Co-occurring Disorders

Goal setting will begin early in your sessions, but keep in mind that it will continue to evolve throughout the treatment. The goals will vary by individual. However, common goals will include controlling or abstaining from substance use and improving psychological and occupational functioning. With the selection of goals, you need to be certain they will be achievable. One objective of setting goals early in the treatment process is to keep the treatment focused on the fundamental goals and keep the treatment directed. The goals set serve as indicators of progress (Luborsky et al. 1995).

Your supportive therapeutic approach should be one of empathy and flexibility with a priority placed on the building of a collaboration with the individual to promote changes in behavior. Goal setting is the bridge to promoting change; goals and objectives of supportive psychotherapy for individuals with co-occurring disorders are summarized in Table 9–1.

Schizophrenia and Substance Use Disorder

Schizophrenia, perhaps especially in public sector patients, is associated with high rates of abuse of alcohol and illicit drugs. According to Dixon (1999), as many as 50% of patients with schizophrenia will also have a co-occurring sub-

Table 9–1.   Goals and objectives for treating patients with co-occurring disorders

Enhance the patient's motivation for change.

Teach the patient how to break the substance use cycle and establish total abstinence from all mood-altering substances.

Teach the patient adaptive coping and problem-solving skills to maintain abstinence in the long term.

Support and guide the patient through trouble spots and setbacks that might otherwise lead to relapse.

Stabilize acute psychiatric symptoms.

Work toward making a positive lifestyle change.

Intervene early in the process of relapse with substances or the psychiatric disorder.

Resolve or reduce problems and improve physical, emotional, social, family, interpersonal, occupational, academic, spiritual, financial, and legal functioning.

Source.   Adapted from Mercer 2001; Washton 2001.

stance use disorder, with the rate of substance use disorder three times that of the general population. The most frequently used substances are alcohol and cannabis.

Patients with schizophrenia in particular can react to confrontation with increased anxiety, emotional withdrawal, and even exacerbation of psychotic symptoms. Too often patients with schizophrenia with concomitant substance use disorder fall between the cracks of existing treatment systems, not treated by the substance abuse system because of the major mental illness and not fully treated by the mental health system because they are told to stop the substance use first.

A supportive psychotherapy approach to the patient with co-occurring schizophrenia and substance abuse is presented in Table 9–2.

Green et al. (2007) have identified four primary theories detailing the high prevalence of substance use disorders in people with schizophrenia. First is the *neural diathesis-stress theory*, which suggests that a neurobiological vulnerability interacts with substance use in vulnerable individuals to trigger the onset of schizophrenia or a relapse of psychosis. Second is the *accumulative risk factor hypothesis*, which posits that persons with schizophrenia may have a greater risk of

Table 9–2. Supportive psychotherapeutic approach to substance abuse in patients with schizophrenia

Include substance abuse in obtaining psychiatric history in the very first session.

Remain aware of substance abuse issues, even with patients who have been abstinent for a long time.

Delay confrontations until the patient can handle them.

Be tolerant of a lack of abstinence, especially at the beginning.

Try an educational approach that does not confront the patient directly.

Make referrals to other treatment modalities after trust has matured.

Reinforce the good side of any ambivalence.

co-occurring disorders because of the cumulative effects of lower cognitive functioning, poverty, and social environments as well as other risk factors. Third, the *self-medication theory* holds that individuals with schizophrenia use substances to decrease the symptoms of schizophrenia and/or reduce the side effects of their psychiatric medications. Finally, Green and colleagues discuss the theory that reward circuitry dysfunction may indicate the possibility of a reward-deficiency syndrome in which the use of substances may help to alleviate the reward circuitry deficit to help the individual have a feeling of normalcy (see Green et al. 1999 and Chambers et al. 2001 for further readings on this theory).

Many individuals with schizophrenia who abuse substances will also experience homelessness and unemployment and will be arrested for petty crimes such as trespassing. Clearly, individuals diagnosed with schizophrenia and substance use disorder are challenging and will require an integrated treatment plan and collaboration with other professionals for them to achieve stability and recovery.

Substance Use Disorders Co-occurring With Mood and Anxiety Disorders

Bipolar Disorder

Mood disorders, including depression and bipolar disorder, are the most common co-occurring disorders among patients with substance use disorders. In many instances, substance abuse in bipolar disorder represents an attempt at self-medication. Alcohol or drugs are used to self-treat manic or hypomanic episodes. Substance abuse as a substitute for mania in patients with bipolar disorder was described in the psychoanalytic literature as early as 1928 (Rado 1928). Various illegal drugs have also been used as an attempt to treat depression.

Addressing the substance use disorder with individuals with bipolar disorder may have to be delayed until these patients are relatively euthymic. As with the patient with schizophrenia, you must develop some tolerance for lack of abstinence, emphasize educational efforts, and nurture a strong sense of trust in the patient before the issues can be addressed fully.

Depression

The role of substance abuse in major depression is complex. As noted earlier, alcohol and drug abuse may be attempts at self-medication of painful affective states, such as depression or dysphoria associated with other conditions. At other times, depression is the result of chronic alcohol or drug abuse (e.g., prolonged cocaine use). Although there are no hard-and-fast rules (and clinicians differ considerably regarding treatment), a clue can often be gained from the pattern of drug or alcohol use. The use of a stable dose of an illicit drug over many years may point to a self-medication of depression as a rationale, while increased use of the drug may point to a vicious circle whereby chronic drug use results in depression, followed by more drug use, and then more depression, resulting in a cycle that you as the therapist will need to assist your patient with breaking (see also Chapter 7).

Anxiety

Supportive psychotherapeutic techniques play an important role in assisting in the relief of anxiety symptoms in persons with co-occurring anxiety and substance use disorder. Suggesting the use of a paper bag for hyperventilation symptoms, medications, and other interventions can be the first step in this process. Careful differential diagnosis, including the diagnosis and treatment of any underlying depression, is essential. The patient may be amenable to addressing the substance use disorder at an earlier stage in treatment. However, anxiety disorders can be profoundly demoralizing, and premature or excessive confrontation will not break through denial as much as it will further demoralize the

Table 9–3. Supportive psychotherapeutic approach to alcohol use disorder in patients with anxiety disorders

Be aware of alcohol use issues and triggers for use.

Delay addressing alcohol use until anxiety is addressed.

Diagnose and treat the anxiety disorder.

Diagnose and treat any underlying depression.

Ask for a diary relating alcohol use and emotional states.

Teach relaxation and other techniques for anxiety relief.

patient and lead to termination of treatment (for a more thorough discussion, see Chapter 8).

A supportive psychotherapy approach to the patient with concomitant alcohol use disorder and anxiety disorder(s) is summarized in Table 9–3.

Cocaine Use

Statistics

The scope of the problem of cocaine use in the United States is discussed in a report by Hughes et al. (2016), which provides therapists, counselors, nurses, and doctors with valuable data on cocaine that they can use to improve their understanding of the breadth of the issues of cocaine use in the country and to provide education and prevention efforts in the community. To summarize the report, the authors reviewed data from the combined 2014–2015 National Surveys on Drug Use and Health.

One out of every 20 young adults across the nation used cocaine in the past year. Among census regions, past-year cocaine use among young adults ranged from 4.22% in the Midwest to 6.06% in the Northeast. At the state level, past-year cocaine use varied from 1.83% in Mississippi to 10.54% in New Hampshire. Cocaine use among young adults increased in 16 states (when combined 2014–2015 estimates and combined 2013–2014 estimates were compared) and three regions. Use remained unchanged for the remaining 34 states and the District of Columbia and for the West. No decreases occurred in any census region or state.

Sigmund Freud on Cocaine

In addition to founding psychoanalysis, Sigmund Freud devoted a significant portion of his professional life to experimentation with drugs. As a medical investigator, he proclaimed cocaine to be an effective treatment for morphine and alcohol addictions as well as ailments ranging from stomach disorders to syphilis. Though many of Freud's beliefs about cocaine have since been discredited, his writings document the medical establishment's early efforts to understand the drug's effect. In *The Cocaine Papers* (Freud 1884/2003), he chronicled his groundbreaking experiments.

According to Mark and Faude (1995), Freud denied he had an addiction despite the fact he used cocaine for 10 years and described it as "a magical substance," and although Freud did recognize the potential of the problems with cocaine, he speculated that the adverse results were related to a personality predisposition and not to any physiological effects.

Supportive Psychotherapy for Cocaine Use

Crits-Christoph et al. (2008) reviewed the outcomes of supportive-expressive psychotherapy and found that it produced considerable improvements in the decrease of cocaine use. Additionally, they found evidence that supportive psychotherapy provided greater results over individual drug counseling alone with changes in family/social problems, particularly for those individuals with more severe complications in this area. The authors also emphasize that if complete abstinence is not achievable, reducing cocaine use is very important. One of the most basic elements of supportive psychotherapy in the context of substance use disorders is that the patient is a person who abuses drugs and not simply an addict. It will be advantageous for you and your patient to have a clear understanding of substance use disorders, whatever the causes, and for you as the therapist to have an understanding of your patient's personality structure (Mark and Faude 1995).

Relapse and Relapse Prevention Strategies for the Therapist

To properly manage relapse, you must assess for clues of relapse. A relapse is an indication for increased treatment interventions. Compton (2001) stresses the need for not only regular monitoring but also reviewing the relapse episode to recognize the triggers of relapse. Compton also notes it is important for the therapist to remind individuals that they have participated in bad behaviors and that they should not think they are "bad or a failure."

The triggers for relapse are numerous. Marlatt and Donovan (2008) describe some of these triggers and use the acronym HALT to assist individuals with the prevention of relapse: Do not get too hungry, angry, lonely, or tired. Without appropriate coping skills, these four feelings could be triggers for relapse.

It is essential, in preventing relapse, for patients to be members of the treatment team and to be allied with their providers (Snow 2015). Snow (2015) addresses the multitude of complications with relapse, including missed appointments, running out of medications, incarceration, emergency department stays, and the loss of support of family and friends. Snow offers some solutions for these setbacks, including scheduling frequent follow-up appointments and addressing both the substance use disorder and the psychiatric disorder at *every* appointment. Clearly, individuals with co-occurring disorders will be challenging and will require you to collaborate with other professionals, including medical, housing, criminal justice, employment, and pastoral.

Case Vignette

A 22-year-old woman arrived at the clinic seeking treatment for depression and substance use disorder. She reported having symptoms of depression "my entire life." She also reported a 4-year history of cocaine, methamphetamine, and ecstasy use. In the past 3 months, she broke up with her boyfriend and her grandmother passed away. She then quit taking her antidepressant medications and began using again. She confided to her therapist that she had been sexually assaulted by four men the previous night after being lured into their apartment with the promise of drugs. Because of her multiple legal problems, she had difficulty finding employment. She was currently on probation. She dropped out of college after one semester.

Her therapist referred her to the emergency room to be seen by a sexual assault nurse examiner. She was also referred to a grief support group and vocational rehabilitation for employment services. She was restarted on her antidepressant medications and referred to a 12-month drug rehabilitation residential program.

Key Points

- The most challenging patients to treat will be those with co-occurring disorders, and their treatment will be enhanced with collaboration.

- The symptoms of the mental disorder and the substance use and behavioral disorder will not improve if only one is treated.

- Treatment plans for co-occurring disorders should include psychoeducation.

- Making a diagnosis may be perplexing because there will be overlapping symptoms.

- All medical conditions must be ruled out.

- It is essential to have knowledge of resources to refer your patients to, including peer support groups.

- The 12-step "one size fits all" theory is not always effective.

- The patient should be included as a member of the treatment team.

References

Alcoholics Anonymous: Historical data: the birth of A.A. and its growth in the U.S./ Canada. 2017. Available at: http://www.aa.org/pages/en_US/historical-data-the-birth-of-aa-and-its-growth-in-the-uscanada. Accessed February 25, 2019.

American Psychiatric Association: Diagnostic and Statistical Manual of Mental Disorders, 5th Edition. Arlington, VA, American Psychiatric Association, 2013

Buddie AM: Alternatives to twelve-step programs. J Forensic Psychol Pract 4(3):61–70, 2004

Cavacuiti CA: Principles of Addiction Medicine: The Essentials. Philadelphia, PA, Lippincott Williams & Wilkins, 2011

Center for Behavioral Health Statistics and Quality: Behavioral health trends in the United States: results from the 2014 National Survey on Drug Use and Health. HHS Publ No SMA 15-4927; NSDUH Series H-50. Rockville, MD, Substance Abuse and Mental Health Services Administration, September 2015. Available at: https://www.samhsa.gov/data/sites/default/files/NSDUH-FRR1-2014/NSDUH-FRR1-2014.pdf. Accessed February 25, 2019.

Chambers RA, Krystal JH, Self DW: A neurobiological basis for substance abuse co-morbidity in schizophrenia. Biol Psychiatry 50(2):71–83, 2001 11526998

Compton P: Treating chronic pain with prescription opioids in the substance abuser. J Addict Nurs 22:39–45, 2001

Crits-Christoph P, Gibbons MB, Gallop R, et al: Supportive-expressive psychodynamic therapy for cocaine dependence: a closer look. Psychoanal Psychol 25(3):483–498, 2008 19960117

Dixon L: Dual diagnosis of substance abuse in schizophrenia: prevalence and impact on outcomes. Schizophr Res 35(suppl):S93–S100, 1999 10190230

Drake RE, Mueser KT: Psychosocial approaches to dual diagnosis. Schizophr Bull 26(1):105–118, 2000 10755672

Freud S: The Cocaine Papers (1884), in Under the Influence: The Literature of Addiction. Edited by Shannonhouse R. New York, Random House, 2003, pp 25–34

Galanter M, Kleber HD, Brady KT (eds): The American Psychiatric Publishing Textbook of Substance Abuse Treatment, 5th Edition. Washington, DC, American Psychiatric Publishing, 2015

Green AI, Zimmet SV, Strous RD, et al: Clozapine for comorbid substance use disorder and schizophrenia: do patients with schizophrenia have a reward-deficiency syndrome that can be ameliorated by clozapine? Harv Rev Psychiatry 6(6):287–296, 1999 10370435

Green AI, Drake RE, Brunette MF, et al: Schizophrenia and co-occurring substance use disorder. Am J Psychiatry 164(3):402–408, 2007 17329463

Hughes A, Williams MR, Lipari RN, et al: State estimates of past year cocaine use among young adults: 2014 and 2015. Rockville, MD, Substance Abuse and Mental Health Services Administration December 20, 2016. Available at: https://www.samhsa.gov/data/sites/default/files/report_2736/ShortReport-2736.html. Accessed February 25, 2019.

Johnson BA: We're addicted to rehab. It doesn't even work. The Washington Post, August 8, 2010. Available at: http://www.washingtonpost.com/wp-dyn/content/article/2010/08/06/AR2010080602660.html. Accessed February 25, 2019.

Lammertink M, Löhrer F, Kaiser R, et al: Differences in substance abuse patterns: multiple drug abuse alone versus schizophrenia with multiple drug abuse. Acta Psychiatr Scand 104(5):361–366, 2001 11722317

Luborsky L, Woody GE, Hole AV, et al: Supportive-expressive dynamic psychotherapy for treatment of opiate drug dependence, in Dynamic Therapies for Psychiatric Disorders (Axis I). Edited by Barber JP, Crits-Christoph P. New York, Basic Books, 1995, pp 131–160

Mack AH, Harrington AL, Frances RJ: Clinical Manual for Treatment of Alcoholism and Addictions, Washington, DC, American Psychiatric Press, 2010

Mark D, Faude J: Supportive-expressive therapy of cocaine abuse, in Dynamic Therapies for Psychiatric Disorders (Axis I). Edited by Barber JP, Crits-Christoph P. New York, Basic Books, 1995, pp 294–331

Marlatt GA, Donovan DM: Relapse Prevention: Maintenance Strategies in the Treatment of Addictive Behaviors, 2nd Edition. New York, Guilford, 2008

Mercer D: Description of an addiction counseling approach, in Approaches to Drug Abuse Counseling. 2001. Available at: https://www.dualdiagnosis.org/resource/approaches-to-drug-abuse-counseling/description/. Accessed February 25, 2019.

Miller SC, Fiellin DA, Rosenthal RN, Saitz R: The ASAM Principles of Addiction Medicine, 6th Edition, Philadelpha, PA, Wolters Kluwer, 2019

Miller WR, Benefield RG, Tonigan JS: Enhancing motivation for change in problem drinking: a controlled comparison of two therapist styles. J Consult Clin Psychol 61(3):455–461, 1993 8326047

National Bureau of Economic Research: Mental illness and substance abuse. 2019. Available at: http://www.nber.org/digest/apr02/w8699.html. Accessed February 25, 2019.

Quello SB, Brady KT, Sonne SC: Mood disorders and substance use disorder: a complex comorbidity. Sci Pract Perspect 3(1):13–21, 2005 18552741

Rado S: The problem of melancholia. Int J Psychoanal 9:420–438, 1928

Secular Organizations for Sobriety: General principles of SOS. 1985. Available at: https://static1.squarespace.com/static/576740f45016e10f9510a056/t/5768d296893fc08c1a44efc4/1466487450589/SOS_Principles.pdf. Accessed February 25, 2019.

Singer V: Dual diagnosis and mental illness (prepared for Lanier Treatment Center). Paper presented at the Training Session for Therapists on Dual Diagnosis and Mental Illness, Gainesville, GA, June 2006

Snow D: What does it take to achieve recovery for persons with severe mental illness co-occurring with substance use disorders? J Addict Nurs 26(4):163–165, 2015 26669222

Washton AM: A psychotherapeutic and skills-training approach to the treatment of drug addiction, in Approaches to Drug Abuse Counseling. 2001. Available at: https://www.dualdiagnosis.org/resource/approaches-to-drug-abuse-counseling/psychotherapeutic-and-skills-training/. Accessed February 25, 2019.

White W, Miller W: The use of confrontation in addiction treatment: history, science, and time for change. Counselor (Deerfield Beach) 8(4):12–30, 2007

Winston A, Rosenthal RN, Pinsker H: Learning Supportive Psychotherapy: An Illustrated Guide. Washington, DC, American Psychiatric Publishing, 2012

Women for Sobriety: WFS New Life Program acceptance statements. 2017. Available at: https://womenforsobriety.org/wp-content/uploads/2018/01/WFS_New_Life_Acceptance_Statements.pdf. Accessed February 25, 2019.

10

Personality Disorders

Everyone has a personality. However, not everyone will present with a personality disorder; these disorders are a variant from well-adjusted, healthy functioning. The most striking and defining aspect of personality disorders is the negative effect these disorders have on interpersonal relationships. For individuals with personality disorders, responses to situations and demands tend to be rigid patterns of thoughts, feelings, and behavior. No exact cause of personality disorders is known. However, it is clear that both biological and psychosocial components have an impact on the development of personality and personality disorders (Hoermann et al. 2013).

In this chapter we outline an approach to supportive work with each of the personality disorders and present greater detail on borderline and histrionic personality disorders. The study of personality disorders has resulted in a massive outpouring of fact and theory, but surprisingly few firm conclusions can be reached. After the existing literature on the treatment of personality disorders is taken into account, however, one reasonable conclusion is that for many of these disorders, patients ought to be treated primarily by supportive psychotherapy. Even those patients having disorders that benefit from psychoanalysis or interpretive therapy often require a component of supportive psychotherapy.

Supportive treatment of personality disorders generally involves a normalization of dysfunctional behaviors. Weak and deficient coping skills must be shored up; tendencies to blame and exploit others must be toned down. Some patients, for example, must learn to give up unrealistic entitlements; others must be urged to overcome obstacles to the entitlements they deserve. Some must become less critical of themselves and decrease the internalization of blame; others must become more objective and stop using externalization as a defense. These goals are set and achieved by a therapeutic relationship and a treatment strategy tailored to the individual patient.

Supportive psychotherapy provides the clinician with the essentials for psychotherapeutic interventions for those with personality disorders and can function as a beginning point for integrating other treatment strategies (e.g., using dialectical behavior therapy [DBT] for patients with borderline personally disorder [BPD]). Supportive psychotherapy is especially applicable in the treatment of most personality disorders because of its focus on bolstering self-esteem and adaptive skills while developing and maintaining a strong therapeutic alliance (Winston et al. 2012). It is important to note that often a person can be diagnosed with more than one personality disorder (Skodol 2018). In fact, as we shall mention in a moment, this is a shortcoming of the current categorical system of diagnosis.

Some words of caution are in order. You should take the time to gain a longitudinal perspective of the patient before concluding that he has a personality disorder. Pharmacological treatments, family therapy, and group therapy may also be indicated. Individual psychotherapy, of any modality, may not be the treatment of choice.

A second cautionary note is that the diagnosing of a personality disorder in children and adolescents should be done with attention to detail because the personalities of patients in this age group are still developing. Indeed, although children and adolescents may present with glaring personality disorder characteristics, it is preferable to defer any personality disorder diagnosis until early adulthood (Skodol et al. 2014).

When individual psychotherapy is indicated, supportive therapy is often preferable to more interpretive treatments. As Perry and Vaillant (1989) note, patients with personality disorders have developed a lifelong homeostatic pattern of adaptive defenses and respond with anxiety and depression when their defenses are breached. These patients will often benefit from social supports and replacement of dysfunctional defenses by alternative ones. Supportive therapy is also indicated when the patient is deficient in coping skills and has the other characteristics described in Chapter 5 (see, specifically, Table 5–1)—for example, a fragile patient with several previous hospitalizations, suicide attempts, self-mutilations, or conflicts with family. The immediate goal with such a patient is to preserve the level of functioning and prevent further regression. In general, a patient with coexisting schizophrenia, or one in an acute medical crisis, will need supportive work and not deep exploration of the personality. Any of these patients may be switched to insight-oriented therapy if you feel it would afford further improvement; however, it is best to start the therapy supportively, because the only fail-safe strategy is not to overestimate the patient's initial stability.

The goals of supportive psychotherapy for your patients with personality disorders will include limiting destructive and disruptive behaviors, maintaining the necessary conditions for treatment, and protecting the therapeutic alliance. Your therapeutic interventions will consist of contracting, limit setting, recontracting, advice, encouragement, and concern (Caligor et al. 2018).

DSM-5 (American Psychiatric Association 2013) divides personality disorders into three clusters. As of this writing, however, the use of dimensional assessments for personality disorders is becoming more prevalent. Indeed, the DSM-5 Personality and Personality Disorders Work Group developed an alternative approach, the dimensional model of personality disorders outlined in Section III of DSM-5, to address the numerous shortcomings of the current approach to personality disorders. For example, the typical patient meeting the criteria for a specific personality disorder frequently also meets criteria for other personality disorders (American Psychiatric Association 2013).

Categorical models are determined by either the presence or absence of symptoms (Hoermann et al. 2019). Dimensional models differ from categorical approaches by classifying the personality disorders based on the degree to which the symptoms impair the patient's functioning (American Psychiatric Association 2013; Hoermann et al. 2018). In other words, instead of making judgments about whether the disorder is present, one asks, "How much is present?"

A dimensional model is based on the theory that disorders consist of a complex interaction of factors over a period of time. The quintessential answer to the diagnosing of the personality disorders, according to Widiger (2007), would be to include the significant components of each of the models. Although Widiger maintains that there is a strong potential for personality disorders to be dimensional, a potential downfall of applying the dimensional model today is that the current DSM-5 and ICD-10 codes are relied on for reimbursement from insurance companies and changes to the coding could prove problematic (Gever 2010).

The Six Personality Disorders for Which There Is the Strongest Evidence Under the Dimensional Model

In this text, we have eliminated reference to categorical clusters of the main text of DSM-5 and have arranged the following six personality disorders based on the dimensional model outlined in Section III of DSM-5. This section includes antisocial, avoidant, borderline, narcissistic, obsessive-compulsive, and schizotypal personality disorders.

Antisocial Personality Disorder

Antisocial personality disorder (ASPD) is distinguished by a pervasive pattern of disregard for the rights of others, and individuals with ASPD often present with hostility and aggression. Deceit and manipulation are common features. Individuals with ASPD usually do not experience genuine remorse for the harm they have caused others. However, when beneficial for them to express remorse, such as in a courtroom, they are very skillful at feigning it. They will often act on impulse with no consideration for the consequences. Their poor impulse control can lead to loss of employment, accidents, and legal problems. Often, they take little or no responsibility for the actions and will frequently blame their victims for the results of their actions. The aggressiveness noted with this personality disorder is distinct from that seen in the other disorders and has a serious impact on society (American Psychiatric Association 2013; Kernberg 2018).

The diagnosis of ASPD should be used cautiously in patients with substance use disorder (SUD). Criminal offenses are not unusual with SUD because of the means used to obtain the illicit substances (American Psychiatric Association 2013; Avery and Barnhill 2018).

Indeed, aggression and violence from a patient can be alarming and dangerous to staff and other patients. Medication and psychotherapy have had significant success in reducing the risk of violence for seriously mentally ill patients (those with schizophrenia, those with bipolar disorder and psychosis). However, the violent impulses of patients with personality disorders are more difficult to treat (Ritter and Platt 2016). It is most likely that violent acts will be seen with BPD and ASPD (Abracen et al. 2014; American Psychiatric Association 2013).

Most of the information available for psychotherapy and interventions for personality disorders is focused on BPD. The development of treatment for ASPD is limited and some in the mental health field are even of the mind-set that this disorder cannot be treated, and thus it is often viewed with ambivalence (Gibbon et al. 2010; Kramer 2016; National Collaborating Centre for Mental Health 2010).

Supportive psychotherapy for patients with ASPD is not as beneficial as it is for those diagnosed with any of the other personality disorders (Kool et al. 2003). However, these authors have found that in a patient with ASPD and depression, supportive psychotherapy might be beneficial.

Avoidant Personality Disorder

Patients with avoidant personality disorder (APD) may be described by others as being shy, timid, and isolated. They are extremely sensitive to what others think about them, and their feelings of inadequacy may cause them to be inhibited and have feelings of being socially inept. These feelings of inadequacy and ineptness can lead to their avoiding any social activity, including work and school. In fact, they will be hesitant to pursue any endeavor for fear of being embarrassed (Bressert 2018a).

The treatment of patients with a personality disorder can be difficult because of their ingrained patterns of thinking. However, patients with APD are good candidates for treatment because their disorder causes them serious anguish, and most do desire to develop relationships with others. This desire can be a motivation for them to follow their treatment plans. The primary treatment for APD is psychotherapy, with the focus of the therapy being to help patients overcome fears and assist them with improved coping skills with social interactions (Cleveland Clinic 2017).

Currently, there is no medication approved by the U.S. Food and Drug Administration for the treatment of any personality disorder. However, off-label use of medications for anxiety symptoms could be helpful: the best pharmacological treatment may be a selective serotonin reuptake inhibitor or a serotonin-norepinephrine reuptake inhibitor (Drago et al. 2016). Not unlike pharmacotherapy for any other mental health disorder, the best results are obtained when medication is combined with psychotherapy (Cleveland Clinic 2017).

Although the avoidant person shares a hypersensitivity to rejection with persons with narcissistic, dependent, and paranoid personality disorders, the person with APD also exhibits anxious and phobic behavior in social relationships. Although avoidant persons can thrive in trusting relationships, they are mistrustful in new encounters and will have difficulty developing a sustained relationship in therapy. You will want to present as a stable, predictable, and available supportive figure, especially focusing on supporting the patient's self-esteem.

Some of the same techniques used in treating social phobias (as described in Chapter 8) can be gently explored with these patients. For example, you can discuss the patient's fears of humiliation and encourage what one might call the "activation energy" for the patient to get over the initial barriers to social contact. When such patients respond to these efforts, however, they do so more slowly than do patients with a social phobia.

Borderline Personality Disorder

Many therapists consider patients with BPD to be the bane of their existence. Such patients are often angry, entitled, and demanding. They will often intrude upon the therapist between sessions in person or by phone. They may be seductive or create countertransference problems and considerable soul-searching in the therapist. They may require, or even demand, hospitalization when it appears to be "medically" unnecessary. Patients with BPD may generate friction among the treatment team through the mechanism of splitting. They can alternate between syrupy thankfulness and outright abuse, and frequently their disorder has a spiraling downward course. Indeed, the patient with BPD will be one of the most difficult you will encounter in your career. You will be challenged with communication skills and will spend a disproportionate amount of your time and resources.

Anger, violence, self-harm, and recurrent suicidality are the most troublesome characteristics of BPD. This disorder is frequently thought to be chronic and resistant to treatment. However, most patients with BPD will have a remission of symptoms, and certain treatments have clearly proven to be effective

(Gunderson 2015). DBT, transference-focused therapy, and supportive psychotherapy were compared in a yearlong clinical trial for BPD. The results demonstrated that transference-focused therapy and supportive psychotherapy led to improvements with impulsivity, depression, anxiety, social adjustment, and anger (Clarkin et al. 2007). In another study, both supportive psychotherapy and mentalization-based psychotherapy were found to be effective in a sample of 58 patients over 2 years (Jørgensen et al. 2013).

The presentations of BPD are variable, often resulting in a misdiagnosis or failure to diagnose. Family members and friends of the patient with BPD have difficulties with coping due to the patient's insecurities, disorganized lifestyle, self-destructive behaviors, and lack of self-awareness (Lockwood 2017). DSM-5 describes BPD as "[a] pervasive pattern of instability of interpersonal relationships, self-image, and affects, and marked impulsivity, beginning by early adulthood and present in a variety of contexts" (American Psychiatric Association 2013, p. 663).

Therapists have developed individual approaches to treating BPD patients, and their methods range across the treatment spectrum, from supportive to insight oriented (expressive). Expressive therapists use a more challenging style, interpret transference issues early, and focus early on the patient's aggression, hostility, envy, and primitive defenses. Supportive therapists play the role of more benign parents, foster positive transference and delay interpretation of it, and focus early on the patient's affective symptoms, self-esteem regulation, and separation-individuation problems. Although supportive psychotherapy is not always fully successful, it can usually reduce the degree of disability caused by this disorder. Supportive psychotherapy with patients with BPD can be difficult, but one can have some comfort in the research that supportive psychotherapy compares favorably with the results of other approaches (Clarkin et al. 2007).

Case Vignette

Karen is a 22-year-old who presented to the outpatient clinic after a 14-day inpatient stay. She was taken to the hospital after she was stopped for running a red light. She was intoxicated and told the police she purposely ran the red light because she wanted to kill herself. She also reported she did not care if anyone else died when she went through the red light. She had a lengthy criminal record, including arrests for shoplifting, DUI, forgery, assault, and attempted burglary. She tested positive for cocaine, alcohol, and marijuana upon admission to the hospital. The report from the hospital described her as being seductive to male staff members and patients. She presented to the outpatient clinic dressed in a low-cut, see-through blouse and extremely short skirt. She has had no substance use treatment. She has had three inpatient treatments after suicide attempts. She reports she has attempted suicide "lots of times." She overdosed on her mother's alprazolam, and her mother found her on the bathroom floor after the two had an argument when she was confronted with taking her mother's credit card. The other two attempts were superficial cuttings to her wrists. Karen stated that she attempted suicide all three times because she felt "picked on." She has had several relationships with men that resulted in breakups. "I have had lots of boyfriends. They were all stupid." She reported, "Once I get drunk and sleep with them, that's it, they dump me." She made excellent grades until her senior year in high school. She was expelled from school when she struck a teacher after receiving a failing grade. "He just did not like me." She stated that she feels "empty" and verbalizes anger because everyone, especially her parents and boyfriend, disrespects her. She has been treated for depression with sertraline, fluoxetine, and venlafaxine. "They did nothing for me except to make me all hyper." She reported she often feels alone and sad and will then feel "on top of the world." She was terminated from three places of employment. "I just can't focus sometimes."

Karen's legal history, reckless behaviors, lack of regard for others, and tendency to blame others could indicate ASPD. However, she reported she had forged checks and stole her mother's credit card to buy cocaine and marijuana. Her sexual promiscuity, substance use, impulsiveness, suicidal gestures, feelings of abandonment, and unstable relationships are more indicative of BPD. The mood swings, substance use, reckless behaviors, poor sleep, and poor concentration could be symptoms of bipolar disorder.

Karen was referred to an intensive outpatient substance use clinic and started on a mood stabilizer. She remained clean and sober for 3 months and had a relapse with alcohol. She joined Alcoholics Anonymous and has now been clean and sober for 4 months. She would often cancel her appointments with her therapist. Her therapist continued to work with her until she was further stabilized and referred her to a DBT therapist. Karen was able to accept this transfer without any anger or feelings of abandonment.

Narcissistic Personality Disorder

According to DSM-5, a person with narcissistic personality disorder (NPD) has a persistent manner of grandiosity and a continuous desire for admiration, along with a lack of empathy. NPD starts by early adulthood and may present in a variety of contexts, as signified by the existence of any five of nine diagnostic criteria (American Psychiatric Association 2013).

A large percentage of patients with NPD will have comorbidity with mood disorders, anxiety disorders, SUD, and other personality disorders (Caligor et al. 2015; Eaton et al. 2017). According to Ronningstam and Weinberg (2013), the most common comorbidity is major depressive disorder, and such patients are very susceptible to SUD because of a need for self-enhancement and chronic disillusionment with self. Frequently, it is not the NPD for which a patient will first seek treatment; it is the comorbid disorder that brings him to the clinic (Caligor et al. 2015). Between 50% and 75% of those diagnosed with NPD are male (American Psychiatric Association 2013).

Persons with NPD believe they are entitled to special treatment and believe they are exceptionally brilliant or attractive. Frequently, they fantasize about their unlimited success and power, superior intelligence, or good looks. A person with NPD will have a lack of empathy and will not be able to recognize the needs or feelings of others. He may not be willing to take risks or to be competitive if there is a possibility of defeat. He may present with an arrogant and haughty attitude. Persons who are in contact with him find his behaviors repulsive, particularly those who feel they have been exploited by him. When the patient with NPD does realize that he has average limitations or is not as special as he has perceived, or that others do not admire him as much as he would prefer, he will often feel devastated and will react with intense anger and shame (American Psychiatric Association 2013; Caligor et al. 2018).

Supportive psychotherapy may be beneficial when addressing the comorbid diagnoses and stabilizing the patient. However, the treatment of NPD requires long-term psychotherapy. Caligor et al. (2015) recommend mentalization-based therapy, which requires specialized training.

Obsessive-Compulsive Personality Disorder

DSM-5 defines *obsessive-compulsive personality disorder* (OCPD) as "[a] pervasive pattern of preoccupation with orderliness, perfectionism, and mental and interpersonal control, at the expense of flexibility, openness, and efficiency, beginning by early adulthood and present in a variety of contexts" (American Psychiatric Association 2013, p. 678). These individuals' preoccupation with rules, regulations, orderliness, perfectionism, and control will interfere with flexibility, acceptance, and efficiency. They will make lists and schedules, and they frequently will disregard any social relationships. They will have difficulty completing projects because they focus too much on details.

The patient who is orderly, obstinate, and parsimonious may evoke much sympathy from the therapist, because these traits can be quite adaptive in the mental health profession. The therapist who anxiously struggles to recall the content of a session in reporting to a supervisor, or who tosses and turns at night reliving a therapeutic blunder, knows what we mean. Although obsessive-compulsive persons are often happy with their adaptations (and will not be seen in therapy), many of them (whom we shall simply call "compulsive") are bothered by their anxiety, indecisiveness, and constricted emotions, and these individuals can be treated supportively for their symptoms.

The patient with OCPD will often present as being caught up in her thoughts and having little expression of emotions. You do not want to try to uncover the emotional tones at first. Instead, as is generally true with supportive psychotherapy, you will begin where the patient is, which means, in this case, focusing on her reasoning, not her emotions. This can be tedious work, but by walking with the patient through the rationalizations and intellectualizations in detail, you can set the climate for the need to realize that there are emotions, too, that are driving the patient.

Patients with OCPD generally are not as in touch with their emotional states as they are with their thoughts. Therefore, you will need to redirect the patient away from describing events and to discuss how the events make her feel. Having her keep a journal will be helpful because such patients sometimes state they do not remember or even know how they felt at the time they did those things. Cognitive therapy approaches are not effective for the patient with OCPD (Bressert 2018c; Skodol et al. 2014).

Schizotypal Personality Disorder

The schizotypal diagnosis covers a broad group of presentations, although it is often assigned to the schizophrenic spectrum. Our suggestions in previous chapters on managing schizophrenia and related disorders may be relevant (see Chapter 6), such as with patients who have ideas of reference.

Patients with schizotypal personality disorder who are well adjusted in isolation and have no other mental disorder are unlikely to seek therapy. Those who come into treatment may do so because of major psychopathology, such as transient psychotic episodes or depression, and one sometimes encounters schizotypal persons who are relatively sociable but disturbed at their inability to relate effectively. Although appearing at first to be cognitively intact, these patients often have odd thoughts, dress, mannerisms, speech, or behavior that is creating social, scholastic, vocational, or occupational problems. You can use the explanatory techniques of supportive psychotherapy, and eventually even some of the directive techniques of earlier chapters, to find ways of altering the oddities or of helping these patients find ways of increasing the acceptance of the oddities in their social environment.

Patients with schizotypal personality disorder will present with perceptual and cognitive distortions and/or eccentric behavior. They may present with odd beliefs. For example, they may believe they can read other people's minds or that their own thoughts have been stolen (American Psychiatric Association 2013; Skodol et al. 2014). They may have related problems with time and thus have difficulty in tolerating separations from their therapists. These patients are also anhedonic. Educational and behavioral interventions are often effective in improving their social mannerisms and eccentric behaviors. You may be required to make very specific suggestions.

Other Personality Disorders Not as Well Supported Under Dimensional Models

The following personality disorders are less established under the dimensional model and may be eliminated in future DSM diagnostic criteria.

Paranoid Personality Disorder

The distinguishing characteristic of the paranoid personality is a lifelong distrust of other people. The paranoid individual assumes that other persons' actions and intentions are nefarious until proven otherwise—and with some of these patients it seems impossible to prove otherwise.

Persons with paranoid personality disorder will go to great lengths to protect themselves and will isolate from others. They are known to attack others whom they experience as perceived threats. They tend to hold grudges, are litigious, and display pathological jealously. Distorted thinking is apparent, and their perception of the environment includes perceiving sinister objectives from genuinely harmless, innocuous comments or behavior, and dwelling on past slights. Therefore, they will not confide in others and do not allow themselves to develop close relationships (Skodol et al. 2014). Other characteristics include sensitivity to criticism, rigidity, hypervigilance, and an excessive need for autonomy (Vyas and Khan 2016).

Because of their mistrust, it is difficult to get close to paranoid patients; nor should you usually try. Rather, you must maintain a predictable distance and refrain from personal remarks. Nevertheless, you must try to establish a trusting relationship. You should avoid crowding the patient and attempt to allow him considerable autonomy. Therefore, you should use directive techniques sparingly, if at all, in the early sessions.

You should not condemn the characteristics that the patient attributes to others with such contempt. Because the attributions to others are often issues of concern to the patient (i.e., projections), you may antagonize the patient if you agree that an attribute is horrible. For example, a patient condemns his coworker for being "money mad." While agreeing with the patient that it is a concern that may be making cooperation with that coworker difficult, you should also indicate that being "money mad" is not especially unusual or blameworthy. While avoiding echoing a revulsion for the characteristics attributed to others, you can empathize with the patient that, given his concerns and vigilance, these are difficult interpersonal situations for the patient.

You will need to be prepared for being the recipient of hostility and negative assumptions. While assuming responsibility for such patients, you need to think through the countertransference aspects of a role in which one is likely to be very frustrated and never appreciated.

There are additional ways to reach the paranoid patient. We have sometimes found that a discussion of mistreatment in childhood can also be a starting point for therapy, because such memories are often accessible to patients and they are willing to talk about them. One patient, who was seen in a forensic setting after assaulting an elderly woman, related how he had been severely beaten by an aunt whom he loved. Another was abandoned by his mother under unexplained circumstances. Throughout his life he had suspicions of women and eventually developed a delusional jealousy. Some paranoid patients also have well-developed, if skewed, senses of humor. Patients may take delight in relating jokes with a sadistic bent, and these can serve as displaced arenas for discussing their own fears and concerns.

Schizoid Personality Disorder

The patient with schizoid personality disorder differs from the patient with schizotypal personality disorder in that the patient with schizoid personality is not fearful of others or relationships but instead may simply have no desire to interact with others.

Individuals with a schizoid personality are often loners, uninterested in socializing and more comfortable with things than with people. They may, however, be highly functional in technical or scientific disciplines. Often, they are stable but marginal, perhaps with steady jobs that offer no career advancement. Perhaps they go home to a brother, sister, or mother, but they never stop for a drink with friends. They are not *unhappy* but merely indifferent and alone. And given the vicissitudes of modern human relationships, some people might even envy their unaffected stoicism!

Patients with schizoid personality disorder will also present with a restricted range of emotion and take little pleasure in life. They may appear to others as being aloof, detached, and cold. Their restricted emotional range and failure to exchange a smile or nod cause them to seem dull or inattentive.

With sufficient trust, you may obtain admission to the person's inner life and strivings and will be able to help your patient make some improvements. Patients with this type of personality, who are capable of close relationships with a very significant other, desire to be loved. In this respect, they are the patient with avoidant personality discussed earlier. The patient with schizoid personality disorder may also suffer from identity diffusion, grandiosity, and sexual inhibition. Eventually, you should try to get in touch with these areas, but initially it may help to share some of the patient's mechanical and abstract interests that are less threatening, such as automobiles and computer systems.

As with many personality disorders, the current definition may cover a heterogeneous population, but the implication for you is that it is important to search for additional needs and desires in the patient that can be made part of a therapeutic agenda. However, you should be careful not to project onto the patient interests that are not there. The primitive nature of the patient's defenses, as well as his suspiciousness, is an indication for an initially supportive approach until you know the patient well enough to develop a treatment plan.

Histrionic Personality Disorder

DSM-5 defines *histrionic personality disorder* (HPD) as "[a] pervasive pattern of excessive emotionality and attention seeking, beginning by early adulthood and present in a variety of contexts" (American Psychiatric Association 2013, p. 667). Frequently, the patient with HPD will be labeled as a "drama queen" (Out of the Fog 2019; SAPA Project Test 2001).

DSM-5 recognizes the historical fact that the diagnosis has predominantly applied to women. As do most other writers, therefore, we shall refer to histrionic patients in this section as female, but the therapeutic strategies presented can be applied with minimal modification to male patients.

The patient with HPD will frequently use statements containing the word *always* or *never*. These patients are often flirtatious or seductive and will dress in a manner that draws attention to themselves. They can be flamboyant and exhibit an exaggerated degree of emotional expression. Yet, at the same time, their emotional expression will be vague, shallow, and lacking in detail. They will often embarrass their friends with excessive ardor and may sob uncontrollably over some minor sentimentality (Out of the Fog 2019).

A helpful mnemonic used to describe the criteria for HPD is "PRAISE ME" (five criteria) (Out of the Fog 2019; SAPA Project Test 2001):

> **P:** Provocative (or sexually seductive) behavior
> **R:** Relationships (considered more intimate than they are)
> **A:** Attention (uncomfortable when not the center of attention)
> **I:** Influenced easily
> **S:** Style of speech (impressionistic, lacks detail)
> **E:** Emotions (rapidly shifting and shallow)
>
> **M:** Made up (physical appearance used to draw attention to self)
> **E:** Emotions exaggerated (theatrical)

We summarize common issues with HPD below.

Emotionality

Emotional expressiveness in the patient with HPD is inappropriately exaggerated, rapidly shifting, and shallow. The patient's style of speech is excessively impressionistic and lacking in detail.

You should encourage your patient to discuss the details of her feelings. Initially, this should be done without regard for the logic or realism of the feelings. Only later in therapy, after the patient can fully describe her feelings, do you slowly edge into the logic or realism of these feelings, using clarifications to help the patient to move from fantasy to reality.

Initially, be tolerant of inconsistencies and the fact that feelings may be diametrically opposed to those expressed in a prior session or even earlier in the same session. Only after your patient seems fully comfortable in describing the details of her emotions should you ask about her changes in attitudes—that is, about the "apparent" inconsistencies. You should not reflect negatively on rapidly shifting attitudes but instead echo the patient's own reason for her changing attitude to begin the discussion. You should use these inconsistencies as a beachhead for the patient to begin understanding her reasoning and the circumstances that changed her feelings. As the patient explores her rapidly alternating feelings, she will improve her understanding of the sequential nature of her thinking.

Depression, Suicidality, and Psychosis

If your patient's emotional distress reaches the level of depression, you can consider use of antidepressant medications, although you should assume there is a suicide potential whenever you write a prescription. Also, although in DSM-III-R (American Psychiatric Association 1987) suicidal behavior was removed from the criteria of HPD, suicidal gestures and efforts are still common.

If the patient's emotionality turns psychotic, the criteria for a brief reactive psychosis will usually be met and the patient will require hospitalization. Experience suggests that the episode will end, suddenly, in a week or two, so management is conservative. You should prepare the hospital staff for the patient's stormy emotional state and to anticipate staff disagreements over diagnosis. (The patient's behavior is often thought to indicate schizophrenia or mania.)

Splitting and Other Manipulative Behavior

During the therapy, your patient's need for attention may take the form of splitting between you and another important person. You should maintain a neutral position, which usually will lead to complaints from the patient of frustration that her needs are not being met. Again, you should explore the details and depths of your patient's feelings and behaviors, often touching on issues of power and powerlessness, before encouraging her to speak of the realistic and logical aspects. In time, she will learn to give the appropriate emphasis to her rational thoughts as well as to her feelings.

A frequent topic that coincides with splitting is the patient's interests in medications such as sedatives and antianxiety agents. One might hear, for example, that a previous physician "told me that I should have Xanax for my fear of flying." However, unless there is a pressing need, you should avoid prescribing medications that can create dependence, such as sedatives or benzodiazepines, because patients with HPD are especially prone to abuse them. Patients may make their medication request a basis for continuing treatment, and if so, it may be necessary to let them become ex-patients rather than iatrogenic substance abusers.

The use of manipulation is goal oriented. Patients will use manipulation to obtain what they want without any regard for the needs or feelings of others. The best way to avoid a power struggle is to not be taken in by their manipulation. Manipulation may be used to avoid taking responsibility for actions, obtain special favors, or avoid unpleasant tasks. The manipulative patient may criticize staff, calling them incompetent or insensitive. A simple response such as "Maybe I am" without any other comment is a good way to handle such an encounter (Ritter and Platt 2016).

Actions

Actions of the patient with HPD are directed toward obtaining immediate gratification, and there is no tolerance for delayed gratification. To treat this aspect, you should explore in detail the feelings of frustration that any delay causes, and you should present a model of appropriate responsiveness to the patient's demands. It helps to give a name to an action so that it is easier to verbalize. The behavior of a patient who keeps getting fired might simply be given the term "getting-fired routine," or the behavior of one who is frequently promiscuously self-destructive might be described as "sexual acting out." Naming the behavior gives the patient a verbal handle to facilitate talking instead of acting.

Your patient is likely to call you frequently, and overuse of this avenue of communication presents opportunities to discuss the patient's frustrations associated with postponing gratification as well as the tendency to exaggerate her needs. In this way, you can set limits on the use of the phone and encourage your patient to discuss her frustrations—for example, her outrage at your "uncaring, unreasonable, and dangerous attitude."

Other means of gratification can also be explored. One substantial area may in some cases be the patient's vocational choice. For example, other factors being equal, your patient may find that being a salesperson for a firm is much more appropriate than working in the accounting office. Selecting an artistic field often well suits individuals with these personalities (i.e., reduces somewhat the need for "adjustments").

Self-Destructive Actions

Your patient may express her anger through inappropriate actions that may be self-destructive. Consistent with the approaches recommended above, the patient should be encouraged to express her anger in detail and to use words in place of actions. You can give positive verbal feedback when the patient uses words rather than actions to express her anger.

When the patient's emotionality, speech, and behavior become satisfactory, supportive psychotherapy may be discontinued. If your patient wants a better understanding of herself, she can then be referred to someone who will provide dynamic psychotherapy. "Better understanding," when it means "Why am I like I am?," is achieved through psychodynamic psychotherapy or psychoanalysis.

Some pointers for supportive psychotherapy with the patient with HPD are given in Table 10–1.

Dependent Personality Disorder

DSM-5 describes dependent personality disorder (DPD) as "[a] pervasive and excessive need to be taken care of that leads to submissive and clinging behavior and fears of separation, beginning by early adulthood and present in a variety of contexts." DSM-5 notes that the "dependent and submissive behaviors are designed to elicit caregiving and arise from a self-perception of being unable to function adequately without the help of others" (American Psychiatric Association 2013, pp. 675–676).

Patients with DPD have the tendency to criticize their abilities and refer to themselves as "stupid." The criticism and disapproval from others provide them with the proof they need of their insignificance, and they lose confidence in themselves. They may avoid obligations and become anxious when they are required to make decisions (Bressert 2018b).

Table 10–1.   Basics of supportive therapy for the histrionic personality

Work on rapport, always. When rapport is lost, histrionic patients become ex-patients.

Despite the preceding guideline, be willing to create an ex-patient instead of losing your therapeutic integrity.

Be prepared for a strong and stormy transference, especially if you are of the opposite gender from the patient.

Discuss the patient's feelings before exploring her rationales.

Attach names to inappropriate behaviors.

Avoid medications that create dependence, but actively treat depression, suicidal behavior, and psychosis.

Prepare to repeat what seems, to you, to be obvious until it becomes obvious to the patient.

Therapy involves a combination of supportive and insight-oriented elements, starting with the former. You may begin to treat such patients by placing them in a dependent role with respect to the therapist and then, almost paradoxically, supporting their self-expression and assertiveness (Perry and Vaillant 1989). Usually, the therapist is fortunate in being able to easily re-create a dependent relationship that can later be interpreted dynamically. This involves both overt and covert dependency as the patient experiences the therapist as a parental figure (Goldman 1956). To facilitate the early development of this dependency, you may sometimes find it helpful to make the patient feel special and offer a few "extras" to the therapy, such as extra time. However, you may feel strong countertransference anger at the patient's entitlements, lack of motivation, and exaggerated helplessness, which may blossom concurrently with the transference. Some therapists will be drained dry by the attention demanded, which (unlike the attention accorded borderline patients) is generally appreciated. However, this early attention nourishes the transference and the early supportive elements of treatment, such as encouraging the patient to overcome the anxiety of decision making and shoring up the patient's reactions to disappointments from his or her protector.

Eventually, the patient will have to be weaned from therapy toward autonomous function. The patient's quest for advice must be partially gratified but titrated with encouragement that the patient make his own decisions and your assurance that it is okay to be wrong. When you encourage the patient's assertiveness and experimentation with new methods of self-esteem development, relationships with peers should naturally supplant the unequal therapeutic dependency. As independence develops, more insight-oriented elements of treatment can be added, if needed, such as interpretation of the patient's ambivalence, anxiety at responsible assertion and decision making, anger, and use of reaction formation against his protector.

Tips for Managing a Therapeutic Process

To build and sustain a consistent therapeutic process with your patients suffering from a personality disorder, all members of the treatment team, including the patient, will be required to put forth some effort. You will find the following fundamentals helpful.

Treatment goals will need to be precisely outlined, with the roles and responsibilities of the patient and all treatment team members specified. Precise management of team members will be required. You should establish a clear description of treatment guidelines and emphasize the importance of adherence to those guidelines. These guidelines include the frequency and duration of treatment and all policies such as consent, treatment team attendance, and confidentiality. The arrangement of a consistent supportive therapeutic environment is crucial (Zweig and Agronin 2011).

Key Points

- Supportive psychotherapy of personality disorders begins with a stabilization of poor coping skills and socially impaired behaviors.

- Patients with personality disorders are often viewed as some of the most difficult to treat and are frequently labeled with derogatory terms such as "drama queen," "manipulative," "toxic to the milieu," or "hateful."

- A diagnosis of a personality disorder should be approached with caution in children and adolescents and deferred until early adulthood.

- The classification of personality disorders is moving from the cluster to the dimensional model.

- Several of the personality disorders (i.e., antisocial personality disorder, borderline personality disorder, narcissistic personality disorder) will require long-term therapy and/or specialized training.

- Supportive psychotherapy will be beneficial in stabilizing patients with personality disorders and to treat commonly co-occurring disorders.

References

Abracen J, Langton CM, Looman J, et al: Mental health diagnoses and recidivism in paroled offenders. Int J Offender Ther Comp Criminol 58(7):765–779, 2014 23640808

American Psychiatric Association: Diagnostic and Statistical Manual of Mental Disorders, 3rd Edition, Revised. Washington, DC, American Psychiatric Association, 1987

American Psychiatric Association: Diagnostic and Statistical Manual of Mental Disorders, 5th Edition. Arlington, VA, American Psychiatric Association, 2013

Avery JD, Barnhill JW: Personality disorders, in Co-occurring Mental Illness and Substance Use Disorders: A Guide to Diagnosis and Treatment. Edited by Avery JD, Barnhill JW. Arlington, VA, American Psychiatric Association Publishing, 2018, pp 83–92

Bressert S: Avoidant personality disorder. October 30, 2018a. Available at: https://psychcentral.com/disorders/avoidant-personality-disorder/. Accessed February 25, 2019.

Bressert S: Dependent personality disorder symptoms. October 24, 2018b. Available at: https://psychcentral.com/disorders/dependent-personality-disorder/symptoms/. Accessed February 25, 2019.

Bressert S: Obsessive-compulsive personality disorder treatment. October 24, 2018c. Available at: https://psychcentral.com/disorders/obsessive-compulsive-personality-disorder/treatment/. Accessed February 25, 2019.

Caligor E, Levy KN, Yeomans FE: Narcissistic personality disorder: diagnostic and clinical challenges. Am J Psychiatry 172(5):415–422, 2015 25930131

Caligor E, Yeomans FE, Clarkin JF, et al: Integrating supportive and exploratory interventions, in Psychodynamic Therapy for Personality Pathology: Treating Self and Interpersonal Functioning. Arlington, VA, American Psychiatric Publishing, 2018, pp 459–496

Clarkin JF, Levy KN, Lenzenweger MF, et al: Evaluating three treatments for borderline personality disorder: a multiwave study. Am J Psychiatry 164(6):922–928, 2007 17541052

Cleveland Clinic: Avoidant personality disorder. November 20, 2017. Available at: https://my.clevelandclinic.org/health/diseases/9761-avoidant-personality-disorder. Accessed February 25, 2019.

Drago A, Marogna C, Sogaard HJ: A review of characteristics and treatments of the avoidant personality disorder. Could the DBT be an option? International Journal of Psychology and Psychoanalysis 2(1):13, 2016

Eaton NR, Rodriguez-Seijas C, Krueger RF, et al: Narcissistic personality disorder and the structure of common mental disorders. J Pers Disord 31(4):449–461, 2017 27617650

Gever J: DSM-V draft promises big changes in some psychiatric diagnoses. February 10, 2010. Available at: https://www.medpagetoday.com/psychiatry/generalpsychiatry/18399. Accessed March 2, 2019.

Gibbon S, Duggan C, Stoffers J, et al: Psychological interventions for antisocial personality disorders. Cochrane Database Syst Rev 16(6):CD007668, 2010 20556783

Goldman GS: Reparative psychotherapy, in Changing Concepts of Psychoanalytical Medicine. Edited by Daniels RS. New York, Grune & Stratton, 1956, pp 101–113

Gunderson JG: Reducing suicide risk in borderline personality disorder. JAMA 314(2):181–182, 2015 26172897

Hoermann S, Zupanick CE, Dombeck M: Personality disorders summary and conclusion. Revised December 2013. Available at: https://www.mentalhelp.net/articles/the-treatment-of-personality-disorders/. Accessed February 25, 2019.

Hoermann S, Zupanick GE, Dombeck M: Personality disorders summary and conclusion. 2018. Available at: https://www.gulfbend.org/poc/view_doc.php?type=doc&id=41589&cn=8. Accessed March 3, 2018.

Hoermann S, Zupanick CE, Dombeck M: Alternative diagnostic models for personality disorders: the DSM-5 dimensional approach. 2019. Available at: https://www.mentalhelp.net/articles/alternative-diagnostic-models-for-personality-disorders-the-dsm-5-dimensional-approach/. Accessed March 1, 2019.

Jørgensen CR, Freund C, Bøye R, et al: Outcome of mentalization-based and supportive psychotherapy in patients with borderline personality disorder: a randomized study. Acta Psychiatr Scand 127(4):305–317, 2013 22897123

Kernberg OF: The differential diagnosis of antisocial behavior: a clinical approach, in Treatment of Severe Personality Disorders: Resolution of Aggression and Recovery of Eroticism. Arlington, VA, American Psychiatric Association Publishing, 2018, pp 197–211

Kool S, Dekker J, Duijsens IJ, et al: Changes in personality pathology after pharmacotherapy and combined therapy for depressed patients. J Pers Disord 17(1):60–72, 2003 12659547

Kramer D: Does treatment based on cognitive behavioral principles reduce recidivism risk in patients diagnosed with antisocial personality disorder? Master's thesis, Utrecht University, Utrecht, 2016. Available at: https://dspace.library.uu.nl/handle/1874/339335. Accessed February 25, 2019.

Lockwood W: Borderline personality disorder. 2017. Available at: https://www.rn.org/courses/coursematerial-125.pdf. Accessed February 26, 2019.

National Collaborating Centre for Mental Health: Antisocial personality disorder: the NICE guideline on treatment, management and prevention. 2010. Available at: https://www.nice.org.uk/guidance/cg77/evidence/full-guideline-242104429. Accessed February 25, 2019.

Out of the Fog: Histrionic personality disorder (HPD). 2019. Available at: http://outofthefog.website/personality-disorders-1/2015/12/6/histrionic-personality-disorder-hpd. Accessed February 26, 2019.

Perry JC, Vaillant GE: Personality disorders, in Comprehensive Textbook of Psychiatry, 5th Edition, Vol 2. Edited by Kaplan HI, Sadock BJ. Baltimore, MD, Williams & Wilkins, 1989, pp 1352–1387

Ritter S, Platt LM: What's new in treating inpatients with personality disorders? Dialectical behavior therapy and old-fashioned, good communication. J Psychosoc Nurs Ment Health Serv 54(1):38–45, 2016 26760134

Ronningstam E, Weinberg I: Narcissistic personality disorder: progress in recognition and treatment. Focus: The Journal of Lifelong Learning in Psychiatry 11:167–177, 2013

SAPA Project Test: Personality disorders. March 2001. Available at: http://www.personalityresearch.org/pd.html. Accessed March 5, 2019.

Skodol A: Expert Q & A: personality disorder. 2018. Available at: https://www.psychiatry.org/patients-families/personality-disorders/expert-q-and-a. Accessed February 26, 2019.

Skodol AE, Bender DS, Gunderson JG, et al: Personality disorders, in The American Psychiatric Publishing Textbook of Psychiatry, 6th Edition. Edited by Hales RE, Yudofsky SC, Roberts LW. Washington, DC, American Psychiatric Publishing, 2014, pp 851–894

Vyas A, Khan M: Case report: paranoid personality disorder. The American Journal of Psychiatry Residents' Journal 11:9–11, 2016

Widiger TA: Dimensional models of personality disorder. World Psychiatry 6(2):79–83, 2007 18235857

Winston A, Rosenthal RN, Pinsker H: Applicability to special populations, in Learning Supportive Psychotherapy: An Illustrated Guide. Washington, DC, American Psychiatric Association, 2012, pp 143–162

Zweig RA, Agronin ME: Personality disorders in late life, in Principles and Practice of Geriatric Psychiatry, 2nd Edition. Edited by Agronin ME, Maletta GJ. Philadelphia, PA, Wolters Kluwer Health/Lippincott Williams & Wilkins, 2011, pp 523–543

11

Crisis Management and Suicidality

The term *crisis* is a systems concept, aptly illustrated in our use of terms like *military crisis, economic crisis, hypoglycemic crisis,* and *crisis of faith.* A *psychological crisis* may be defined as an unstable situation with uncertain outcome in which an individual's coping capacity is temporarily overwhelmed. Such crises may be generated by external events or intrinsic processes, or by a combination. Many will resolve favorably without intervention. However, because a psychological crisis embodies a high risk of adverse outcome, a short period of therapy is often beneficial. It is advantageous for therapists to have a solid understanding of the approaches and methods of crisis practice. Additionally, therapists will need to develop a compassionate and empathic perspective of the individual in crisis.

Overview of Supportive Therapy for Individuals in Crisis

We believe that supportive treatment is indicated for nearly all persons in crisis. Although it is true that previously healthy people can usually tolerate the additional stress of confrontational interpretations and therapeutic style, supportive therapy is appropriate for them because it increases the time for individuals to process the crisis and enables them to readapt using their own resources. Those in crisis are also unlikely to be made dependent by brief periods of support. Despite the risk of creating dependency on the therapist, supportive therapy is obviously also indicated for previously vulnerable and psychologically impaired people, because in the short term they are at greater risk of decompensation with defense-weakening approaches. We shall use the term *crisis intervention* to refer to this supportive mode of treatment.

Crisis resolution is often conducted as a team effort involving various providers and decision-makers. However, let us approach it from the standpoint of a therapist who is called upon to see a patient individually. Usually, this occurs after an initial assessment has established that there is a crisis warranting further treatment. The first meeting with the therapist may take place the day after a no-admit decision is made in a general hospital emergency room, or after a telephone self-referral during which the therapist has gotten a brief idea of the patient's condition. Other modalities of treatment, such as hospitalization, crisis groups, or family therapy, may have been considered already or may be assigned as necessary.

Unlike the intake of a patient who has been waiting some time to begin long-term individual therapy, the first interview in crisis must be telescoped for both assessment and therapeutic purposes. Thus, this first interview shares many characteristics with the second interview in long-term therapy, concentrating less on a detailed reconstruction of the patient's history and more on talking comfortably about the here-and-now issues that have brought the patient to therapy. Possibly the patient will continue with long-term therapy, but there is no guarantee. Because most crises are self-limited, the patient may not even return for a second meeting.

As noted by Roberts and Ottens (2005), it is critical in the beginning to establish rapport while assessing lethality and discovering the triggering events. Furthermore, it is important to identify the main presenting problem and mutually agree on short-term goals. Roberts and Ottens reiterate that crisis intervention therapy includes identifying failed coping skills and then helping the individual to replace them with adaptive coping skills

Each session in brief supportive crisis therapy can be thought of as a movement in a symphony. Each needs its own structure and some closure; at the same time, some themes should be introduced that will be taken up in later sessions. The musical listener may not know what he is about to hear, but he usually expects to learn in advance a few things, such as the composer, the key, and the number of movements. Likewise, the therapist should provide the patient with some advance structure.

The patient is also a collaborator and not a totally passive listener in this composition; she should usually be allowed to talk freely and introduce the themes for 10 or 15 minutes. The therapist should follow the rule of "listen more at first and talk more at last," an approach based on empirical studies of success in crisis-resolution interviews (Rusk and Gerner 1972). This is because the patient comes to the therapist with dual expectations of finding someone who will listen and someone who will help. Sometimes, listening alone appears to provide relief. Usually, the therapist will actively provide some relief in the first session and work on developing a future that provides hope.

History and Development
of Time-Limited Crisis Support

Programs of crisis support, although they may transition into long-term therapy, are themselves time-limited. However, crisis intervention differs considerably from brief psychotherapy. For example, patients are carefully selected for the latter by their suitability for interpretive work, but patients will seek treatment on their own for the former because of immediate need.

The principles of crisis support were first developed by Erich Lindemann in the aftermath of the 1942 Cocoanut Grove nightclub fire, which killed 492 people (Lindemann 1944). Lindemann's work was primarily concerned with bereaved patients, both those with and those without preexisting psychiatric illness.

Another psychiatrist considered to be a founder of crisis intervention is Gerald Caplan, who augmented Lindemann's crisis theory and described and documented the four stages of a crisis reaction: rise of tension from the crisis, increased disruption of daily living, rapid increase in tension with the failure to resolve the crisis, and a point at which the individual goes into a depressed state or may partially resolve the crisis by using new coping methods (Roberts and Ottens 2005).

MacDonald (2016) recognizes the importance of Caplan and Lindemann's pioneering work in the development of crisis intervention but maintains it is not sufficient for describing present-day mental health crises that may evolve with no single triggering event or preexisting mental health issues. MacDonald discusses the three domains of crises that are relevant for today's therapists as follows. First is the developmental crisis, which is the result of an ordinary life occurrence like a pregnancy or graduation. While these may be routine happenings, they may need monitoring to safeguard the individual's return to his or her previous level of functioning. The second domain is a situational crisis. This is the most common form of crisis you are likely to encounter. Examples of situational crises include rape, sudden death of a loved one, grief, and a motor vehicle accident. The third domain—existential crisis—is common when an individual reaches a milestone birthday such as age 30, 40, or 50 and begins to question if his life has meaning, purpose, or value.

Current crisis intervention strategies have been expanded from Caplan and Lindemann. Roberts and Ottens (2005) describe the seven-stage crisis intervention model as follows:

1. Plan and conduct a thorough biopsychosocial and lethality/imminent danger assessment;
2. Make psychological contact and rapidly establish the collaborative relationship;
3. Identify the major problems, including crisis precipitants;
4. Encourage an exploration of feelings and emotions;
5. Generate and explore alternatives and new coping strategies;
6. Restore functioning through implementation of an action plan;
7. Plan follow-up and booster sessions.

The Supportive Therapy Patient in Crisis

Crisis for the patient in supportive therapy often means the further breakdown of coping abilities in a person with already weakened skills. The patient may react, as any other person would, with anxiety or panic and regression as more mature defenses are lost. However, crisis also can represent the loss of a job or community placement that has taken months or years to achieve, contributing to the patient's distorted belief that he is incapable of making it in the community. This is an example of a person in an existential crisis. As in the formerly high-functioning patient, crisis may represent the obvious actions of environmental stressors or mental illness, but a new possibility is added: the crisis may be primarily a result of the therapy. Even when the therapy has been going well, the patient may blame the therapist for the decompensation.

As the therapist, you must undertake the task, often left untouched by hospitalization, of learning from the experience and strengthening the patient against future crises. Because previous hospitalizations may have provided the patient relief, the patient may also view the crisis as a respite from family stress that will place her in the cocoon of an intensively supportive environment.

To the extent that interchange of information is legally permissible, the therapist ought to assist other providers in giving the patient the best possible care in the least restrictive setting. While you cannot and should not make decisions for the other providers, you should provide them with the kind of information on which such decisions are based. Knowing the patient better than any other care providers, you may feel obliged to take the awkward position of arguing for or against hospitalization. When you are making such arguments, it helps to have objective measures (e.g., palpable examples of disturbances of behavior in the home), as opposed to therapeutic impressions that are difficult for someone who does not know the patient personally to evaluate.

While some disturbances are absolute indications for intensive measures and/or hospitalization (e.g., assault or suicide attempt with a lethal weapon), the change from baseline behavior is also important. Some patients hallucinate frequently, while others will use alcohol or drugs regularly. A new therapist meeting such a patient is sometimes inclined to hospitalize him on the spot but may decide not to when the previous therapist calls up and explains that the patient has been functioning quite well despite the symptoms. Obviously, a major change in mood or loss of judgment, the appearance of command hallucinations that the patient has trouble resisting, or an escalation of substance abuse is relevant to emergency disposition. Previous physical and neurological findings as well as current medications may need reconsideration; for example, subjective and motor restlessness may be caused by akathisia, a side effect of high-potency antipsychotic medications that has been linked to suicide.

Another reason for this interface with other professionals is to learn what (if anything) has gone wrong with the therapeutic relationship. Like consultants, emergency personnel can provide fresh observations or perspective on the treatment. On some occasions, it may also be important to discuss the opinion of emergency personnel that the therapist has been handling the patient badly—an impression that is sometimes conveyed to the patient.

Sometimes patients deliberately seek other sources of help even when the therapist is readily available. These occurrences merit special attention. The patient, although not in genuine crisis, may appeal for crisis support elsewhere to emphasize her distress to therapist or family. This type of pseudo-emergency can unfortunately escalate into a genuine emergency when a determined patient feels she is not being taken seriously. Birk and Birk (1984) acknowledge that it is indeed a challenge to assist persons in crisis in managing the crisis and protect them from undue risk without encouraging dependency on the therapist.

Regardless of whether the crisis is genuine, the therapist should consider the following possibilities: You may have mistakenly rebuffed the patient's request for help or decided it was not serious. Rage or anxiety may have been precipitated by threat of loss, such as your announcement of vacation or termination, leading the patient to seek reassurance elsewhere that someone will continue to care for him. To most patients, crisis is a sign of failure that they may not wish to tell you about. Patients may blame either themselves or their therapists for it. The crisis may have been created from an obvious therapeutic error (e.g., a critical or sadistic remark), or the crisis may have resulted from an unaddressed psychodynamic change (e.g., development of a psychotic transference).

Because some patients cannot tolerate excessive closeness with one person (usually their therapist), it may be beneficial for them to have other providers to turn to briefly. Such patients may be intuitively "diluting" their personal transference to the therapist by seeking out the impersonal institutional transference to a psychiatric emergency room, which also suggests that they would benefit from outpatient services provided by *different* therapists on successive visits. One way of finding this out is to let someone else do the crisis therapy and share observations later. In any case, when the patient returns to the first therapist, the two should discuss the evolution of the crisis and the proper use of the therapist for support, such as availability for telephone calls or unscheduled sessions.

Suicide

Statistics

Firearms are used in nearly 50% of all suicides. In 2015 the total number of deaths by suicide with the use of a firearm was 22,018. The total number of deaths by suicide this same year, 44,193, is more than the capacity of the Philadelphia Phillies' home stadium. The National Suicide Prevention Lifeline receives more than 1 million calls for help each year. In the weeks after a call, less than one-quarter of the callers are seen by a behavior health provider (Substance Abuse and Mental Health Services Administration News Letter 2014).

Most suicide victims will have seen a primary care physician rather than a mental health clinician prior to their death. As many as 45% of those who died from suicide were seen by a primary care physician in the month before their death, whereas only 20% were seen by a mental health professional (Luoma et al. 2002).

These statistics are clearly an indication that clinicians should be aware of suicide and of the need to assess every patient for suicidality and to educate as many people as possible, including primary care providers. Additionally, it is evident that there is a need for collaborative care with these fragile and vulnerable individuals.

Predicting Suicidality

Scores of studies have attempted to determine predictive factors that would justify the employment of suicide-preventing measures in a vulnerable patient, and many researchers have developed rating scales to assess imminent suicide potential. Unfortunately, there is still no reliable way to predict long-term suicide potential in an individual patient. The ability to predict whether an individual will commit suicide has not improved over the past 50 years according to an exhaustive analysis of suicide research (Franklin et al. 2017). As Joseph Franklin of Harvard University, the lead author of the study, notes:

> Our analyses showed that science could only predict future suicidal thoughts and behaviors about as well as random guessing. In other words, a suicide expert who conducted an in-depth assessment of risk factors would predict a patient's future suicidal thoughts and behaviors with the same degree of accuracy as someone with no knowledge of the patient who predicted based on a coin flip...This was extremely humbling—after decades of research, science had produced no meaningful advances in suicide prediction. (quoted in Sliwa 2016)

Franklin cautions that the findings of the study do not invalidate the risk guidelines and recommends these guidelines remain in use. However, he asserts that there is an urgent need to evaluate these guidelines within longitudinal studies (Sliwa 2016).

Suicide Risk Factors and Warning Signs

It is important to understand the difference between warning signs and risk factors. Warning signs are specific symptoms or behaviors, such as feelings of hopelessness, social isolation, and substance use, and can be addressed with interventions. Warning signs signify an immediate risk of suicide and are unique to an individual, whereas risk factors are found in individuals and groups/demographics. Risk factors are not modifiable and include factors such as being a white male, having previously attempted suicide, and having a family history of suicide (American Foundation for Suicide Prevention 2019; Suicide Prevention Resource Center 2017).

There is no single cause for suicide—it occurs when stressors exceed the coping skills of an individual who is suffering from a mental health condition. Depression is the most common disorder associated with suicide. Most people who take their lives will present with warning signs (American Foundation for Suicide Prevention 2019). Table 11–1 lists risk factors and warning signs of suicide. For further reading on risk factors in relation to method of suicide, age group, gender, and other demographics, refer to the article by O'Neill et al. (2018).

It is crucial for all mental health clinicians to recognize the difference between risk factors and warning signs. It is equally important for clinicians to speak of these factors. Talking about warning signs will assist family and friends in knowing what actions can be taken to help someone who is a current suicide risk. Educating about risk factors will help those in the community to understand what changes may be needed to decrease suicide risks (Suicide Prevention Resource Center 2017).

Supportive Psychotherapy for the Potentially Suicidal Patient

Supportive psychotherapy for the potentially suicidal patient must, first and foremost, address the signs and symptoms, such as depressive affect or illogical

Table 11–1.   Risk factors and warning signs of suicide

Risk factors

Recent discharge (within 1 month) from an inpatient setting

First 6 months in the treatment of depression

First few years after diagnosis of a schizophrenic illness

Prior suicide attempt

Family history of suicide

Mood disorders

Personality disorders

Access to lethal means

White male

Warning signs

Speaks of being a burden to others

Speaks of feeling trapped

States there is no reason to live

Is experiencing unbearable physical pain

Speaks of killing self

Increases use of substances

Isolates from others

Gives away prized possessions

Conducts online searches for a way to kill self

thinking, that can lead to suicide and, if possible, treat the underlying psychiatric or social disorder, such as depression, substance abuse, or family discord. Even with the most isolated patients, there will be other sources of care, and you must clarify who is responsible for monitoring symptoms and taking action. One or more of these responsible agents must have the power to hospitalize the patient. It should be made clear who is responsible in the absence of the primary psychiatrist or therapist, and this secondary caregiver should be able to see the patient rather than simply be available. The roles of others in the patient's environment should be clarified, such as by designating a relative who is responsible for removing potentially lethal medications. The patient and significant others should therefore have a clear idea of the procedures to follow when help is needed outside the therapy sessions. However, when contacting significant others, you must clarify in advance what is being communicated and why, so that the patient does not feel betrayed. If suicide or dangerous suicidal gestures are likely, hospitalization is usually indicated. The more acute the suicidality, the more pressing is the indication. That is, there is some tendency to avoid hospitalization in those patients whose suicidality is chronic and unchanging. A supportive therapeutic agenda that, within this context of a properly structured setting, should help reduce any future risks is listed in Table 11–2.

Suicide Prevention and No-Harm Contracts

It is helpful in planning interventions to determine the patient's motives. You should strive to achieve empathy with the patient's feelings to the maximum degree practical, since a patient can be moved nearer to suicide by feeling that her hopelessness is beyond what anyone else can understand. The patient's specific motives then provide a basis for symptom-directed therapy. For example, the therapist might show that there is no "need" for suicide or suicidal gestures by discussing other means of obtaining the same goals. This may require some advocacy outside the session, such as obtaining pain medication from the physician treating the patient's cancer or assisting the patient in obtaining Social Security payments. The downgrading of unattainable life goals in the young person with schizophrenia, the patient recovering from depression, or the person with early dementia is another frequent need.

One noticeable omission from the above is no-harm contracts, which many therapists, including the authors of this text, feel are more frequently than not expedient substitutes for the therapist's time instead of adjuncts to effective psychotherapy. In the past, no-harm contracts, known by many names, including contracts for safety and no-suicide contracts, were very common, with as many as 70% of psychiatrists and 80% of psychologists using this tool (Joiner et al. 2009). In lieu of no-harm contracts, the recommendation is to use *safety*

Table 11–2. Therapeutic agenda for the suicidal or previously suicidal patient

Treat the symptoms and underlying psychiatric disorder, if possible.

Even if the patient does not address them, ask questions about suicidal thoughts, including

- The most recent suicide attempt.

- Past history of suicidal thoughts and actions.

- Family history of suicide (some patients may feel they are playing a family role attempting suicide).

- Key anniversaries, such as death of a spouse, and the feeling that suicide will lead to reunion.

Elicit the motives and use them in therapy.

Explore the meaning of death, suicide, and its outcome fantasies (i.e., how others are expected to react).

Address the patient's tendency to "solve" problems through substantive actions.

Clarify recent losses, including therapy losses, such as resignation from the clinic of someone important to the patient.

Minimize the presence of agents of suicide (i.e., firearms, medications, etc.) and disinhibiting/depressive agents (i.e., alcohol and drugs).

Attempt to provide missing elements of social support (i.e., employment, family ties).

If prescribing medications:

Avoid refills and lethal total dosages.

Know the treatment of overdoses of the medications in use.

Clarify necessary absences well in advance whenever possible and explain to patients that they will be seen by another therapist—that is, they are to keep the appointment.

Strive to know the meaning of a suicide attempt so that you can attempt to find substitutes for it.

plans, also called *crisis plans.* Joiner et al. (2009) refer to this intervention as a part of "Commitment to Treatment Statements." An example of such a statement can be found in the article by Rudd et al. (2006) that compares the two interventions.

The safety plan differs from the no-harm contract in that the former places a priority on what a person *will do.* For example, the safety plan includes relaxation techniques; physical activity to reduce stress; access to support systems, including family members and the therapist; and emergency phone numbers. It is important to note that although safety plans are the recommended intervention for the prevention of suicide, only anecdotal evidence exists regarding their success in reducing suicide risk (Kirkwood and Bennett 2017). Additionally, there is no legal protection for clinicians with the use of a no-harm contract, and there is no one standard form for such a contract (Kroll 2000). Clearly, there is a need for further research regarding interventions in the prevention of suicide.

September 10 is World Suicide Prevention Day. The purpose of this observance is to encourage worldwide movement to prevent suicides with various activities to raise awareness that suicide is preventable. Despite the progress in suicide prevention, obstacles remain. Additionally, there is debate regarding the legitimacy of preventing suicide (Arensman 2017; De Leo 2002; World Health Organization 2010). There will be multiple opportunities for you to be involved in this worldwide movement, and the references noted at the end of this chapter provide ideas for involvement both locally and globally.

Supportive Therapy After a Suicide Attempt

Supportive psychotherapy for your patient who has attempted suicide is imperative. A psychological assessment should be completed as soon as possible after the incident so your patient can relate the most detailed account of the progression of events leading to the suicide attempt. The essential features of intervention after an attempted suicide are an early therapeutic alliance, narrative interviewing, psychoeducation, and collocation with other personal and safety planning (Michel et al. 2017).

A common reaction of the patient who has attempted suicide is shame. The feelings of shame may coexist with an impulse to hide or leave the hospital, and a fear of seeking help. The feelings of shame experienced by the patient can be relieved if you approach the patient in a kind, respectful, and nonjudgmental manner. Being mindful of the possible shame reaction after a failed attempt will allow you to interact with your patient in a way that could make it easier for her to accept and benefit from therapy after a suicide attempt (Wiklander et al. 2003).

Supporting Those Left Behind by Suicide

The loss of a loved one to suicide could result in feelings of guilt, shame, confusion, anger, and sadness for those left behind. According to Schneidman (1969), for every successful suicide there will be six survivors who suffer with significant grief. Supportive psychotherapy for the loved ones left behind will be critical.

One group of survivors that is far too often overlooked is siblings, who are referred to as "the forgotten mourners." As many as 25,000 people each year will become sibling survivors of suicide. Those who lose a sibling to suicide can suffer from depression, posttraumatic stress disorder, and thoughts of taking their own lives (Sibling Survivors 2014; Weinstock 2017). A study in the United Kingdom revealed that 6% of bereaved young people had attempted suicide, and 67% of these individuals had not sought help. Of those who did seek help, the most common source was a general practitioner. Twenty percent received no mental health support. Additionally, in this study, people bereaved by suicide received less support than those bereaved by other causes of sudden death (Pitman et al. 2017). Supportive psychotherapy will be advantageous to guide the siblings through this traumatic, life-changing, and overwhelming crisis.

Clinicians who treat those at risk for suicide are subject to losing a patient to suicide. In 1997 the Clinician Survivors Task Force was developed, under the auspices of the American Association of Suicidology, to provide mental health clinicians with a support system for their loss. It is estimated that as many as one in five therapists and as many as one in two psychiatrists will lose a patient to suicide. The personal emotional reactions of a mental health provider are not that different from those of family members: shock, grief, and disbelief. Professionally, the clinicians involved in care may question what they may have missed, what they should have done, or why they did not do more when their patient was hospitalized. In some cases, the loss of a patient by suicide may be so devastating to the clinician that it ends his or her career in the mental health field (American Association of Suicidology 2012).

The range of emotions experienced by the mental health professional with the loss of a patient by suicide must be addressed. Gitlin (1999) suggests three methods of coping with a patient's suicide. First, decrease the sense of isolation by speaking to trusted friends, family members, colleagues, or one's own therapist. In some cases, meeting with and grieving with the family members of the patient will be beneficial. Second, make efforts at reparative, constructive behavior. This may be accomplished by helping others cope with similar experiences— for example, present a case at grand rounds or write a case report. Third, use specific cognitive defenses. These could include understanding that the suicide of a patient is an occupational hazard for mental health clinicians and that there is no way to predict suicide for any individual.

Bereavement, Grief, and Mourning

Bereavement, the meaning of which is derived from an Old English word meaning "to rob," is a common and unavoidable reaction to the death of a loved one, but it often creates a crisis that requires professional support. Although definitions vary, bereavement may be divided further into its intrapersonal component, *grief,* and its social expression, *mourning* (Dubin and Weiss 1987).

According to Sadock and Sadock (2003), grief is the subjective feeling brought about by the death of a loved one, and the term is used interchangeably with *mourning*. However, mourning is the process by which grief is resolved. The expression of grief includes a wide range of emotions that is dependent on cultural norms and on the circumstances of the loss (e.g., sudden death in contrast to one that is anticipated).

Survivors normally react with depression to the death of a loved one in the process of uncomplicated bereavement, which can take a year or more to resolve. The wish to be dead is often present, but not a specific suicidal plan. Survivors may focus on things they could have done to save the deceased person, ways in which they mistreated the deceased, or simply the difficulty of living without the deceased. Somatic symptoms (e.g., anorexia, insomnia) of the kind found in a major depressive disorder are often present, but more severe symptoms suggest a major depressive disorder and a pathological grief reaction.

An eclectic supportive agenda for dealing with the immediate consequences of grief is presented in Table 11–3.

Case Vignette

Ms. Carson, a 31-year-old patient with a well-controlled schizoaffective disorder, a history of limited-symptom panic attacks, and obvious dependent personality traits, has lived for 6 years with Mr. Miller, 10 years her senior, in a relationship that was stable and provided many satisfactions. Mr. Miller had always had a seizure disorder, but one day Ms. Carson got a call from the hospital and learned that Mr. Miller had had a seizure at work and died. She immediately called her case manager. The case manager talked to her at length on the phone and had her come in immediately for counseling. The following day, Ms. Carson's therapist arranged to see her every few days for the next week. Ms. Carson also met with the other people in the clinic who knew her well so that they could express their condolences and also so that she would be comfortable mourning in their presence. This included the other patients who shared the afternoon clinic with her. Ms. Carson was assured that someone would be available every day to talk to if she needed it.

In therapy, the therapist listened for the themes of Ms. Carson's crisis. There was her sense of loss at Mr. Miller's unexpected death. However, the therapist also sensed that Ms. Carson's concern about her own problems was actually more importante. She had been reliant on Mr. Miller's income to pay the rent, and they had no savings. Mr. Miller had an insurance policy, but Ms. Carson was not legally married to him. Now she was angry that they had never gotten married. The therapist noted how long their relationship had been and how it seemed reasonable to expect part of the insurance, because "he [Mr. Miller] would have wanted it that way." Negotiations were arranged with Mr. Miller's family to see if they would give part of the insurance to Ms. Carson. They did. The loss of Mr. Miller was approached now as an opportunity for Ms. Carson's growth. She could expand her hours in the clinic's work program and interview potential roommates referred by the clinic. At first, she was reluctant to take on the additional work. The case manager offered to visit her at work if any problems arose, but this was not necessary. Within 6 weeks, she had made a significant adjustment to her bereavement and was back to her biweekly schedule of therapy.

This vignette illustrates many points. The preexistence of an institutional transference was useful in providing multiple sources of support without increasing the patient's dependency on any one provider; this was especially important because the patient had a long history of dependent behavior. Informal group sup-

Table 11–3.   Supportive agenda for grief

Ventilation (except in chronic grief): avoid stereotyped reassurances

Review of the circumstances surrounding the death

Acceptance of patient's unrealistic attitudes in the immediate aftermath of grief (e.g., self-reproach, identification phenomena, yearning for return)

Assistance in current activities that patient is truly unable to perform

Assistance in developing new relationships

Medication (when necessary)

Improvement of patient's defenses and shoring up of vulnerabilities

Encouragement of rituals of mourning

Placement in extended context[a]

Addressing patient's anger toward deceased and desires for revenge, if present

[a]Examination from philosophical, religious, and social perspectives; outside biographical readings may help; support groups are sometimes useful but may encourage chronic grief.

port was available in the clinic setting. The crisis was also *reframed* as an opportunity for growth, change, and further steps toward independence. The clinic team worked together and made adaptations to assist the patient, which is not unusual with someone like Ms. Carson, who was well liked to begin with. However, the total additional time was not excessive, and it was offered during regular clinic hours. Perhaps the time with some other patients was shortened because of Ms. Carson's crisis. Such adjustments are both possible and appropriate in a public mental health setting that provides supportive therapy to many patients.

A final psychodynamic point is worth noting. Perhaps Ms. Carson's grief was more shallow than expected because of her own psychiatric problems. But often the opposite occurs, and a chronically ill psychiatric patient is devastated by a major loss (especially of one's mother). In this case, however, the therapist was aware that it would be unwise to make Ms. Carson feel obligated to grieve too much.

Unresolved Grief and Bereavement

Whether or not the patient, like Ms. Carson, has a preexisting psychiatric disorder, long-term psychotherapy is often necessary to deal with unresolved issues. Although Lindemann (1944) implied that normal bereavement was usually resolved in a few months, further observations on the process, such as Zisook et al.'s (1985) study of unresolved grief, substantiate that grief may become chronic, inhibited, or delayed, and that even "normal" grief may take years to resolve. Various predictors of difficulties have been offered. In a classic study, Parkes (1965) found that "self-blame" and "difficulty in accepting the fact of loss" were present more frequently in bereaved patients who presented to psychiatric clinics as opposed to those persons located at home. Failure to progress through the appropriate stages, the sudden death of the deceased, and the close relationship of the lost person are useful guidelines in predicting future difficulties. Long-term therapy will often be required to reach the cognitive and affective completion mentioned above. Psychiatric symptoms such as depression and somatization may also require treatment.

Counseling the bereaved patient who is already in supportive psychotherapy requires an additional understanding of the interaction of the patient's psychiatric problems with the grief reaction. Ambivalence toward the "lost object" is especially evident in patients with schizophrenia. Some will have difficulty grieving because of this. On the other hand, patients who were essentially not invested in the lost person may not need to grieve, and there is no point in getting them to do so. The major problem in many dependent patients—as Lindemann, in his original formulation, notes— may be the loss of behaviors that were sustained by the deceased person. Additional social support will be necessary to "replace" the lost person and prevent regression.

Bereavement and the Loss of a Child

Research on bereavement and the loss of a child is scarce. Most research on bereavement has been centered on the loss of a spouse. Hendrickson (2009) notes that the literature that does exist shows conflicting data and evidence supporting that parents who are grieving the loss of young children are at increased risk for suicide.

The death of a child is the most devastating and overwhelming loss a person could ever suffer. This heartbreak is like no other, and parental grief differs from grief over other losses in that it is intensified, exaggerated, and lengthened. The death of a baby who dies from sudden unexplained infant death (SUID) poses grieving components that are without equal. Parents are left to cope with an unexpected and unexplained death, no time for good-byes, and no anticipatory grief. Often, the parents are young and are experiencing a death for the first time (Anastasi 2011).

SUID usually occurs before the age of 1 year and is the most frequent cause of death after the first month of life. Parents will struggle with guilt, wondering if the death could have been prevented. Anger and irritability are common and can be directed to family members, health professionals, and God. It is not uncommon to experience low self-esteem, self-blame, and depression (Christ et al. 2003).

Two peer support groups for parents who lose a child and their families are The Compassionate Friends (www.compassionatefriends.org) and Bereaved Parents of the USA (www.bereavedparentsusa.org).

Key Points

- Supportive psychotherapy is an effective crisis intervention and is even more effective when there is collaboration with other disciplines.

- Although crisis intervention is time-limited, it may transition into long-term therapy.

- Developmental, situational, and existential are the three domains of crises the therapist may encounter with his or her patients.

- The therapist will be faced with the task of helping the patient to learn from the crisis and strengthen his or her coping skills for any future crisis.

- There is no way to predict suicide, and losing a patient to suicide will be the most difficult situation to deal with in a mental health career.

- The statistics on suicide are staggering, and the fact that as many as 20% of those who died from suicide had been seen by a mental health professional 1 month prior to their death is a clear indication of the need to assess every patient for suicidality.

- There is no one single cause for suicide. However, in most cases, the patient at risk for suicide will present with warning signs.

- It is important to know the difference between warning signs and risk factors.

- An occupational hazard for the mental health professional is the suicide of a patient.

- Few resources are available for clinicians who lose a patient to suicide, and it is imperative for clinicians to seek out others to process the complex emotions associated with this loss.

- Supportive psychotherapy will be beneficial for bereaved patients who may also present with depression and anger.

- An assessment after a suicide attempt should be performed as soon as possible, with the fundamental goal being to determine the risk of further self-harm.

- The emotional impact of the death of a child from sudden unexplained infant death is overwhelming, and limited literature is available to clinicians on the subject.

References

American Association of Suicidology: Clinicians as survivors of suicide: basic information. February 28, 2012. Available at: http://pages.iu.edu/~jmcintos/basicinfo.htm. Accessed February 26, 2019.

American Foundation for Suicide Prevention: Risk factors and warning signs. 2019. Available at: https://afsp.org/about-suicide/risk-factors-and-warning-signs. Accessed February 26, 2019.

Anastasi JM (ed): The death of a child, the grief of the parents: a lifetime journey, 3rd edition. National Sudden and Unexpected Infant/Child Death and Pregnancy Loss Resource Center at Georgetown University. 2011. Available at: https://www.ncemch.org/suid-sids/documents/SIDRC/LifetimeJourney.pdf. Accessed February 26, 2019.

Arensman E: Suicide prevention in an international context. Crisis 38(1):1–6, 2017 28256167

Birk L, Birk AW: Managing emergencies in the practice of psychotherapy, in Emergency Psychiatry: Concepts, Methods, and Practices. Edited by Bassuk EL, Birk AW. New York, Plenum, 1984, pp 373–382

Christ GH, Bonanno G, Malkinson R, et al: Appendix E: Bereavement experiences after the death of a child, in When Children Die: Improving Palliative and End-of-Life Care for Children and Their Families. Edited by Institute of Medicine (US) Committee on Palliative and End-Of-Life Care for Children and Their Families; Field MJ, Behrman RE. Washington, DC, National Academies Press, 2003, pp 201–212. Available at: https://www.ncbi.nlm.nih.gov/books/NBK220798/. Accessed February 26, 2019.

De Leo D: Why are we not getting any closer to preventing suicide? Br J Psychiatry 181:372–374, 2002 12411260

Dubin WR, Weiss KJ: Emergency psychiatry, in Psychiatry, Revised Edition, Vol 2. Edited by Michaels R, Cavenar JO, Cooper AM. Philadelphia, PA, Lippincott, 1987, pp 201–212

Franklin JC, Ribeiro JD, Fox KR, et al: Risk factors for suicidal thoughts and behaviors: a meta-analysis of 50 years of research. Psychol Bull 143(2):187–232, 2017 27841450

Gitlin MJ: A psychiatrist's reaction to a patient's suicide. Am J Psychiatry 156(10):1630–1634, 1999 10518176

Hendrickson KC: Morbidity, mortality, and parental grief: a review of the literature on the relationship between the death of a child and the subsequent health of parents. Palliat Support Care 7(1):109–119, 2009 19619380

Joiner TE Jr, Van Orden KA, Witte TK, et al: Commitment for treatment statements (CTS) instead of no harm contracts, in The Interpersonal Theory of Suicide: Guidance for Working With Suicidal Clients. Washington, DC, American Psychological Association, 2009, pp 92–93

Kirkwood A, Bennett L: The shift from "no harm contracts" to "safety plans" for suicide prevention and treatment: a literature review. 2017. Available at: https://www.bcbe.org/cms/lib08/AL01901374/Centricity/domain/121/suicide%20prevention/SSAFETY%20PLANS%20FOR%20final%20.pdf.pdf. Accessed February 26, 2019.

Kroll J: Use of no-suicide contracts by psychiatrists in Minnesota. Am J Psychiatry 157(10):1684–1686, 2000 11007726

Lindemann E: Symptomatology and management of acute grief. Am J Psychiatry 101:141–148, 1944

Luoma JB, Martin CE, Pearson JL: Contact with mental health and primary care providers before suicide: a review of the evidence. Am J Psychiatry 159(6):909–916, 2002 12042175

MacDonald DK: Crisis theory and types of crisis. June 2016. Available at: http://dustinkmacdonald.com/crisis-theory-types-crisis/. Accessed February 26, 2019.

Michel K, Valach L, Gysin-Mallart A: A novel therapy for people who attempt suicide and why we need new models of suicide. Int J Environ Res Public Health 14(3):E243, 2017 28257071

O'Neill S, Ennis E, Bunting B: Factors associated with suicide in four age groups: a population-based study. Arch Suicide Res 22(1):128–138, 2018 28166461

Parkes CM: Bereavement and mental illness, Part 1: a clinical study of the grief of bereaved psychiatric patients. Br J Med Psychol 38:1–12, 1965 14300775

Pitman AL, Rantell K, Morgan P, et al: Support received after bereavement by suicide and other sudden deaths: a cross-sectional UK study of 3432 young bereaved adults. BMJ Open 7(5):e014487, 2017 28554915

Roberts AR, Ottens AJZ: The seven-stage crisis intervention model: a road map to goal attainment, problem solving, and crisis resolution. Brief Treatment and Crisis Intervention 5:329–339, 2005

Rudd MD, Mandrusiak M, Joiner TE Jr: The case against no-suicide contracts: the commitment to treatment statement as a practice alternative. J Clin Psychol 62(2):243–251, 2006 16342293

Rusk TN, Gerner RH: A study of the process of emergency psychotherapy. Am J Psychiatry 128(7):882–886, 1972 5009269

Sadock BJ, Sadock VA: Human development throughout the life cycle, in Kaplan and Sadock's Synopsis of Psychiatry: Behavioral Sciences/Clinical Psychiatry, 9th Edition. Edited by Sadock BJ, Sadock VA. Philadelphia, PA, Lippincott Williams & Wilkins, 2003, pp 16–65

Schneidman ES (ed): On the Nature of Suicide. San Francisco, CA, Jossey-Bass, 1969

Sibling Survivors: Sibling grief. 2014. Available at: http://www.siblingsurvivors.com/sibling-grief. Accessed February 26, 2019.

Sliwa J: After decades of research, science is no better able to predict suicidal behaviors. November 15, 2016. Available at: http://www.apa.org/news/press/releases/2016/11/suicidal-behaviors.aspx. Accessed February 26, 2019.

Substance Abuse and Mental Health Services Administration News Letter: Preventing suicide: following up after the crisis. 2014. Available at: https://www.samhsa.gov/samhsaNewsLetter/Volume_22_Number_2/preventing_suicide. Accessed February 26, 2019.

Suicide Prevention Resource Center: Understanding risk and protective factors for suicide: a primer for preventing suicide. 2017. Available at: http://www.sprc.org/sites/default/files/migrate/library/RiskProtectiveFactorsPrimer.pdf. Accessed February 26, 2019.

Weinstock CP: After a suicide, sibling survivors are often overlooked. 2017. Available at: http://www.npr.org/sections/health-shots/2017/08/25/545554065/after-a-suicide-sibling-survivors-are-often-overlooked. Accessed February 26, 2019.

Wiklander M, Samuelsson M, Asberg M: Shame reactions after suicide attempt. Scand J Caring Sci 17(3):293–300, 2003 12919465

World Health Organization: Towards evidence-based suicide prevention programmes. 2010. Available at: http://www.wpro.who.int/mnh/TowardsEvidencebasedSPP.pdf. Accessed February 26, 2019.

Zisook S, Shuchter S, Schuckit M: Factors in the persistence of unresolved grief among psychiatric outpatients. Psychosomatics 26(6):497–499, 503, 1985 4011815

PART III

Interactions and Special Settings

12

The Medically Ill Patient

Medical and psychiatric illnesses often overlap. The medically ill patient may present with a decreased self-esteem and poor coping skills. Your roles as a supportive psychotherapist include therapist, teacher, and researcher. Additionally, you will be responsible for the management of the psychosocial, behavioral, and social aspects of medical illness and its effects, with the intention of promoting better health. One of your most demanding tasks as a therapist is to help treat the patient who has serious medical illness as well as mental illness. Attempts to distinguish between organic and functional disorders can be baffling. This is especially true when delirium or dementia complicates medical illness in the hospitalized patient. Too often delirium is underdiagnosed. Nursing notes from a 3-year study of hospitalized older adults contained enough data to make a diagnosis of delirium 85% of the time, yet this information was almost never used to make the diagnosis of delirium (Trzepacz 1996). Indeed, it is critical to recognize delirium and differentiate it from cognitive decline, depression, and other conditions. For additional reading on recognizing the differences, see the review by Insel and Badger (2002) and Chapter 9 of this manual.

Agitation, assaultive behaviors, and verbal outbursts may lead to appeals from medical staff to move the patient to a psychiatric unit. As you take on the role of consulting therapist, questioning, evaluation, and clinical observations are your tools for diagnosis. We can broadly conceive of three categories in which your patients may have difficulty with or complaints about their bodies:

- The patient's problem may be limited to a physical illness (as previously coded on Axis III of DSM, which is now combined with other illnesses in DSM-5; American Psychiatric Association 2013), in which case the patient would be treated in a general medical facility.
- The patient may have a disorder with both physical and psychological manifestations, such as Alzheimer's disease or an alcohol-induced delirium. Treatment may take place in a psychiatric facility or in a medical facility with psychiatric consultation.
- The patient may present with one of many somatic symptoms and related disorders, the category of which includes somatic symptom disorder, illness anxiety disorder, conversion disorder (functional neurological symptom disorder), psychological factors affecting other medical conditions, factitious disorder, other specified somatic symptom and related disorder, and unspecified somatic symptom and related disorder. These disorders are found in many patients who have somatic complaints without a reasonable organic basis. Such patients may eagerly seek somatic treatment but refuse psychiatric consultation.

General Considerations of Support in Acute and Chronic Illness

Each of the disorders mentioned above indicates a disturbance—to some degree organically or psychologically based—in bodily function. In these, there is the interplay of psychological defenses with the patient's physical condition. Depending on the course and chronicity of the disease, the patient's adaptation may be relatively stable or labile, but supportive psychotherapy can usually improve the outcome. Freudenrich et al. (2008) stress the importance of identifying your patients' main coping mechanisms and then increasing their range of coping skills, including emotion-based coping, problem-based coping, and attitudinal-based coping.

Despite the profound differences between, for example, a patient with conversion disorder with paralysis and a patient with genuine paraplegia, there are practical reasons to approach such patients similarly. First, both patients will present in a medical setting, not a psychiatric one. Second, in many illnesses (e.g., chronic fatigue syndrome), the etiology may be unknown. Third, both patients may be unwilling to entertain a psychiatric component to their condition. Fourth, in a truly biopsychosocial approach, the clinician should recognize that no disease is purely biological, psychological, or social in origin.

According to Bhagar and Pisano (2006), the suggestion of a psychological cause for the patient's symptoms could cause disbelief, resistance, or denial. They offer a five-step approach for validating somatic symptoms in addition to supportive psychotherapy. The first step is for you to allow the patient the time to summarize his physical symptoms without interrupting him. Ask about prior workups. Step 2 involves acknowledging the difficulty of having the symptoms. Maintain good eye contact, express concern, and give undivided attention. At Step 3, encourage the patient to work out solutions or help him recognize ways past coping mechanisms have worked. At step 4 you will provide a tentative suggestion but leave it to the patient to put it into action when he is ready. For example, if he complains of dizziness, suggest that he get up from a sitting or lying position slowly to decrease dizziness. Ask the patient if the suggestion sounds logical and how difficult it would be to do. Finally, step 5 may involve starting with what the patient presents as a solution and discussing feasibility. For example, the patient may not be receptive to interventions and may want a referral to a specialist or to see you more often.

Differences Between Supportive Therapy and Psychiatric Consultation

Supportive psychotherapy for patients with physical illness is often indicated in hospital settings, with the initial need being determined upon psychiatric consultation. The practice of consultation-liaison medicine itself involves a variety of skills, including the psychiatric assessment of frequently uncooperative patients, the clarification of nebulous consultation requests to improve the patient's behavior, the resolution of complex medical/pharmacological issues, and the assessment of staff-patient interactions. For these aspects of the work, the reader is referred to the comparison of two psychiatric service approaches by Lucke et al. (2017) and the handbook on consultation-liaison psychiatry edited by Leigh and Streltzer (Leigh 2015). In addition, you must recognize psychological defenses and the reactions of your patients to their physical illness, topics addressed later in this chapter.

The decision to undertake psychotherapy (as opposed to a brief consultation or series of consultations for patient management) obviously depends on the patient's own wishes, the course of the disease, and the anticipated length of stay. However, as listed below, there are several potential differences between psychiatric consultation and supportive psychotherapy in the medical setting, especially when the illness is not life-threatening (for a discussion of these issues, see Certa 2017):

- Supportive therapy focuses on improving the patient's adaptation to illness and ability to make the best possible decisions about medical care; it should not be given specifically to improve the patient's behavior.
- Ideally, supportive therapy should be arranged so that it can continue when the patient is discharged.
- Supportive therapy can focus on long-term issues.
- The supportive therapist may be engaged independently by the patient as an independent care provider and with complete confidentiality.

In addition, according to Leigh (2015), two functions are provided by the consultation-liaison therapist: that of the specialist providing expert advice for the patient and that of a liaison. An essential skill for the supportive therapist is to have the ability to recognize the psychological defenses and the various reactions to the categories of physical illness.

Personality Types and Reactions to Illness

Reactions to medical illness vary considerably; you are likely to encounter many of the reactions shown in Table 12–1. Many of these reactions to illness are unavoidable, and most can be partly adaptive by protecting the patient from a further breakdown of coping skills. The diagnosis of a chronic medical illness could elicit a challenge to self-esteem, fear of loss or injury to body parts, fear of pain, and fear of the unknown. Additionally, the patient may have to

Table 12–1.   Typical reactions to serious medical illness

Anxiety

Panic

Denial

Dependency (sometimes exaggerated into helplessness)

Depression

Loss of control

Acknowledgment of limitations and mortality

Guilt over causal role in the illness, resulting in dependency

Entitlement

Relief or resignation

Impulsive, aggressive, or violent behavior

Compensation for loss (e.g., exaggeration of sexuality)

Counterphobia (e.g., becoming an expert on the disease)

Regression (e.g., loss of sexuality, resurgence of oral needs)

Displacement: focus on lesser, minor, or unrelated problems

Projection/externalization: blame on others and doctor

Cognitive distortion and disorientation

Delusion

adjust her lifestyle and perhaps lose employment or make a change in employment placement.

Mentally ill patients with a new diagnosis of a chronic medical illness are likely to be very vulnerable. Often, they can become abusive, demanding, or seductive and exhibitionistic to staff. They may flout safety rules, refuse to accept standard therapies, or sign out against medical advice. In the outpatient setting, noncompliance with treatment or the ineffective overutilization of medical resources often occurs. For further reading on psychiatric reactions to medical illness and coping skills, see the article by Falcone and Franco (2006).

Stages of adaptation to medical illness are summarized in Table 12–2. It should be noted that denial, although often a maladaptive response, can be adaptive under some circumstances, allowing a patient to lead an active life while deemphasizing a poor prognosis or the likelihood of severe side effects. As discussed later in this chapter, denial need not be addressed unless it is causing problems.

You will need to help your patient through the appropriate stages of adaptation to illness by assessing the patient's overall defensive pattern, addressing it in a style that the patient accepts, and selectively improving better defenses in the hope of supplanting more dysfunctional ones.

Although interventions must be guided by the specific illness, the therapist must always understand how to adapt techniques to the personality of the patient. Even a person who functions with relatively little conflict in the "outside world" can be knocked flat both physically and psychologically by hospitalization and medical treatment. Patients with preexisting personality disorders, lacking insight into their long-standing maladaptive defenses, are especially likely to experience (or create) difficulties in a medical setting. For further reading on supportive psychotherapy when faced with a patient's defenses, see the article by Hoffman (2002).

The proper pattern of supportive interventions for different personality types follows the three levels of technique discussed in our chapters on technique (Chapters 3 and 4). For example, at the first level (i.e., basic communication), you may need to convey the message (which would lose effectiveness if made explicit) that your patient is important and does not have to act out, leave the hospital, or seduce the staff to establish his or her masculinity or femininity. At the second level, you may need to confront maladaptive behavior with your patient. At the third level, you may need to provide modified interpretations to strengthen your patient's more adaptive defenses. Additionally, Falcone et al. (2014) suggest that the therapist ask permission to discuss the illness with the patient, then begin with an open-ended question, and reflect back the patient's opinion, exposing the ambivalence.

Controlling, compulsive patients react variously to hospitalization. Some can enjoy the enforced dependency that they do not allow themselves when they are well. Others, more rigid in their need for continuous control, cannot tolerate the imposed discipline. Some of their needs can be satisfied by developing an opportunity for them to exercise as much control as possible over

Table 12–2. Stages of adaptation to medical illness

Stage	Common maladaptive responses
Stage 1: Acknowledgment of illness	Denial
	Panic
	Psychosis
Stage 2: Regressive dependency	Noncompliance
	Signing out against medical advice
	Overdemandingness
	Confusion and agitation
Stage 3	
A. Return to normal functioning	Premature return to functioning
	Reluctance to return to functioning
B. Return to a permanently reduced level of functioning	Inability to adapt to disability
	Maladaptive compensations for disability
C. Terminal (i.e., failure to recover)	Inability to complete personal, financial, and family business

Source. Adapted from Perry and Viederman 1981. We have added Stages 3B and 3C.

their medical regimens. Some can take a part of their outside lives or businesses into the hospital room and maintain an island of control in the sea of medical chaos. Others will find it satisfying to participate in organized recreations such as word puzzles and model building. Insight-oriented methods of therapy, which would seek to diminish their isolation of affect and cognition, can sometimes be successful but may need to be modified by buttressing with self-esteem–maintaining interpretations (e.g., "This is a difficult time for an organized and methodical person like yourself, because some things cannot be predicted."). Indeed, these patients' indecisiveness is often exacerbated by illness, and the therapist must find ways to thwart their inherent tendency to balance each side of an issue equally.

Attention-demanding patients may have histrionic or narcissistic traits. Limit setting is necessary but can also be supportive. The mere availability of a therapist to listen to them is a gratification that may lessen their demands on other staff, because it maintains their needed belief that they are interesting, likable people despite the medical disfigurements they may undergo. Such patients may be concerned with the effect of illness on sexual attractiveness or physical strength. Quite unlike compulsive patients, they may neither want nor need detailed explanations for their illness, because their psychological defenses come from emotional, not cognitive, sources.

Paranoid or schizoid patients suffer most from the invasion of personal space or the sense of assault brought on by hospitalization or medical procedures. A therapist who is not the primary care physician has an advantage in dealing with such patients because she does not represent the oppressive forces of the establishment and can appear to side *with* the patient against the unfeeling attacks of the medical world, while at the same time trying to mitigate the perceived threats. Pseudo-biological explanations (e.g., "You're angry because you are sick") help to validate the patient's suspicious *feelings* but weaken the perception that the staff is deliberately trying to be injurious. Illness itself also reinforces paranoia: the patient believed that the world was out to get him and it *did*. This reinforcement offers some mildly paranoid patients a strength in their adversity, and you should not necessarily undermine it. Rather, the patient can be complimented: "You're strong enough to put up with all this stuff without making a fuss." In other cases, however, the paranoia may be excessive, and you must moderate it with reality testing. It helps to imply that the patient is sick and that he is suffering but that it is nobody's fault. However, therapeutic failure and hostility will undoubtedly follow from interpretations such as "You're blaming others for something that has just happened to you for no reason."

Self-defeating or masochistic patients view illness as a justified punishment and receive some gratification from it that should not necessarily be dissipated by interpretation. Therefore, the therapist should sympathize with their complaints but prevent them from extending their disability or utilizing it for secondary gain. Such patients may also develop somatoform pain disorder, somatization disorder, or hypochondriasis.

Borderline patients, with their inherent difficulties in separation/individuation and abandonment, also achieve some gratification from the constant presence of caregivers but invariably demand too much of them. As in outpatient treatment, limit setting is required, and it is important to prevent these patients from viewing the therapist as omnipotent, because disappointment and flight from treatment are the usual consequences.

Typical reactions of personality styles and supportive techniques for working with different personality styles are summarized in Table 12–3.

Supportive Therapy in Life-Threatening Illness

Physical illness creates stress, and the recognition that one is gravely ill may create a crisis. Therefore, many aspects of grief counseling can be applied to medical illness (see Chapter 11).

Whereas grief primarily focuses on a past event, the stress of illness is an ongoing process, and researchers have found that there is an evolving pattern of reactions that depends upon the type of illness and the patient's understanding of the illness. Two of the most useful loss-of-health models are from Kübler-Ross (1969) and Griffith (2007). Griffith provides an overview of brief supportive psychotherapy for a patient who is dying. From work with the terminally ill, Kubler-Ross emphasizes the predominant modes of reaction as denial, anger, bargaining, depression, and acceptance. Griffith's model derived from work with a patient with schizophrenia who was admitted into hospice after his pulmonary and cardiac disease rapidly progressed. Although patients may not evolve through the "typical" sequence of stages, it is more important for you simply to be aware of what stage the patient is in, or if he is experiencing reactions typical of several stages at once.

When you are treating a mentally ill patient with life-threatening medical illness, you will need to be prepared with specific communication skills, compassion, and an understanding of palliative care. The World Health Organization (2019) has defined palliative care and its components. Palliative care promotes the quality of life of patients and their families who are confronting the obstacles associated with life-threatening illness. Palliative care provides relief from pain and other distressing symptoms, regards dying as a normal process, intends to neither hasten nor postpone death, combines the psychological and spiritual aspects of patient care, and offers a support system to help the family cope during the patient's illness and in their own bereavement. In addition, coordination of care with medical providers and family is essential.

Table 12–3.   Therapeutic techniques for personality styles

Personality	Patients who	Often feel	Are helped by
Dependent	Ask lots of questions Often disappoint you	You will find them unworthy You will not care for them	Offering regular brief sessions Setting limits
Obsessive	Are insistent Are detail oriented Are demanding	They must control their illness, the staff, or the schedule	Offering detailed explanations Providing choices and the reason for each choice Using patient input collaboratively
Narcissistic	Are self-centered Criticize others and the qualifications of doctors	Fearful, threatened, and vulnerable They must protect themselves from injury	Avoiding confrontation Keeping informed Stressing that they deserve the best care staff can provide Benign reinforcement of narcissism
Suffering victim[a]	Always have symptom and require attention Think of themselves as undeserving victims or martyrs May not follow recommendations	Suffering is their role Illness punishes them (and sometimes their doctor) Someone should care for them	Frequent visits Praise for their suffering
Paranoid	Refuse to participate in plans Nontrusting Are litigious	They are being taken advantage of by others, purposefully neglected, or harmed	Staying calm Not arguing Avoiding your fear of litigation Offering understanding Giving clear instructions

Table 12–3. Therapeutic techniques for personality styles *(continued)*

Personality	Patients who	Often feel	Are helped by
Histrionic	Are flirtatious Want to call the doctor by first name	Illness will invalidate them or make them unattractive They need to be special	Encouragement to verbalize concerns Setting boundaries Remaining courteous and objective
Schizoid	Are very lonely Avoid medical care	Doctors are invading their privacy	Making them part of treatment planning (a good idea for most patients)
Not really ill or antisocial	Have Munchausen's syndrome Have factitious disorder Receive secondary gain from illness	You will find out the truth	Regular matter-of-fact care Avoiding countertransference anger

[a]This may be better represented in the dimensional model of personality disorders as a combination of dependent and other narcissistic traits.

Source. Based on Falcone et al. 2014, modified and with the last category added.

For further readings on supportive therapy with mentally ill patients with chronic medical illness and its scope, definition, and benefits, see the articles by Baker (2005) and Trachsel et al. (2016).

Therapy with the patient dealing with dying involves some commonsense principles as well as some sophisticated ones. Cassem and Stewart's (1975) eight essential C's of patient management ask for competence, cheerfulness, and consistency of the physician; and concern for, comfort of, and communication with the patient, allowing the presence of children and fostering family cohesion and integration.

Is denial an obstacle for your therapeutic interventions? Because denial can be initially adaptive in major illness, as Hackett and Weisman (1969) showed in their landmark study, it should be treated with salutary neglect unless it is creating problems. As a corollary, it follows that engaging the patient in discussions about death may uncover more anxiety than is necessary. Some of your patients may never progress past the stage of denial and will doctor shop until they find a provider who acknowledges their idea that nothing is wrong with them. Whether denial is adaptive or maladaptive will hinge on whether your patient continues to comply with treatment even while denying the prognosis.

Zimmermann (2007) analyzed 30 articles in palliative care, nursing, general medicine, and psychiatry journals and found that denial is seen by many professionals as an obstacle to palliative care. Zimmermann, however, is of the belief that denial may be seen as integral to coming to terms gradually with impending death.

- *Interpret idiosyncratic reactions to the illness to help your patients achieve comfort.* Most obvious are those reactions of guilt or personal responsibility for illness in which the patient's behavior played a role (e.g., drunk driving and an auto accident, smoking and cancer). In the long run, modification of such behaviors improves survival, but in the acute situation you should accept that the damage is already done and not reinforce the patient's guilt. Less obvious are guilt feelings that the illness is a deserved punishment for some wrongdoing, and it may take considerable time before the patient is willing to express these to you. In this connection, you must be comfortable in talking about the patient's religious conceptions, for they may embody attributions of guilt that are worsening the patient's current condition. (See

Chapter 17 for more comments on the importance of being familiar with the values of one's patients.)

- *Foster a realistic understanding of the disease and its consequences.* Such an understanding usually includes a reasonable account of the prognosis, which should obviously be determined by the primary physician treating the illness. Although a fatal prognosis might seem to be the worst imaginable thing about an illness, often there are other factors that cause the patient even more discomfort. These include unfounded fantasies about the illness and its progression; realistic but avoidable problems of early abandonment by one's family; and excessive pain, suffering, disfigurement, and loss of dignity. For example, amputation is traumatic for physically active young adults, but (after the denial stage) they need specific reassurance that they can continue to be physically active and athletic. Or a postmastectomy patient can be reassured, somewhat abstractly, that "most men do not feel less love for their wives as a result of the operation." Such generalizations provide intellectualizations for the patient to use against dysphoric affect. Many of your patients who have been diagnosed with cancer may see their diagnosis as a death sentence involving debilitating treatments and thoughts of a long and painful dying process. Lederberg and Holland (2011) affirm that supportive psychotherapy for patients with cancer is the most important tool of the therapist. Although their discussion is directed toward therapy with cancer patients, the information provided applies equally to patients with other life-threatening illness.
- *Be prepared to discuss the effect of the illness on the completion of the patient's life plan or work.* Supportive psychotherapy for your patient with a terminal illness will have some differences. First, it will be more time-limited and focused. Second, your patient's goals will be much simpler and uncomplicated. Third, the treatment of your dying patient will require collaboration with medical, nursing, and pastoral professionals.

  The goals of therapy for your patient with a terminal illness are, first, to provide a transparent information about the illness; second, to encourage the expression of emotions and assist with managing the emotions; third, to maintain a rapport with your patient to allow her to have the feeling of support in her battle with death; and, finally, to intervene on your patient's behalf with family, friends, and medical staff (Culkin 2013).
- *Offer environmental interventions to aid the patient's adaptation.* These interventions include working with the patient's family members so they can

relate to the patient in a way that addresses her needs most effectively. Some gratifications can be provided to patients with strong dependency needs. You will have limitations regarding how much you will be able to assist your patient, and referring your patient to support groups will also be effective once he has developed past the denial stage. Today, most cities have support groups for terminal illnesses, including cancer, heart failure, AIDS, and other serious terminal illnesses. You may have a patient who finds speaking in groups to be stressful. In this case, a referral to complementary therapies such as art, music, mediation, or yoga could be helpful. Provide for continuous care. Indeed, those with mental illness are known to have a shorter life span and to be more chronically medically ill (De Hert et al. 2011). Clearly, approaching your patient's care with a multidisciplinary team and plans for follow-up is crucial. Other brief admonitions for the therapist developing a supportive technique with medical patients are presented in Table 12–4.

Medical Illness Causing Disfigurement

Body image is a significant psychosocial issue for patients with a medical illness causing disfigurement. Your role will be to assist these individuals with the impaired coping mechanisms of denial, avoidance, and projection and to help them develop more useful ways of reacting. Those born with congenital disfigurements will not have different psychosocial responses or needs than the individual with a traumatic disfiguring injury (Bradbury 2012). The following case vignette incorporates supportive therapy for a patient with a severe disfigurement caused by neurofibromatosis, a genetic disorder that causes tumors to form on nerve tissue (Mayo Clinic 2017).

Case Vignette

Mr. R. is a 35-year-old man with the diagnosis of neurofibromatosis. All his siblings also suffered from this genetic disorder. However, he had a more severe case, and his body was completely covered with large, grotesque tumors. He was admitted to an assisted living facility when his family could no longer care for him. His sisters reported he had quit bathing and refused to eat. They informed staff: "He was always a talkative and kind-hearted soul with a great sense of humor. He just got very depressed and quit talking to us. We can't pick

Table 12–4. Therapist do's and don'ts in medical illness

DO learn about the patient's specific illness and its etiology, course, treatment, and prognosis.	DON'T use the illness as your only guide to therapy.
DO establish yourself as the patient's ally.	DON'T neglect the patient's family.
DO determine the meaning of the illness for the patient.	DON'T assume the illness means the same for the patient as it would for you.
DO explore hidden issues such as related guilt.	DON'T attempt interpretations of deeper or threatening material.
DO work out a rationalization or meaning for the illness, including the patient's role in it.	DON'T give a facile explanation or dismissal of the illness.
DO allow the patient to express religious concerns.	DON'T turn into a religious advisor.
DO expect to satisfy some dependency needs.	DON'T give in to all demands for gratification.
DO deliver your interpretations in the patient's defensive style.	DON'T be placed in the role that the patient demands of you.
DO explore the realistic potential of somatic treatments and engender hope.	DON'T overdo it to the point of losing credibility.
DO try to address as much of the patient's dysfunction as possible.	DON'T forget about possible organic factors in the patient's psychiatric condition that cannot be addressed by therapy (e.g., electrolyte imbalance, toxicity, remote tumor hormonal effects).
DO explore compliance or noncompliance with treatment.	DON'T assume the patient's treatment decisions are wrong because they differ from the ones you would make.
DO determine the patient's stated agenda for therapy.	DON'T assume the patient has put the total agenda on the table.

him up and put him into the shower." After his admission to the skilled nursing facility, he remained in his bed facing the wall and would not leave his room for any of the activities. His meals sat on the bedside table untouched. He would not respond to the nursing assistants when they offered to take him to the shower. The nursing assistants were complaining of the foul odor in his room and were frustrated that their efforts to communicate with him were ineffective. When approached by the therapist, he would minimally respond but was cooperative. When the subject of him leaving his room to join in activities was approached by the therapist, Mr. R. responded that he did not want to be around anyone. "I am just fine here by myself. I am too ugly for anyone to see me. I don't need anyone."

Mr. R.'s therapist researched neurofibromatosis and recognized that Mr. R. was severely depressed. The therapist listened to Mr. R.'s feelings of "being ugly" and provided him with additional information on his disorder. He acknowledged to Mr. R. that the disease could be "ugly" but that Mr. R. had many good qualities that could benefit others in the home and that Mr. R. himself was not "ugly." The therapist informed Mr. R. he had a lot to offer the older residents in the facility—his youth and his humor, among other things—and relayed to Mr. R. that his participation would be very beneficial to the group. The therapist met with Mr. R. several times, and Mr. R. began to respond more and even made a few jokes. Two weeks later, Mr. R. allowed the nursing assistants to help him shower and he joined a bingo game. He was well accepted within the group. He continued to thrive and entertained the older residents with his jokes and antics and educated the residents on his disorder.

Cancer

A diagnosis of cancer can be terrifying for your patient, who will be challenged with the threat of death, the fear of disfiguring treatments, pain and discomfort from other side effects of treatments and medications, and an unpredictable prognosis. You can expect to assist your patients with the challenges that this life-threatening illness will have on their lives. It will, of course, be impossible for you as the supportive psychotherapist to know everything about every cancer. However, it is crucial for you to have an understanding of your patient's prognosis and treatment, disease progression, usual side effects of the treatment, and the effect on your patient's comorbid conditions. Depression and anxiety are common reactions with any chronic or life-threatening illness. For a more in-depth discussion on these two emotional reactions, see the chapters on anxiety disorders and mood disorders (Chapters 7 and 8) in this manual.

The likelihood of psychological implications of cancer is described by Jevne et al. (1998, p. 215) as follows:

a. *a silent onset:* "If cancer can come unannounced, then it can return unannounced." The knowledge that cancer can return lingers even in patients where the prognosis is excellent.
b. *delayed diagnosis:* "If the medical profession didn't believe me once, maybe it will not believe me again." Undiagnosed malaise, resulting in test after test of "we found nothing," lowers trust in the science where patients look for treatment and survival.
c. *invasive, disfiguring treatment:* Cancer treatment is often demanding physically and emotionally. Patients dread the treatment as much as, if not more than, the disease itself, leading them to question both the process and outcome.
d. *multiple losses:* Body image or body function changes, loss of existential security, loss of predictability, loss of social acceptability, and role changes are among everyday losses of the cancer patient.
e. *association with death:* For many patients, a cancer diagnosis is a death sentence and may be their first encounter with mortality.
f. *chronic, unpredictable course:* Confronting the fear or the reality of the disease, and dealing with challenges over an extended period, despite resources.

Supportive psychotherapy for patients with cancer has been found to be very effective (Lederberg and Holland 2011). One study revealed that 62.2% of 300 cancer patients experienced depression and anxiety. This study also revealed the importance of counseling for depression and anxiety as a means of improving patients' psychological disorders, which would ultimately improve the quality of medical care (Khalli et al. 2016). Another study found that those who had been diagnosed with breast or stomach cancer had the highest levels of depression and anxiety among all cancer patients (Nikbakhsh et al. 2014). For further readings on depression and anxiety in cancer patients, see the article by Jacobsen and Jim (2008).

Lederberg and Holland (2011) provide both the beginning and the experienced supportive psychotherapist with the essential foundations of supportive psychotherapy for patients with cancer and indicate that many of these techniques will also apply equally to your patients with other life-threatening illnesses. Lederberg and Holland have identified the following key factors in providing therapy:

1. *Location.* Location can include outpatient, inpatient, or home care, or delivery by telephone or email. The most important issue is that your patient knows you are there for her.

2. *Timing.* Some sessions may need to be shortened because of the patient's fatigue or level of illness. Even if your interaction may be brief, the session may be meaningful, especially when your patient is very ill.

3. *Frequency.* Again, this will vary on the basis of the level of your patient's illness. As your patient recovers, outpatient visits can be scheduled with the same regulations and procedures as those followed with your physically healthy patients. However, be aware that with each medical setback the cycle will restart.

4. *Sense of urgency.* Often, your patient may feel his time is limited and have a need to resolve his problems rapidly. You must give special attention to the time frame within which the goals may be reached.

5. *Flexibility of approach.* Your patient's concerns can change rapidly as she deals with fears, anger, the illness, treatments, and family issues. The course of cancer will have sudden episodes that will interrupt your patient's stable periods.

6. *Understanding of the disease process.* As noted earlier, you will need to understand the disease process. Your initial evaluation should include the diagnosis, staging, prognosis, current treatment, and side effects of the treatment. Without an understanding of the medical issues, it will be impossible for you to provide the needed psychological support (Lederberg and Holland 2011).

Key Points

- Your roles with the medically ill psychiatric patient will include those of therapist, teacher, and researcher.

- Planning care with a multidisciplinary team approach is crucial.

- Delirium or dementia could confound the medical diagnosis and requires a sound understanding of all the signs and symptoms.

- Supportive psychotherapy, regardless of the patient's adaptation and coping skills, can improve the outcome of his or her acceptance of the illness and improve coping skills.

- It is important to remember the psychiatric patient with a medical illness is vulnerable; therefore, the supportive therapist will need to understand should the patient become abusive and/or demanding.

- To assist your patient through the adaptation stages of a medical illness, you must first assess his or her defense pattern.

- It is not unusual for a patient to experience grief with a medical diagnosis.

- The terminally ill patient will require not just an education on her illness but also encouragement and management of her emotions.

References

American Psychiatric Association: Diagnostic and Statistical Manual of Mental Disorders, 5th Edition. Arlington, VA, American Psychiatric Association, 2013

Baker A: Palliative and end-of-life care in the serious and persistently mentally ill population. J Am Psychiatr Nurses Assoc 11(5):298–305, 2005

Bhagar HA, Pisano M: 5-step "listen therapy" for somatic complaints. Curr Psychiatr 5(5):110, 2006

Bradbury E: Meeting the psychological needs of patients with facial disfigurement. Br J Oral Maxillofac Surg 50(3):193–196, 2012 21440966

Cassem NH, Stewart RS: Management and care of the dying patient. Psychiatry Med 6(1–2):293–304, 1975 11664585

Culkin J: Psychotherapy with the dying person. 2013

De Hert M, Correll CU, Bobes J, et al: Physical illness in patients with severe mental disorders. I. Prevalence, impact of medications and disparities in health care. World Psychiatry 10(1):52–77, 2011 21379357

Falcone T, Franco K: Treating psychiatric reactions to medical illness. Curr Psychiatr 5:105–119, 2006

Falcone T, Dickstein L, Sieke EH, et al: Coping with chronic medical illness. 2014. Available at: https://teachmemedicine.org/cleveland-clinic-coping-with-chronic-medical-illness/. Accessed February 27, 2019.

Freudenrich O, Kongtos N, Querques J: Support patients coping with medical illness. Curr Psychiatr 7(13):76–76, 2008

Griffith LJ: Brief supportive psychotherapy for a patient with chronic schizophrenia who is dying. Psychiatry 4(12):49–54, 2007 20436764

Hackett TP, Weisman A: Denial as a factor in patients with heart disease and cancers. Ann N Y Acad Sci 164:802–817, 1969 5263110

Hoffman RS: Working with a patient's defenses in supportive psychotherapy. Psychiatr Serv 53(2):141–142, 2002 11821542

Insel KC, Badger TA: Deciphering the 4 D's: cognitive decline, delirium, depression and dementia—a review. J Adv Nurs 38(4):360–368, 2002 11985687

Jacobsen PB, Jim HS: Psychosocial interventions for anxiety and depression in adult cancer patients: achievements and challenges. CA Cancer J Clin 58(4):214–230, 2008 18558664

Jevne RF, Nekolaichuk CL, Williamson FH: A model for counselling cancer patients. Canadian Journal of Counselling 32:213–229, 1998

Khalli A, Faheem M, Fahim A, et al: Prevalence of depression and anxiety amongst cancer patients in a hospital setting: a cross-sectional study. Psychiatry J 2016:3964806, 2016 27752508

Kübler-Ross E: On Death and Dying. New York, Macmillan, 1969

Lederberg MS, Holland JC: Supportive psychotherapy in cancer care: an essential ingredient of all therapy, in Handbook of Psychotherapy in Cancer Care. Edited by Wilson M, Kissane D. Hoboken, NJ, Wiley, 2011, pp 3–14

Leigh H: The function of consultation-liaison psychiatry, in Handbook of Consultation-Liaison Psychiatry, 2nd Edition. Edited by Leigh H, Streltzer J. New York, Springer, 2015, pp 11–14

Lucke C, Gschossmann JM, Schmidt A, et al: A comparison of two psychiatric service approaches: findings from the consultation vs. liaison psychiatry-study. BMC Psychiatry 17:1171–1174, 2017 28068983

Mayo Clinic: Neurofibromatosis. 2017. Available at: http://www.mayoclinic.org/diseases-conditions/neurofibromatosis/home/ovc-20167893. Accessed February 27, 2019.

Nikbakhsh N, Moudi S, Abbasian S, et al: Prevalence of depression and anxiety among cancer patients. Caspian J Intern Med 5(3):167–170, 2014 25202445

Perry S, Viederman M: Management of emotional reactions to acute medical illness. Med Clin North Am 65:3–14, 1981 7206897

Trachsel M, Irwin SA, Biller-Andorno N, et al: Palliative psychiatry for severe persistent mental illness as a new approach to psychiatry? Definition, scope, benefits, and risks. July 2016. Available at: https://bmcpsychiatry.biomedcentral.com/track/pdf/10.1186/s12888-016-0970-y?site=bmcpsychiatry.biomedcentral.com. Accessed February 27, 2019.

Trzepacz TP: Delirium: advances in diagnosis, pathophysiology, and treatment. Psychiatr Clin North Am 20:(3)429–448, 1996 8856810

World Health Organization: WHO definition of palliative care. 2019. Available at: http://www.who.int/cancer/palliative/definition/en/. Accessed February 27, 2019.

Zimmermann C: Death denial: obstacle or instrument for palliative care? An analysis of clinical literature. Sociol Health Illn 29(2):297–314, 2007 17381818

13

The Older Patient

The aging and longevity of the population in the United States, among other factors, have led to increasing emphasis on geriatric mental health as a subspecialty interest requiring special expertise. Acquiring that expertise can take years. However, the basic techniques of supportive psychotherapy can be readily applied to elderly patients, provided one is aware of the special attitudes and adaptations that the therapist should make to serve that population more effectively.

Approximately one in five older adults in the United States suffers from a mental health disorder—the most common being anxiety, severe cognitive impairment, and mood disorders. Depression among the elderly is too often not recognized and consequently untreated or undertreated. Older adults are more likely to focus on their physical issues and less likely to report psychiatric symptoms (Centers for Disease Control and Prevention 2014).

Mental Health and Aging

It is helpful to review the age-related psychological changes that individuals typically undergo. Cognitive functions in typically aging individuals do not decline significantly enough to require major changes in therapy technique; however, some individuals may begin to experience a "benign" forgetfulness of recently acquired information and difficulty encoding new information, especially if it does not have intrinsic meaning.

A common source of worry for older adults and their family members is memory loss. The range of severity is from mild forms to severe impairment that may represent Alzheimer's disease (Blazer and Steffens 2014). Impairment of short-term memory is the most frequently reported concern of older adults and the most common cause for cognitive evaluation, and too often the difficulties related to cognitive impairment are dismissed by family members or providers as normal aging (Weiner 2014).

Except for dementia and depression, there is limited knowledge about common mental disorders in the elderly. Indeed, there is both a need for diagnostic assessment tools that are adapted to the cognitive capacity of the elder population and a need to raise awareness of psychosocial problems among the older population to provide a higher quality of mental health services (Andreas et al. 2017).

Typical adaptational responses of elderly patients are listed in Table 13–1, illustrating how a limitation in available outlets may result in a channeling of maladaptive defenses into psychiatric symptoms instead of action.

The mental health and well-being of your elderly patient are just as essential as those of your younger patients. The population worldwide is aging rapidly, with the proportion of individuals over 60 expected to increase from 12% to 20% between 2015 and 2050. More than 20% of adults 60 years or older suffer from a mental or neurological disorder. Problems related to mental health are often unrecognized by health care professionals and the older adults. Additionally, the stigma surrounding these conditions creates a reluctance in people to seek help (World Health Organization 2017b).

Barriers to Mental Health Care for Older Adults

Stigma

Unfortunately, stigma toward those with mental illness is still common today and strips these individuals of their self-respect in addition to adding to their

Table 13–1.   Some adaptational responses in older patients

Withdrawal (with or without depression)

Physical and affective isolation

Manipulative and passive-aggressive tactics

Clinging dependency

Entitlement

Denial

Projection

Externalization

Somatization and/or hypochondriasis

Focusing on past successes

Obsession with past memories and lost opportunities

Limitation of social contacts to those that are reinforcing

Selective perception and rejection of dissonant messages

Devaluation of new developments in technology or culture

Interest in religion and/or the ritualistic aspects of religious observance

current harmful patterns of isolation and hopelessness. The consequences of stigma can be more debilitating than the mental illness. Clearly, the need exists to educate mental health providers and the community on ways to overcome stigmatizing behaviors (Henderson et al. 2014). *Stigma*, according to Charles and Bentley (2016), refers to "having some condition or characteristic that is perceived by others as a particular token of shame, disgrace, and social unacceptability" (p. 149). Those authors also identify the need to continue with practices that reduce stigma.

Among professionals in all areas of health care, stigmatization and discrimination against people with mental illness exist (Henderson et al. 2014). This suggests the need to decrease stigmatizing of mental health patients by mental health providers in the early career stage and among those providers who may be experiencing burnout.

Stigma has been chronicled as the primary cause of negative attitudes toward older adults (De Mendonça Lima 2004). Older adults may be embarrassed to reveal any emotional or mental health problems they may be experiencing. This reluctance is understandable when one recognizes that this group of people came of age in an era when the topic of psychiatric disorders was considered taboo. Family members, friends, and caregivers may also have some of the same attitudes and beliefs and will not offer support or assistance with seeking mental health care. Consequently, older adults will gravitate to their primary care providers for all health problems, including covert and overt mental health disorders (Morris 2001).

Ageism

Older adults seeking mental health care may be burdened with the barrier of ageism. The World Health Organization (2019) defines *ageism* as "the stereotyping and discrimination against individuals or groups on the basis of their age; ageism can take many forms, including prejudicial attitudes, discriminatory practices, or institutional policies and practices that perpetuate stereotypical beliefs." Indeed, the report suggests that ageism may now be even more pervasive than sexism and racism.

Ageism may hinder a family's or even a therapist's understanding of normal aging and mental disorders in older adults. For example, the symptoms of depression may be perceived as normal in the older adult by family members, and they may believe that nothing can be done to alleviate the depression. Health professionals may also have the same misconceptions and not properly diagnose the depression (Morris 2001). Eighty percent of people age 60 or older reported experiencing ageism such as others surmising that problems of memory and physical impairments were due to their age (Dittmann 2003). The common negative stereotypes of ageism include such terms as "cranky," "childlike," "helpless," and "unapproachable." The resulting physical health consequences of ageism include increased stress, a decreased will to live, and an impaired recovery from illness (Seegert 2016).

Financial Barriers

Access to mental health care has always been a problem in the United States because of the cost (Rowan et al. 2013). The steep deductibles, services not covered, and cost of prescription medications can make a difference between getting help and not (Connolly 2017). Even though Medicare provides coverage, older adults in the United States face higher financial barriers to healthcare than older adults in 10 other high-income countries. One-quarter of the U.S. elderly say that they often worry about having adequate finances to cover food and housing. Of these older adults, 31% will skip care because of costs (Osborn et al. 2017). Despite health care reform and Medicare coverage, financial barriers still exist because of the inadequate reimbursement rates by insurers (Bishop et al. 2014).

Geriatric Psychotherapy

Baby boomers are aging, and the demand for mental health services by these older adults will increase. One question for therapists working with the elderly is: Will therapy change when you are working with older adults? The answer is yes, or we would not have this chapter, but there is more to it. Therapists will need to adapt psychotherapy when working with elderly patients, but not because of their age per se. The change in therapy will be needed not because of developmental differences but because of context effects, cohort effects, and specific challenges that are common in later life. The context effects involve changes in living arrangements such as long-term care or a retirement community. Cohort effects will involve modifications because of the differing skills, values, and life experiences of the younger cohorts. The specific challenges of the older adults require specific knowledge and therapeutic skills, not because of the patient's age, but because of the problems they present to the patient (Knight 2009).

Table 13–2 presents suggestions for adapting supportive psychotherapy for older patients. We suggest that therapy with the older patient proceeds best if you *not* imagine that the patient wants what you and other mental health providers have—youth and unlimited opportunities.

The full benefits of psychotherapy in the elderly have gone underappreciated. Among older adults, the acceptance of psychotherapy has increased. The cognitive status of the patient and the mental health disorder will determine the eligibility for psychotherapy (Ansari and Grossberg 2016).

Frequent Issues and Concerns in Geriatric Psychotherapy

With aging, there will be an increased focus on physical health and a necessity for mental health providers to have the skills to provide age-specific ser-

Table 13–2.   Adaptations of technique for older patients

Adjust therapy sessions to accommodate for sensory and cognitive deficits (Wyman et al. 2011).

Adopt a slower pace of treatment and present material over multiple meetings (Wyman et al. 2011).

Adapt techniques to the patient's medical, physical, and sensory deficits (Wyman et al. 2011).

Expect that a larger percentage of time will appropriately be spent discussing past events rather than the present, and that this emphasis may reflect not a defensive avoidance of current decisions, as it might in younger patients, but an appropriate review and setting in place of experience.

Be more willing to accept the patient's tendency to somatize some psychological difficulties.

Be able to safely give more gratifications without creating the difficulties that would ensue with some younger patients.

Pay more attention to environmental supports (e.g., a companion for isolation, a meal delivery service, the use of pets), using the setting of therapy to plan with the patient and encourage a socialized program of ongoing activities.

As with supportive therapy for younger patients, consider utilizing specific interpersonal, cognitive, or behavioral techniques (for a brief review, see Moberg and Lazarus 1990).

vices, including those related to physical, cognitive, and functional disabilities (Zechner et al. 2018).

Older patients will often struggle with self-esteem. You will need to discover how your patient maintains self-esteem with the consequences of the biophysical losses associated with aging and build upon those coping skills. You should recognize that older patients often seek approval and support from their therapist. The older patient will often rely on the therapist for confirmation of competency and normalcy and for restoration of feelings of mastery and self-esteem (Atiq and Gilling 2006).

Dealing with loss will be a common issue in therapy with elderly patients. Older patients will likely suffer multiple losses of spouses, friends, and relatives as well as a loss of functions and independence. Losses could trigger a fear of future losses. The multiple changes that come with aging, including dependency on others for care and the fear of dependency related to physical illnesses, can be frightening. Psychotherapy provides the older patient with the opportunity to explore and respond to these frightening feelings in a safe manner that is life-enhancing rather than stagnating (Atiq and Gilling 2006).

Empathy, Transference, and Countertransference

Most therapists understand that previous generations held a variety of myths about aging that have been somewhat dissipated by factual knowledge. For example, current research tells us that gender-specific attitudes and roles continue throughout life; older persons may of necessity (e.g., when widowed) assume traditional roles of the other sex, but they do not become asexual, and they continue to be interested in both physical and sexual activity unless illness supervenes.

Despite the availability of sound research on the aging process, problems of empathy will persist in both younger and older therapists. For example, it is difficult for the much younger therapist to appreciate the life experience of an elderly person who has grown through a different set of economic, cultural, and military upheavals. From the therapist's point of view, the patient's problems may be attributed to doggedly retained but outdated attitudes, a situation conducive neither to sympathy nor to empathy in the therapist. Thus, you might find insufferable the elderly woman's perceived role as secondary to her husband, or the elderly man's insensitivity to his wife's social needs.

Empathy

Understanding what the other person is experiencing is *empathy*. Empathy is not synonymous with sympathy. *Sympathy* is described as feeling sorry for someone and is an automatic, emotional response. Empathy requires us to understand the other person's point of view. Today, clinical empathy is being overshadowed by the need for efficiency. For example, touching of patients has declined and physical barriers between patients and providers have increased in medical services because of technology. Nurses once held a patient's hand or arm to take a pulse, but this task is now replaced by a probe attached to a patient's finger. Computerized medication carts on wheels also create a physical barrier (Dean 2017).

Empathy involves your ability to be alert, listen, and become involved with your patient and to correctly interpret what your patient is verbalizing. The communication of empathy to your older patients will leave them with the feeling that they are understood. The use of reflective statements will be helpful. For example, you may say, "It seems you are very frustrated with your increased need for assistance with getting dressed" or "It sounds like your son is causing you some frustration." The use of reflective statements is to confirm your understanding of what your patient is saying to you. Another tactic is to begin your reflective statements with "If I understand you correctly, you feel…" You do not want to use the phrase "I know exactly how you feel." Such a response does not convey empathy or an understanding of your patient's feelings.

Transference and Countertransference

Transference is the result of a patient experiencing the therapist as an important person from the past with whom he had a meaningful relationship. The feelings, beliefs, assumptions, and experiences regarding the therapist are projections from the patient's earlier relationships, displaced onto the therapist (Atiq and Gilling 2006; Winston et al. 2012). *Countertransference* is defined as the therapist's experience of the elderly patient (Atiq and Gilling 2006). Countertransference does not inevitably foster ageism, although the two are often intertwined (Semel 2006). Moreover, transference does not "age" as fast as the patient. The elderly patient may develop transferential love for the therapist or experience the therapist as a punitive parent; the female patient may fantasize about having a child by the therapist as if he were her husband, despite a 50-year age difference. This is a consequence of our earlier observation that minds do not age in the way that bodies do, and that affective experience transcends history and chronology. However, because of the patient's longer life span, the sources of transference are more likely to include significant others in later life, such as spouse or friends, as well as the patient's parents.

Despite the ability of most elderly persons to adapt to significant changes in life circumstances, many will lose psychological resiliency. For example, in Mark Twain's *The Adventures of Tom Sawyer*, after Becky Thatcher initially spurns him, Tom is afflicted with thoughts of death:

> The boy's soul was steeped in melancholy.… It seemed to him that life was but a trouble at best, and he more than half envied Jimmy Hodges, so lately released. It must be very peaceful, he thought, to lie and slumber and dream for ever and ever, with the wind whispering through the trees and caressing the grass and the flowers over the grave, and nothing to bother and grieve about,

ever any more.... She would be sorry someday —maybe when it was too late. Ah, if he could only die *temporarily*! (Twain 1876[1875]/1981, pp. 56–57)

But Tom cannot sustain the mood for long, and he returns to his other machinations, for, as Twain notes, "the elastic heart of youth cannot be compressed into one constrained shape long at a time" (p. 57).

Compare Tom Sawyer's resilience with Ivan Ilyich's inescapable realization that he is going to die:

> He could not understand it and tried to dismiss the thought as false, unsound, and morbid, to force it out of his mind with other thoughts that were sound and healthy. But the thought—not just the thought but, it seemed, the reality itself—kept coming back and confronting him.
>
> And one after another, in place of that thought, he called up others, hoping to find support in them. He tried to revert to a way of thinking that had obscured the thought of death from him in the past. But, strangely, everything that had once obscured, hidden, obliterated the awareness of death no longer had that effect. (Tolstoy 1886/1981, p. 94)

In matters of advice, it is especially important for the younger therapist not to play the role of younger therapist. The inherent prestige and authority of "therapist" or "doctor" usually outweigh the perception of immaturity associated with "young" until evidence to the contrary presents itself. Playing the role of younger therapist can give rise to countertransference problems opposite to the devaluations discussed earlier. The therapist, inhibited by respect for elderly persons (e.g., modeled after that for his or her own grandparents), may become too timid to effectively explore and direct the therapy (Yesavage and Karasu 1982).

Depression and Suicide Among the Elderly

Certainly, we need to learn as much as we can about the causes of suicide among the elderly, although there seems to be a relative lack of understanding in this area. This could be a result of the mind-set that the older adult is too wise to act on suicidal thoughts or assuming older adults are happy in their retirement years. However, the rates of suicide among the elderly are alarming (see Chapter 11 for suicide and Chapter 7 for depression). A study of homebound older adults receiving home-delivered meals found high rates of reports of depression and suicidal thoughts; one-third of these homebound older adults were taking antidepressants (Sirey et al. 2008).

In 2012, there was about one elderly suicide every 80 minutes. The rate of suicides among the elderly was 15.4 per 100,00. Firearms were the most common means for completing suicide (American Association of Suicidology 2014). Clearly, every elderly patient must be asked about suicidal ideation.

Supportive Psychotherapy in Dementia

The World Health Organization (2017a) defines *dementia* as a syndrome that is chronic or progressive in nature with a deterioration in memory, thinking, behavior, and the ability to perform everyday tasks. The guidelines in Table 13–2 will be particularly useful when you are working with the patient with dementia. We have, of necessity, expressed some concerns about patients whose memories are too impaired for them to learn from the processes in psychotherapy.

You may be saddled with the responsibility of informing your patient of her diagnosis of dementia. There is no consensus among physicians and psychiatrists on how or when a patient should be informed of the diagnosis. Psychotherapy is based on honesty, providing the patient with an understanding of his disorder and its prognosis and management. You will find that the principles of supportive psychotherapy will allow for the building blocks for a therapeutic discussion (Junaid and Hegde 2007).

Death and Dying

The elderly face a reality that cannot be ignored or overlooked: approaching end of life. For those with inadequate coping skills, the prospect of death can be extremely difficult. End-of-life discussion is a subject many are uncomfortable with, but it is a necessary part of supportive psychotherapy for the elderly.

Most people report that talking to loved ones about death is important, but much fewer have accomplished this task. Eighty percent of people stated that they would want to discuss impending death with their doctor about treatment toward end of life, yet only 7% reported having had this conversation (Institute for Healthcare Improvement 2016). Clearly, these alarming statistics highlight the significance of approaching the subject of death and dying with your elderly patient.

Key Points

- Psychotherapy for older persons has a large and relevant research and teaching literature. The therapist should continue his or her own lifelong education in that area of expertise.

- Nearly 20% of older persons suffer from mental illness disorders and depression. Often these needs will go unrecognized and untreated.

- Barriers to obtaining treatment for mental health problems include stigma, ageism, and inadequate financial resources.

- Supportive psychotherapy for older patients is similar to that for younger patients, but some adaptations are needed.

- Frequent issues encountered in therapy with older persons include physical and cognitive decline, decreased self-esteem, and grief and loss. Empathy is of value with all patients but is of particular importance when working with older patients. Concerns of transference and countertransference will be more prominent with older patients.

- Difficult subjects to approach patients about include suicide and death and dying.

References

American Association of Suicidology: Elderly suicide fact sheet. 2014. Available at: http://ccsme.org/wp-content/uploads/2017/01/B2-Older-Adults-Fact-Sheet.pdf. Accessed February 28, 2019.

American Psychiatric Association: Diagnostic and Statistical Manual of Mental Disorders, 5th Edition. Arlington, VA, American Psychiatric Association, 2013

Andreas S, Schulz H, Volkert J, et al: Prevalence of mental disorders in elderly people: the European MentDis_ICF65+ study. Br J Psychiatry 210(2):125–131, 2017 27609811

Ansari IJ, Grossberg GT: The growing role of psychotherapy in the elderly. J Gerontol Geriatr Res 5:272, 2016

Atiq R, Gilling PM: Common themes and issues in geriatric psychotherapy. Psychiatry (Edgmont) 3(6):53–56, 2006 21103186

Bishop TF, Press MJ, Keyhani S, et al: Acceptance of insurance by psychiatrists and the implications for access to mental health care. JAMA Psychiatry 71(2):176–181, 2014 24337499

Blazer DG, Steffens DG: Treatment of seniors, in The American Psychiatric Press Textbook of Psychiatry, 6th Edition. Edited by Hales RE, Yudofsky SE, Roberts LW. Washington, DC, American Psychiatric Publishing, 2014, pp 1233–1261

Centers for Disease Control and Prevention: The state of mental health and aging in America. 2014. Available at: https://www.cdc.gov/aging/pdf/mental_health.pdf. Accessed February 28, 2019.

Charles JLK, Bentley KJ: Stigma as an organizing framework for understanding the early history of community mental health and psychiatric social work. Soc Work Ment Health 14(2):149–173, 2016

Connolly D: High costs prevent people from seeking mental health services. February 2, 2017. Available at: http://thehill.com/blogs/pundits-blog/healthcare/320727-high-costs-prevent-people-from-seeking-mental-health-services. Accessed February 28, 2019.

Dean S: Are our busy doctors and nurses losing empathy for patients? January 12, 2017. Available at: http://theconversation.com/are-our-busy-doctors-and-nurses-losing-empathy-for-patients-68228. Accessed February 28, 2019.

De Mendonça Lima CA: The reduction of stigma and discrimination against older people with mental disorders: a challenge for the future. Arch Gerontol Geriatr Suppl 9(9):109–120, 2004 15207405

Dittmann M: Fighting ageism. 2003. Available at: http://www.apa.org/monitor/may03/fighting. Accessed February 28, 2019.

Henderson C, Noblett J, Parke H, et al: Mental health–related stigma in health care and mental health–care settings. Lancet Psychiatry 1(6):467–482, 2014 26361202

Institute for Healthcare Improvement: The conversation project. 2016. Available at: https://theconversationproject.org/. Accessed February 28, 2019.

Junaid O, Hegde S: Supportive psychotherapy in dementia. Adv Psychiatr Treat 13:17–23, 2007

Knight BG: Psychotherapy & older adults resource guide. 2009. Available at: https://www.apa.org/pi/aging/resources/guides/psychotherapy. Accessed February 28, 2019.

Moberg PJ, Lazarus LW: Psychotherapy of depression in the elderly. Psychiatr Ann 20:92–96, 1990

Morris DL: Geriatric mental health: an overview. J Am Psychiatr Nurses Assoc 7(suppl):S2–S7, 2001

Osborn R, Dotyn MM, Moulds D, et al: Older Americans were sicker and faced more financial barriers to health care than counterparts in other countries. November 15, 2017. Available at: http://www.commonwealthfund.org/publications/in-the-literature/2017/nov/older-americans-sicker-and-faced-more-financial-barriers-to-care. Accessed February 28, 2019.

Rowan K, McAlpine D, Blewett L: Access and cost barriers to mental health care by insurance status, 1999 to 2010. Health Aff (Millwood) 32(10):1723–1730, 2013 24101061

Seegert L: How ageism can negatively affect the health of older adults. June 9, 2016. Available at: https://healthjournalism.org/blog/2016/06/how-ageism-can-negatively-affect-the-health-of-older-adults/. Accessed February 28, 2019.

Semel VG: Countertransference and ageism: therapist reactions to the older patient, in Strategies for Therapy With the Elderly, 2nd Edition. New York, Springer, 2006, pp 223–235

Sirey JA, Bruce ML, Carpenter M, et al: Depressive symptoms and suicidal ideation among older adults receiving home delivered meals. Int J Geriatr Psychiatry 23(12):1306–1311, 2008 18615448

Tolstoy L: The Death of Ivan Ilyich (1886). Translated by Solotaroff L. New York, Bantam Books, 1981

Twain M: The Adventures of Tom Sawyer (1876[1875]). New York, Bantam Books, 1981

Weiner MF: Neurocognitive disorders, in The American Psychiatric Press Textbook of Psychiatry, 6th Edition. Edited by Hales RE, Yudofsky SE, Roberts LW. Washington, DC, American Psychiatric Publishing, 2014, pp 815–850

Winston A, Rosenthal RN, Pinsker H: Learning Supportive Psychotherapy: An Illustrated Guide. Washington, DC, American Psychiatric Publishing, 2012

World Health Organization: Dementia fact sheet. December 12, 2017a. Available at: https://www.who.int/news-room/fact-sheets/detail/dementia. Accessed February 28, 2019.

World Health Organization: Mental health of older adults. December 12, 2017b. Available at: https://www.who.int/mediacentre/factsheets/fs381/en/. Accessed February 28, 2019.

World Health Organization: Aging and life-course. Frequently asked questions: ageism. 2019. Available at: http://www.who.int/ageing/features/faq-ageism/en. Accessed February 28, 2019.

Wyman MF, Gum A, Arean PA: Psychotherapy with older adults, in Principles and Practice of Geriatric Psychiatry, 2nd Edition. Edited by Agronin ME, Maletta GJ. Philadelphia, PA, Wolters Kluwer Health/Lippincott Williams & Wilkins, 2011, pp 179–202

Yesavage JA, Karasu TB: Psychotherapy with elderly patients. Am J Psychother 36(1):41–55, 1982 7081516

Zechner MR, Birkmann JC, Sperduto J, et al: Sensitizing inpatient mental health staff to the challenges of aging. J Psychosoc Nurs Ment Health Serv 56(4):12–16, 2018 29328357

14

Special Populations

In this chapter we discuss guidelines for working with special populations and considerations to be kept in mind when working in special settings. The universe of potential psychiatric patients includes all of us. And the ability of the therapist to recognize the humanity and needs of patients is the key skill required to provide quality care to the patients, representing a wide variety of personality types, backgrounds, and ethno-cultural characteristics, we encounter. Patients also come to us from various settings. In this chapter we look at two populations that come to therapy with unique needs because of the settings in which they are found and the attitudes of society toward them: 1) people in prisons, jails, and detention centers and 2) intellectually disabled people.

The commonalities between these groups are, perhaps, few in terms of their needs and psychiatric diagnoses, although there is certainly some overlap. But at least one feature is common and that is that their care and their autonomy are very much controlled by others. People in jails and prisons may access psychiatric care in many institutions, but their access to certain services and medications may be limited by policy, funding, and attitudes of the management of their facility, with little choice in provider or therapeutic setting. The intellectually disabled, by contrast, are often served by a wide variety of caregivers, social workers, and medical and mental health providers, but they may have minimal privacy and often little control over the services they receive.

Individuals in Jails, Prisons, and Detention Centers

In this section we address supportive psychotherapy issues in special populations involving patients who are in residential settings involuntarily. The settings discussed—jails, prisons, and detention centers—are ones that, unfortunately or fortunately depending on your perspective, have become increasingly important for therapists. It is unfortunate that so many people are now seen in such settings, but fortunate that attention is now being directed to their needs, which was not always the case a generation ago. The one often "involuntary setting" not covered directly here is the inpatient behavioral health unit. There is so much specialized literature on these settings that we will not attempt to teach therapists how to perform psychotherapy in general but concentrate instead on the adaptations of supportive psychotherapy in such settings. Most correctional settings provide in-service training for new and continuing employees. National accrediting agencies such as the National Commission on Correctional Health Care (www.ncchc.org) have a wealth of resources, including information on regional conferences and certification for health care workers and publications.

Most therapists learn from their first day that residents of special settings can run the gamut of psychopathology from fairly normal "guy next door" to "serial killer psychopath." In such settings, it may be possible to learn something about the person who is going to become your patient and also to modify your therapy as your knowledge base evolves. The one behavior that constantly surprises therapists is that patients in such settings, especially those with antisocial personalities, frequently lie even when they know their lies will be discovered. And when confronted about their lies, they do not exhibit the normal reactions of guilt or remorse. Patients who have this pattern of lying are often those with ASPDs, and group therapy with their peers is the best therapy for those patients.

However, not all criminals have antisocial personalities, and distinguishing between persons with antisocial personalities and persons who have performed antisocial acts will often open up therapeutic possibilities for residents, who can make changes in their lives, even within prison.

Working in a correctional setting can be sad, challenging, and rewarding all at the same time. You will have to learn the correctional jargon and always be fully aware of your surroundings. The awareness of transference and countertransference is of utmost importance in this setting. For example, you may be required to address the needs of a rapist or child molester. If this proves to be difficult for you and your feelings, you must address it or speak with your supervisor and request to be reassigned. This setting calls for you to be firm but polite, as you may find yourself being tested by inmates. Overcrowding of inmates and high turnover of staff are common problems. Observing humans in ankle and waist chains can be distressing. The important thing to remember is that the safety of the inmates and staff is a primary concern, and you must defer to correctional officers' directions. We have, of course, spoken a lot about countertransference earlier, in Chapter 2. A quick summary of your possible countertransference reactions in these settings is given by one expert (Brown 2007) and might prompt you to classify yourself as having one or more of the following:

- Fear
- Denial of fear
- Becoming the advocate
- Becoming the puppet of the inmate
- Inability to trust
- Desire to punish
- Guilt
- Disdain and emotional separation

But now we will just review a few facts and survey the domain of corrections. A jail is a facility where one is incarcerated short-term, usually less than a year (although some stays are longer). Persons may be detainees waiting for trial or prisoners serving a short sentence. Jails usually fall within the jurisdiction of the city or county. Jails will vary in the number of inmates, ranging from only a few to several thousand depending on the size of the city or county. Consider the size of the city of Los Angeles, California, or Chicago, Illinois, compared with the small town of Avon, Indiana. Prisons are under the jurisdiction of the state or federal prison systems and inmates may be serving sentences from 1 year to a life sentence with no parole. The term *detention center* is often used interchangeably with *jail*. That is because such facilities often house presentence *detainees* as well as sentenced *inmates*. However, detention centers are often referred to as places of confinement for illegal immigrants or refugees. No matter where the detainees or inmates are housed, they have a constitutional right to treatment of their medical and mental health needs.

In the 1800s two volunteers, Louis Dwight and Dorothea Dix, were repulsed to find that the mentally ill were housed in jails or prisons or wandering the streets. Dwight organized the Boston Prison Discipline Society, which spurred the Massachusetts legislature to advocate for all mentally ill inmates in jails and prisons to be transferred to Massachusetts General Hospital. As a result of Dwight's tireless efforts, the incarceration of mentally ill individuals was declared illegal. In 1833, the State Lunatic Asylum at Worcester opened, and more than half of the first patients were admitted directly from jails. Dix followed Dwight and uncovered horrendous conditions. She pressured politicians with dogged determination for changes in the treatment of the mentally ill. Dix is remembered for establishing 32 psychiatric hospitals by 1880 ("Breaking the Tragic Cycle" 2005; Gollaher 1995). Regrettably, we have come full circle and are now once again housing the mentally ill in jails and prisons. Ask some of the inmates and they will tell you it is considered a crime to be mentally ill.

A report by Torrey et al. (2011) uncovered the depths of the regression of the treatment of the mentally ill in the United States. In 2010 the percentage of persons with serious mental illness (SMI) in jails was equal to that in 1840. Currently there are about 35,000 state psychiatric beds in the United States (Torrey 2016), and 2 million people with mental illness are booked into jails each year (National Alliance on Mental Illness 2019).

The movement of the 1970s to provide treatment in the least restrictive environment has resulted in many cases of persons receiving no treatment at all. The deinstitutionalization movement has led to what is known as *transinstitutionalization*: the movement from psychiatric hospitals to another institution, such as a nursing home, shelter, or jail (Mowbray et al. 2002). Usually, when those with mental illness are arrested, the charges are minor, such as trespassing (looking for a place to sleep), lewdness (urinating in public), open container violations, retail theft (stealing food), or jaywalking. Placing a person with an SMI in a $10' \times 10'$ cell can be very traumatic for the individual.

Case Vignettes

Rhonda is a 25-year-old woman seen on the suicide watch unit of a large county jail in the western United States. She is naked except for a suicide blanket. She denies wanting to harm herself or kill herself. When she was brought in, her legal charge was assault. Rhonda was living in a group home and was diagnosed with intellectual developmental disorder, severe. Her records indicated she had the functioning capability of a 3-year-old. She became upset in the home when a staff member turned the television off and told Rhonda to "wash up for supper." Rhonda cried and struck the worker. The police were called to the home, and she was taken to jail when the police noted the worker had a blackened eye. Rhonda is tearful, frightened, and unable to comprehend why she is in jail with no clothes.

Martin is a 42-year-old man seen on the suicide watch unit after being brought into the same jail with a charge of improper use of 911. He had phoned 911 twelve times in 3 hours. The police responded to his apartment three times; the third time he was arrested. Martin phoned 911 because he believed his neighbor had placed a camera in Martin's smoke detector to spy on him. When he realized there was a camera in his cell, he became more paranoid and delusional. He began banging his head on the door and screaming. He was unable to follow the correctional officer's orders to move away from his door and sit on his bunk. He was extracted from his cell. Forced medication of haloperidol 5 mg, diphenhydramine 50 mg, and lorazepam 2 mg was given intramuscularly, and he was medically treated for a wound to his head.

Clearly, these two cases could have had very different outcomes in a hospital setting from what occurred in a correctional setting.

Giving advice can be problematic in some circumstances but especially in correctional environments, even though you might think the choices in those environments are limited (see Table 14–1). Examples of advice we think are correct in all environments include recommending to a patient with alcohol use disorder and/or a substance use disorder that he cut down and, in most instances, preferably stop using alcohol or illegal substances. You should be able to point out that returning to drug-using environments is much more conducive to relapse than returning to drug-free settings. You may also point out to the person with an alcohol use disorder that living in an alcohol-free home is much better than living in one with ready availability of alcohol. Advising a detainee to utilize faith-based coping using her established faith seems to be fair advice and is in fact part of the treatment plans in facilities where we have practiced. Giving advice to change religions is absolutely not. Advice to think about one's religious orientation may be appropriate if it stems from problems that the patient has raised in therapy. If the patient is making a choice between religions, you can ask him to clarify his reasons for deciding to choose and so forth, and then allow him to come to his own decision. In correctional environments, however, it is best to refer patients to the chaplain for religious doctrinal questions.

Case Vignette

A 32-year-old male detainee from a Central American country was in an immigration detention facility being evaluated for asylum under provisions of the Convention against Torture. He was receiving psychotherapy for various issues, including posttraumatic stress disorder (PTSD). He had gotten into some minor fights with other detainees and had a problem with anger and frustration tolerance. One day he was lining up to go to the recreation yard and for some reason, the previous group was staying longer than expected and there was a wait of about 15 minutes. Suddenly, he ran to the front of the line, grabbed a soccer ball, and ran toward the soccer field. Of course, the other detainees started yelling at him, and the detention officers confronted him and told him he should go back in line or else face discipline. He refused to go back in line and was handcuffed behind his back to be taken to disciplinary housing. Immediately, he began hyperventilating loudly and noisily.

The officers escorting him diverted immediately to the medical triage room. Mental health personnel were called, and a therapist who knew him was available. The therapist gave him calming instructions on how to relax, by thinking of something pleasant or a pleasant scene (e.g., guided imagery techniques). Then the therapist starting counting breaths and told the detainee to synchronize his breathing with the numbers. The counting slowed down, and the detainee slowed his breathing and began to breathe normally.

The therapist conferred with the detention officers and all agreed that the detainee was in no condition to be taken to disciplinary housing at that time, and he was instead placed in a mental health observation room in the medical clinic. The therapist checked on him several times, and to the therapist's surprise, after a few hours the detainee said that he was better and requested to go back to housing. Normally in a disciplinary situation he would have been sent as in the original plan to disciplinary housing, but the custody officers conferred with the shift lieutenant and decided that he would be sanctioned using other measures, such as loss of privileges, but not by confinement. He returned to his usual housing.

Table 14–1. Giving advice in special settings

Become intimately familiar with the legal and documentation requirements of your setting.

Be aware that correctional settings can be highly litigious environments and that therapists are frequently sued or referred to medical and psychology boards because of complaints from detainees even about the giving of "wrong advice." Therefore, any advice giving should be carefully documented with qualifications such as "Based on your history, you would be a good candidate for the anger management group, but only if you're sure you can handle the stress. Don't sign up for it unless you've really thought about it and you're always going to be responsible for your own behavior." (Prisoners have sued for advice to join a group in which, for example, they could not control their anger and assaulted another prisoner) The majority of practice-standard or legal complaints are eventually dismissed as frivolous, but it can be extremely stressful to the therapist while they are being reviewed or adjudicated.

Be mindful of how difficult it will be to practice in such environments and decide for yourself if you want to do so or move on if you find you do not want or cannot handle the stress. We are familiar with some correctional environments where we feel it is impossible to practice psychotherapy in any meaningful sense, since psychotherapy (of all types) involves some level of positive relationship between therapist and patient.

Never give advice that could be construed as outside your field of expertise—for example, advice that is legal or quasi-legal in nature about filing applications for benefits and so forth.

Phrase advice in terms of probabilities and document it as such (e.g., "You would probably be better off getting a day job because you have had problems staying awake when you are on the night shift, don't you think?").

If your setting is too toxic for advice giving yet you still want to work there, then stop giving advice and qualify all your "advisory" statements as such: "I can't give advice on this, so you'll have to make your own choice. All I can tell you is what I know about XYZ."

In his next therapy session, he told the therapist that he had been taken prisoner and tortured frequently in his home country, and furthermore, when they came to his cell to torture him, he was cuffed behind his back and taken to the torture room. He said that the incident while waiting to enter the recreation yard had triggered his memories of torture. Therapy for his PTSD continued to address the effects of his PTSD on his current behaviors, and there were no further incidents for the rest of his stay in the facility.

This vignette shows the mixture of correctional-type issues with psychotherapy processes in a detention facility, and the need for changing decisions and accommodations for mental health problems. It is typical of the complex issues faced by therapists in those settings. The therapist may be involved in settings other than a traditional office. There is the need to respond to emergencies. Also needed is the skill of interacting and even negotiating outcomes with custody officers. Therapists in those settings often say that "custody, not medical, runs the institution" and that the outcome may not always meet the wishes of the therapist. In the previous incident, the outcome was a good one. The detainee did not get a "free ride" for his behavior, but he did receive treatment and accommodation in the disciplinary process.

In most correctional institutions, mental health personnel give input in the disciplinary process, since it is well known that mentally ill persons have difficulty tolerating the isolation and other sanctions typically imposed in discipline. A balance needs to be achieved to keep holding patients responsible for dangerous behaviors while still addressing the vulnerabilities of mentally ill persons to the typical disciplinary processes. The need to strike such a balance is certainly leading to much creative thinking about alternative modes of discipline. However, when discipline is imposed, the supportive therapist has the task of addressing the patient's reactions to and toleration of the process. The priority in all institutions is assessing for risk of self-harm or harm to others, often on a daily basis. But an added task is obviously to improve the patient's ability to cope with the discipline. For example, this may involve suggesting activities that the patient can engage in to pass the time, planning ahead for the future, and so forth. Even being able to give paper handouts for education or blank papers for writing and journaling is helpful and should be allowed in correctional settings. Boredom is to be avoided when at all possible.

Supportive therapists in correctional settings often struggle with ethical issues when they try to help patients strengthen coping skills and defenses. How does one, or should one, shore up a patient who experiences remorse over his crime? On the other hand, how does one address the patient who has no remorse? It should help to explore the patient's value system and see if this is reasonable and conventional or too extreme to work with. You should find areas where you can work productively using conventional values, or areas that are value-free. The patient may have interests to pursue, relationships to discuss, and plans to make. If he is not amenable to therapeutic assistance, then he will not be a candidate for therapy. This problem often solves itself, as many patients who find therapy unhelpful reject the service anyway. However, the following vignette illustrates some ethical issues.

Case Vignette

A 37-year-old man was apprehended crossing the border from Mexico into the United States. He had actually spent much of his childhood in the United States but was deported at the age of 27 because of an outstanding deportation order. Since then he had tried to return covertly on several occasions. Because this was his third return to the United States, he was sentenced to 6 months in a U.S. federal correctional institution. He was assigned to a therapist. He related to the therapist his fears of being raped in prison. For the first time, he said, he wanted to tell someone that he had been raped when he was 12 years old by a "friend" of the family and at age 27 by a gang of men in Mexico. The therapist worked with him on a safety plan to avoid being in situations where he could be vulnerable. This worked out well. On one occasion, while working in the laundry room, another man grabbed his chest, and he pushed the man away. A pushing match ensued, but he was not injured, and the officers intervened.

The prisoner developed confidence, even in the prison environment, that he could look out for his own safety, and he was not further molested during his sentence. However, at the end of the sentence, he began to wonder if he would be deported again. The therapist asked him to speculate what would happen if he were, and the patient said he would definitely not remain in Mexico but would return to the United States illegally. The therapist had expected to hear this and commented, "You just have to learn NOT to get caught!" Later, the therapist felt guilty that he had condoned illegally entering the United States. He wondered if he should have qualified his remark with something like "Well, I can't condone illegal immigration...but..." Perhaps he should have said, "I know you could always return illegally, but your track record on that is not great. If you return to Mexico, can't you get a visa to some other country and apply to be a resident?" (The answer to that question is actually positive.)

Correctional institutions are immersive environments. The most immediate and overwhelming impression of persons who enter such environments is that they are prisoners themselves and surrounded by inmates. Indeed, except for high-security environments, inmates do the majority of routine cleaning and maintenance work of facilities and (despite the requirement of frequent counts) are up and about throughout the day. The impression people have that inmates are locked in cells all the time is basically true only in regard to high-security environments. Corrections environments are also physically and psychologically dangerous. Inmates frequently make unjustified complaints of abuse against staff members. Awareness of the problems and dangers should be part of your training and decision making about professional placement and actions.

When psychotherapists are treating patients within the institution, there are many activities (therapeutic, quasi-therapeutic, and simply nontherapeutic but assigned to therapists) that are found in correctional or residential institutions (see Table 14–2).

Therapists in correctional settings often are subject to what is called "manipulation" by inmates. However, the tendency to call an inmate manipulative should lead to an examination of the inmate's own adaptation to meet his needs in the correctional setting. To be sure, however, therapists in those settings will frequently be accused (by custody staff) of "coddling" the inmates. Learning one's own reasonable responses to special requests will take time. One of the experts in the field does suggest the following guidelines for responding to requests for special privileges (Appelbaum 2010, p. 103):

- Explore alternatives to granting privileges.
- Base privileges on objective data.
- Use privileges mostly for patients with serious mental disorders.
- Involve custody staff in special privilege decisions.

Telepsychiatry

Telepsychiatry is often used in jails and prisons to augment care delivered by on-site providers. Considering that most prisons are in rural areas and access to clinicians is insufficient or nonexistent, the use of telepsychiatry is an asset for inmates and corrections staff. The scheduling of appointments is no different from that in an on-site clinic. Most inmates and staff will be comfortable with the videoconferencing, as many have used programs and apps such as Skype and FaceTime and participated in video courts. However, telepsychiatry or telemedicine differs from connecting with others on Skype or FaceTime

Table 14–2. Activities of psychotherapists in correctional or residential settings

Deliver psychotherapy.

- Individual or group therapy for sleep hygiene
- Cognitive therapy for insomnia
- Guided imagery and relaxation therapy
- Mindfulness
- Suicidality assessment and postattempt therapy

Develop safety plans to reduce risk of suicide.

Assess culpability for discipline within institution or mitigation of punishment.

Determine suitability to be placed in restrictive housing (formerly called "segregation units" and, by inmates, "the hole")—so-called baseline stable evaluations to determine if a mentally ill inmate was responsible for his or her actions.

Provide input to the facility disciplinary committee.

Participate in risk management for release.

Participate in risk management for parole.

Determine need for placement in institution infirmary, crisis unit, external hospital, or special mental health facility.

Release to a lower level of care.

Determine risk of re-offense.

Determine need for one-on-one sitter during suicide watch.

Evaluate an individual on hunger strike.

Provide group interventions in hunger strikes.

Determine safety and need for staff companions during travel.

Determine safety to see outside consultant.

Placement after PREA (Prison Rape Elimination Act) allegation.

Assess risk of retaliation after PREA allegation.

Determine safety and suitability for work assignment (e.g., should this inmate with schizophrenia be allowed to work in the kitchen?).

Table 14–2. Activities of psychotherapists in correctional or residential settings *(continued)*

Respond to request for cell, cellmate, or unit change.

Determine whether placement in a single cell (a major perk in most institutions) is warranted.

Recommend special allowances for blanket, mattresses, or equipment.

Grant "lay-in" (day off work) for mental health reasons.

Determine suitability for rehabilitation classes.

Determine whether individual is malingering.

Serve as a "gatekeeper" to prescribers of medicine.

Get referrals from other staff members for specialized assessments or psychological testing.

Request certificate showing completion of classes.

Make recommendations for or against involuntary commitment for mental health reasons.

As a staff member, provide escort or discipline in, for example, transfer of inmates and during meetings.

Respond to emergency medical, fire, disaster, or security codes.

Train in the use of firearms in case of riot.

Train and prepare for hostage situations.

Participate in preparedness for institutional lockdowns.

Wear protective clothing when interviewing dangerous inmates.

Do a takedown on an inmate.

Apply restraints to an inmate.

Interview and conduct some sort of psychotherapy with inmates in cells, suicide watches, or 5-point restraints.

"Talk down" and defuse violence in agitated and dangerous inmates.

Report inmate misconduct (dealing with confidentiality issues and duty to report vs. right to confidentiality).

• Report staff misconduct.

because there are requirements that must be met to ensure that HIPAA guidelines are fulfilled. The agency you work for will help ensure the secure arrangement of the system. Depending on the setting and equipment of the facility, the inmates' charts may be faxed, emailed, or accessed electronically.

Individuals With Intellectual Disabilities

Developmentally disabled individuals in the United States—those people defined as having severe physical or neurological problems that affect their development in the years before age 22—make up about 3% of the population. Individuals with intellectual disabilities may account for up to a third of the developmentally disabled population (Baxter and Cain (2006). Until the 1970s, it was thought that psychiatric and psychological treatment of persons with intellectual disabilities would have little to no effect and, indeed, that such individuals were incapable of participating in most types of psychotherapy. In past centuries, most of these individuals would have been placed in institutional settings. With deinstitutionalization and the increasing integration of the developmentally disabled into the community—with family, in group homes, or through transitioning to independent living   services to and research about this particular population have increased dramatically. It is now increasingly common for the developmentally disabled to be referred to and receive psychotherapy if needed. The prevalence of mental disorders in the intellectual disability population is most likely similar to that in the general population (Baxter and Cain (2006), although many would estimate that number higher (Došen and Day 2001).

Complicating the access to services for people with intellectual disabilities and mental disorder is that they need both social services and mental health resources, which are often two different channels of resources to pursue. In addition, because of their intellectual disabilities, including verbal limitations, intellectual deficits, and behavioral characteristics, diagnosis of mental disorders can be difficult.

In Chapter 9, we discussed *co-occurring diagnosis* issues, referring to patients with substance use disorders and mental illness. Another use of that term applies to persons with intellectual disability and mental illness. Supportive psychotherapy is ideally suited to this population, since it does not require some of the levels of abstraction, denial of gratifications, impulse control, and behavioral restraint that we typically associate with psychodynamic psychotherapy.

A good introduction to supportive psychotherapy in this population has been provided by Gentile and Jackson (2008), who identified five cardinal points:

- Patients with intellectual disabilities may have a higher rate of psychiatric disorder than the general population.
- They are often referred for services because of disruptive behavior, verbal or physical aggression, or destruction of property.
- They are often acutely aware of their disability and have had a lifetime of shame and embarrassment from being told about it.
- They often have a life history of separation from families and unresolved grief and loss reactions.
- Because of their disabilities, they have often developed "learned helplessness," which can be offset somewhat if the therapist can develop treatments in which they have some control over aspects of their lives.

In addition to the specific challenges of dealing with psychiatric patients with intellectual disabilities themselves, the fact that they are most often dependent on professional or family caregivers for both their physical care and legal custodianship means that ethical issues such as privacy and self-determination are often complicated and have both therapeutic and emotional implications. Caregivers are often protective of their clients, and there may be some "turf war" conflict with mental health and other providers, as well as some reluctance to trust the patient's growing autonomy. In addition, the caregiver is used to having a great deal of information about his or her client, and this may conflict with the privacy concerns of the therapist (Hollins 2001, pp. 29–30).

Supportive Techniques for Intellectually Disabled Patients

Because supportive therapy techniques have a strong component of patient education and coordination with the patient's community, they are well suited to work with intellectually disabled patients. Such individuals may present with disruptive behavior that may, in part, be caused by a limited ability to cope with frustrations as well as neurological and other biological problems that limit their coping mechanisms (Gardner 2000, pp. 1–4).

Keller (2000, pp. 27–47) presents an overview of the processes needed to successfully involve intellectually disabled clients and their caregivers in psychotherapy. The process begins with explaining the value and techniques of therapy with those involved. Therapy itself should begin, as does all therapy, with the therapist establishing a relationship with the patient. Intellectually disabled patients are most often referred to therapy by service providers or family members. The patient enters therapy, often confused, with a negative view of previous contact with mental health professionals who have been involved with evaluating their disabilities, and with a lack of understanding of the process. As Keller notes, the first step in beginning therapy is to provide the patient with emotional support before educating him about psychotherapy, why it is used, what happens, and what the patient's and therapist's roles are. Patients with intellectual disabilities may present with a lack of verbal abilities and may require pictures and diagrams to assist with describing their feelings and experiences (Keller 2000, p. 33).

The Royal College of Psychiatrists (RCP) (2006) conducted a systematic review of the need for psychotherapy for disabled individuals in which they called for a widening of understanding of emotional and psychological matters in people with learning disability, through efforts ranging from providing individual therapy to facilitating psychotherapeutic understanding by caregivers and other service providers who have continuous involvement in the life of their clients. The RCP study surveyed service providers and therapists about a broad array of concerns and recommendations about therapy for learning disabled patients. The study authors concluded from their findings that psychotherapy is widely supported as an important tool in the care and treatment of such populations. Therapies that show promise include cognitive-behavioral therapy, psychodynamic therapy, and art, music, and drama therapy, along with family/systemic therapies. Underlying all of these is the emotional support and engagement of patients in understanding their feelings and learning coping skills and behavioral strategies that help them assert their independence (see also Prout et al. 2000).

Burke (2013) has developed a manual of psychotherapy for working with patients with learning disabilities for service providers in Ohio. In addressing the mental health needs of the intellectually disabled population, Burke begins by describing symptoms and characteristics of such individuals that may differ from the general population. For example, depressed individuals may talk out loud about their concerns and be irritable rather than sad. Anger, aggression, and self-injury may also be indicative of depression.

In beginning therapy with persons with intellectual disabilities, aspects to be considered include the following (Burke 2013, p. 16):

- Intellectual functioning
- Presenting symptoms
- Changes in behavior or emotion
- Existing stressors
- Past experience and skills in coping with similar problems

Such patients may have trouble expressing themselves verbally, so the therapist should be sensitive to affect and body language. Patients will likely respond to specific questions of a concrete nature rather than hypothetical questions. Using simple concrete language and taking a slower approach with shorter sessions are important to progress. Such patients will also benefit from direct education and a directive approach. Repetition of information and homework and other patient activities (such as art, role-playing, music) can be very useful.

Patients are helped to focus on identifying their own strengths and working on using those strengths in coping with their problems and to develop feelings of hopefulness. The goal of supportive therapy is to help individuals overcome feelings of depression, anxiety, fears, or other symptoms that reduce their ability to function. Supportive therapy involves creating an environment of increasing self-awareness and developing strategies for improved feelings of self-worth. Baxter and Cain (2006, p. 123) identify ways in which the supportive therapist can assist:

1. Decreasing external stressors by increasing support by the patient's community
2. Recommending and developing effective strategies for increasing pleasurable activities
3. Helping the patient feel more secure in therapy and in his or her community
4. Providing guidance and recommendations for dealing with problems
5. Helping the patient to verbalize strong emotions in order to relieve anxiety and depression
6. Assisting the patient in developing and implementing coping strategies

It goes without saying that working with patients who are also intellectually disabled requires specific strategies to take into consideration their limitations. Morasky (2007) describes four parameters that the therapist should keep in mind:

1. *Speed of thought processes.* Speed of thought processes is one indication of intellectual ability.
2. *Number of problems.* Intellectually disabled patients may be dealing with physical, mental, and emotional issues related to past history and current symptoms as well as their intellectual coping.
3. *Abstraction versus concrete thinking.* Intellectually disabled patients tend to be more concrete in their thinking, and therapists may need to help with learning abstract concepts.
4. *Complexity.* Many of the decisions of daily life have layers of complexity that can be difficult to interpret. When a particular decision has ramifications that the patient cannot predict or understand, the task of decision making can be daunting.

Intellectual activities that are difficult and may be more challenging for persons with intellectual disabilities as well as psychological diagnoses include memory, reasoning, decision making, planning, and problem solving. Supportive psychotherapists will need to work with patients to improve their coping skills with these intellectual limitations in mind.

A wide variety of caregivers and medical service providers interact with people who have intellectual disabilities. Harvey and Cloud (1998) provide a useful summary of the skills required of all such providers that are particularly relevant to counseling and therapy, including rapport building, respect, reliability, attention, active listening, attending, reflection, paraphrasing, empathy, and goal setting. Working with persons with dual diagnoses, the therapist needs to be aware of the therapeutic moment in which to use these skills, such as when the patient is confused or facing negative events, and help the patient to understand his or her feelings in the moment.

In this vein, Perkins (1999) discusses the conditions necessary for effective therapy with intellectually disabled patients. These include empathic understanding, respect, therapeutic genuineness, and specificity so that the patient understands and is able to deal with issues that the therapy is trying to affect.

Key Points

- Supportive psychotherapy can be adapted for work with people in prison, jails, and detention centers and people with intellectual disabilities.

- Although there are limitations to supportive psychotherapeutic work in correctional settings (e.g., regarding advice-giving and directive therapy), which can be physically challenging and litigious environments, there are many positive reasons to choose work in those environments.

- Knowledge of the personal histories of patients often provides the understanding of their behaviors and their therapy.

- Correctional environments have many complex and cooperative features, as illustrated by the admonition "Custody, not medical, runs the institution." The better the therapist understands the multidisciplinary nature of these environments, the better off he or she will be and the better the patient can be treated.

- Intellectually disabled people also present therapists with special challenges, but the concrete and directive methods of supportive psychotherapy are ideally suited to working with persons who lack higher abilities of abstractive and introspective thought.

- Supportive therapy, with its strong components of patient education and coordination with the patient's community, is well suited to work with intellectually disabled patients and can help them make better decisions and enjoy their lives more.

References

Appelbaum KL: The mental health professional in a correctional culture, in Handbook of Correctional Mental Health. Edited by Scott CL. Washington, DC, American Psychiatric Publishing, 2010, pp 91–118

Baxter JT, Cain NN: Psychotherapeutic interventions, in Training Handbook of Mental Disorders in Individuals With Intellectual Disability. Edited by Cain NN, Holt G, Davidson PW, et al Kingston, NY, NADD Press, 2006

Breaking the tragic cycle. Frontline (PBS), May 10, 2005. Available at: https://www.pbs.org/wgbh/pages/frontline/shows/asylums/special/reentry.html. Accessed February 28, 2019.

Brown GP: Countertransference in correctional settings, in Correctional Psychiatry: Practice Guidelines and Strategies. Edited by Thienhaus OJ, Piasecki M. Kingston, NJ, Civic Research Institute, 2007, pp 11-1–11-11

Burke T: Overview of Therapeutic Approaches for Individuals With Co-occurring Intellectual/Developmental Disabilities and Mental Illness for Direct Support Staff and Professionals Working in the Developmental Disability System. Cleveland, Ohio Mental Illness/Developmental Disability Coordinating Center of Excellence, 2013

Došen A, Day K: Epidemiology, etiology, and presentation of mental illness and behavior disorders in persons with mental retardation, in Treating Mental Illness and Behavior Disorders in Children and Adults With Mental Retardation. Edited by Došen A, Day K. Washington, DC, American Psychiatric Press, 2001, pp 3–24

Gardner WI: Behavioral therapies: using diagnostic formulation to individualize treatment for persons with developmental disabilities and mental health concerns, in Therapy Approaches for Persons With Mental Retardation. Edited by Fletcher RJ. Kingston, NY, NADD Press, 2000, pp 1–25

Gentile JP, Jackson CS: Supportive psychotherapy with the dual diagnosis patient: co-occurring mental illness/intellectual disabilities. Psychiatry (Edgmont) 5(3):49–57, 2008 19727299

Gollaher D: Voice for the Mad: The Life of Dorothea Dix. New York, The Free Press, 1995

Harvey K, Cloud L: Counseling skills for the paraprofessional. NADD Bulletin I(3):2, 1998

Hollins S: Psychotherapeutic methods, in Treating Mental Illness and Behavior Disorders in Children and Adults With Mental Retardation. Edited by Došen A, Day K. Washington, DC, American Psychiatric Press, 2001, pp 27–44

Keller E: Points of intervention: facilitating the process of psychotherapy with people who have developmental disabilities, in Therapy Approaches for Persons With Mental Retardation. Edited by Fletcher RJ. Kingston, NY, NADD Press, 2000, pp 27–47

Morasky RL: Making counseling/therapy intellectually attainable. NADD Bulletin X(3):3, 2007

Mowbray CT, Grazier KL, Holter M: Managed behavioral health care in the public sector: will it become the third shame of the states? Psychiatr Serv 53(2):157–170, 2002

National Alliance on Mental Illness: Jailing people with mental illness. 2019. Available at: https://www.nami.org/learn-more/public-policy/jailing-people-with-mental-illness. Accessed February 28, 2019.

Perkins DM: Counseling and therapy, revisited. NADD Bulletin II(2):3, 1999

Prout HT, Chard KM, Nowad-Drabik KM, et al: Determining the effectiveness of psychotherapy with persons with mental retardation: the need to move toward empirically based research. NADD Bulletin III(6):1, 2000

Royal College of Psychiatrists: Psychotherapy and Learning Disability. London, Royal College of Psychiatrists, 2006

Torrey EF: A dearth of psychiatric beds. February 25, 2016. Available at: http://www.psychiatrictimes.com/psychiatric-emergencies/dearth-psychiatric-beds. Accessed February 28, 2019.

Torrey EF, Kennard AD, Enslinger D, et al: More mentally ill persons are in jails and prisons than hospitals: a survey of the states. January 28, 2011. Available at: https://community.nicic.gov/blogs/mentalhealth/archive/2011/01/28/more-mentally-ill-persons-are-in-jails-and-prisons-than-hospitals-a-survey-of-the-states.aspx. Accessed February 28, 2019.

15

Community and Family Involvement

Whether delivered in a private setting or as part of a clinic, hospital, group home, or school, therapy is at its core a community process. The patient, and the therapist for that matter, are part of a community: family, work, social, clinical—all contribute to the patient's circumstances and affect the patient and are affected by the patient. You may recall a book titled *It Takes a Village* (Clinton 2006), which is about community involvement with children. It is also true of your patients. They were children of their community, families are part of their community, they have jobs and go to school in their community, and you and your clinic are a community enterprise.

Much of what we have discussed so far has been focused on the patient-therapist relationship. But as practitioners, we know that there are several other players in the therapeutic process, including families, treatment teams, social workers, and medical professionals. While the relationship of therapist and patient is the core of supportive therapy, much of the process, especially in a clinic or inpatient facility, will involve other professionals. Indeed, the entire clinical structure of case manager, therapist, social worker, family, and other resources is designed to be supportive of the patient and provide the tools the patient needs to improve health, participation in the community, and self-confidence through therapy, training, and resources. For example, the principal therapist might be a psychologist working with a psychiatrist or nurse practitioner who is managing prescribing of psychiatric medicines, and with social workers and case managers who are helping with such efforts as job training and housing. Family and the staff of residential facilities, if appropriate, are involved in the treatment process, often recommending admission to an inpatient unit or clinic enrollment, and are certainly concerned with and vital to success of treatment and posttreatment care.

The supportive psychotherapist usually interfaces frequently with other clinic staff and periodically with professionals from outside agencies and with family and social connections of the patient. The coordination of information is key to helping the patient achieve the goals of treatment and maintain better mental health even after the therapy has concluded.

While we prefer our definition of supportive psychotherapy, presented in Chapter 1, with its focus on therapy that is empirically based, many clinicians see the process from different perspectives (Brenner 2012; Edenfield and Saeed 2012):

- Supportive psychotherapy consists of the fundamental elements of all psychotherapy.
- Supportive psychotherapy is one end of the spectrum of dynamic psychotherapy.
- Supportive psychotherapy is a distinct set of directly helpful psychotherapy interventions.
- Supportive psychotherapists often encourage clinic colleagues to accept therapists who practice other empirically based psychotherapies (e.g., meditation and one of its subtypes, mindfulness).

Overall, the aim of psychotherapy in general, and supportive psychotherapy specifically, is to resolve patients' distress, restore and enhance function, and facilitate further progress. Treatment planning, particularly in a hospital, clinic, or other organization, allows the participants to move in a coordinated fashion to develop a comprehensive approach to caring for the patient (Makover 2016; Mariush 2002).

Inside Interfaces

In many clinics and inpatient settings, a patient is treated by representatives of several mental health professions who constitute a treatment team. In such settings, the therapist should understand that other mental health professions have different training; they experience and invest their roles differently; and they often achieve different satisfactions from them. For example, the psychiatrist may be open to innovative or paradoxical interventions. Another team member may perceive such efforts as "experimenting with my patient." Indeed, the question "Whose patient is it?" is present, sotto voce, behind many staff disagreements.

Often the patient, living with an institutional transference, knows that the clinic will outlast any member of the treatment team. Psychiatric residents, in particular, may find that their pharmacological and therapeutic expertise is accepted more readily than their treatment planning suggestions, on the rationale that they will not have to live with the long-term consequences of their treatment plans. In addition, suggestions from psychiatric residents regarding treatment planning may be taken less seriously because the residents are often the least experienced members of the treatment team. In such cases, it is important to emphasize common bonds, such as the desire to improve the quality of patient services and the conditions of society (Barton and Barton 1983). Indeed, patients receiving care at teaching hospitals show improved outcomes because of the resources and expertise available and the coordination of such expertise in patient care (Dashoff 2017).

Interfaces with other staff serve many essential functions. Whether or not the patient has a single case manager whose job it is to ensure the maximally effective, coordinated, continuous services of several agencies, the therapist can make contributions to the many case management functions (Table 15–1).

Selection of Patients at Risk for Relapse, Neglect, or Social Breakdown

You should help determine which patients are offered therapy, what approach the therapy should take, and what goals are to be achieved. You should also contribute to the screening criteria. Patients are sometimes wrongly assigned to a level of service solely on the basis of a chart review, resulting in inadequate or inappropriate services—or an inevitable shifting of the patient between departments. Therapists bring a holistic approach to understanding the patient's

Table 15–1.   Some common functions of therapy and case management

Inside interfaces (intra-agency functions)

Selection of patients and triage

Assessment of patient's needs, strengths, weaknesses, and goals for treatment

Treatment planning, coordination, review, and updating

Monitoring of patient's participation and progress

Advocacy to obtain needed services

External interfaces

Engagement with and linkage to outside services

Coordination of inpatient-outpatient services (continuity of care)

Discharge planning

Involvement of family in assessment, treatment, and follow-up (includes helping the family to work with the patient after discharge)

Source.   Adapted from Intagliata et al. 1986; Kanter 1989; Lamb 1982.

status that may add needed expertise to chart review findings. All staff should contribute to the clinic's selection and assignment policies.

Assessment of Patient's Needs, Strengths, Weaknesses, and Goals for Treatment

Similarly, you may have a unique perspective of the patient's strengths and weaknesses, knowing the patient "from the inside," whereas the case manager sees the patient's objective successes and failures "from the outside," looking primarily at the physical and social functioning of the patient rather than internal conflicts. Neither perspective is right or wrong; together, as we will see below, they can provide the most complete picture of the patient for use in treatment planning. Too, the therapist is likely to have had longer sessions with the patient about motivations and goals.

Treatment Planning, Coordination, Review, and Updating

When many professionals are involved in a patient's care, treatment planning may be formal with other staff and agencies or more informal with family, peer groups, and the patient or any combination of participants. The process has a common theme: communication (Mariush 2002; Sun et al. 2013).

You should not prematurely raise issues in therapy that generate inappropriate activity by other staff, such as sending a patient for job placement when she is not ready. This happens when therapists are unwilling to confront patients with reality. Instead of saying, "We really ought to discuss this," they may say, "Talk about getting a job with your rehabilitation counselor. I have nothing to do with that decision." Conversely, failure to address important issues (sometimes because the patient conceals them) will impede the progress of therapy. In supportive psychotherapy, perhaps more so than in other types of psychotherapy, you should not assume that the patient will "automatically" talk about important issues when they become pressing enough.

Despite efforts to prescribe only treatments that will be successful, it should be borne in mind that many patients are conflicted about treatment goals that will make them more independent. For example, they may accept work assignments but sabotage them either consciously or unconsciously. When faced with such conflicts, you might take what Kanter (1985a) calls a "passive managerial attitude" (p. 84) and a "gradual trial-and-error approach" (p. 85) for the months and even years it takes the patient to become independent.

Monitoring of Patient's Participation and Progress

Team reviews of individual patients are a standard feature of clinic programs, and such meetings should also be used for broader purposes to generate a positive attitude toward the work and to prevent staff burnout. As Menninger (1984) notes, case presentations often reveal, contrary to preexisting opinion, that a patient has made significant progress. If this has not been the case, an outside consultant may introduce a new perspective or facilitate the staff's changing their assumptions about the best mode of treatment for a specific patient or generally.

Advocacy to Obtain Needed Services

Advocacy helps to further the patient's goals, but it is also a characteristic of supportive psychotherapy in general. Even a single effort to act on the patient's behalf can convince the patient that you have a genuine commitment to his interests. Although the therapist cannot serve as the patient's legal advocate and may oppose the patient on some issues, opportunities for straightforward advocacy arise that will increase the patient's tolerance of the inevitable differences of opinions.

Because the therapist knows the patient best, Lamb (1982) has argued that therapists are best suited to serve as case managers. Although the therapeutic aims mentioned so far, as well as the general goals of supportive therapy (e.g., the maintenance or improvement of the patient's function), overlap those of case management, we believe that the roles have evolved distinctly and that it usually serves therapy to keep them separate. In addition, many therapists lack the training to perform case management activities or the willingness to perform community outreach (Schwartz et al. 1982). In public clinics and other institutional settings, caseloads may mean that therapists simply do not have the time to handle all aspects of a patient's program. For example, in discussions with patients about their legal resources, you might want to suggest that they be very clear as to their wishes but leave it up to their attorney as to how to achieve those wishes. Restated, their attitude should be "What" is their role? "How" can their attorney help them?

Differences of Opinion

Although we have emphasized the benefits of interfaces with other staff, special problems do arise, such as when treating patients with a diagnosis of borderline personality, in whom the phenomenon of splitting may be common. *Splitting*, identified by Freud and elaborated by Melanie Klein and others, refers to the separation of mental contents into all-good and all-bad compartments. In individual therapy, the patient may see the therapist as sometimes good and sometimes bad, and is unable to maintain an integrated representation of the therapist as a fallible, sometimes flawed, but nevertheless supportive human being.

As a patient interacts with more than one staff member, she may turn some into idealized individuals and others into hated enemies. These individuals in turn will sometimes live up to their roles because of unconscious dynamics that have been termed *projective identification* (done by the patient) and *counter-identification* (done by the staff member). Gabbard (1989) notes that the *therapist* is usually the idealized figure, unaware of the possibility of disruptive and destructive activities of the patient outside the therapy. This situation is more likely to arise when the therapist is out of touch with the patient's real life. As discussed earlier in this book, a cardinal rule of supportive therapy is to know what has happened in the patient's real life and to provide an environment in which the patient feels free to report what happens. Of course, this does not always occur as desired, and the talked-to therapist may still be misinformed. Some splitting is unavoidable, and it may be both necessary and beneficial. If so, it can be used productively, allowing the maintenance of a positive transference with the therapist while the patient projects negative feelings onto the clinic or other staff. For example, as Weiner (1982, p. 138) notes, one of the advantages of a therapist-administrator split is the ability to designate the coercive work, such as legal steps to treat the patient involuntarily, to the latter. In that way, a therapist can disclaim control over the patient's involuntary hospitalization or medication, fostering the therapist alliance. On the other hand, the patient may realize that the therapist had an influence on such matters, and thus the deliberate use of this can erode the patient's trust of therapy or result in a perception of herself as a helpless patient with a helpless therapist fighting an all-powerful administrator (Worden 1951). However, this type of split is especially useful in achieving an alliance with psychotic patients and in treating specific problems that patients have in relation to authority figures.

Conflicts can also arise from discipline-specific roles and theoretical or ideological predilections; examples are the perspectives of short-term "reformers" and long-term "traditionalists," medicators and nonmedicators, hospitalizers and community treaters, and family and professionals (Seeman et al. 1982). Sometimes such conflicts arise from splitting, diagnostic uncertainty, or differing theories of psychopathology. A more apt approach is an open acknowledgment of staff differences and willingness to experiment with treatment strategies that will give the patient more opportunity to develop responsibility without being blamed for failure.

Some team members may think that coercive treatment cannot work. The supportive psychotherapist should counter such thinking, as it is not true and limits what can be offered patients. Most patients receiving involuntary treatment become voluntary patients within weeks of being involuntarily treated (Keisling and Peele 1980). Many patients treated involuntarily will thank the treatment team later. Patient and family education programs that explain symptoms, causes, and treatment processes, as well as provide strategies for coping and for achieving patients' goals, are being adapted by many inpatient and clinic settings and have proven successful in this regard (Cole 1993).

Despite the potential for disagreement, the differing perspectives of members of the treatment team are generally synergistic in improving the patient's treatment. Differences of opinion among the clinic's staff may stimulate fruitful discussion and increased objectivity, leading to innovative solutions to the patient's needs. It is not unusual for differences to be resolved by making the treatment plan more comprehensive.

Staff differences can increase an understanding of the patient, as the following cases (modified from Novalis 1989) illustrate.

Case Vignettes

A family that has been seen frequently by a case manager for a year is engaged in family therapy. The 22-year-old daughter admits to the new therapist on the second visit that she is heavily into cocaine but says she will not tell her case manager because the latter "is just like my mother" and thinks too highly of her.

A 24-year-old borderline patient avoids seeing his case manager every time he suffers a setback at work because the case manager calls it "self-defeating" behavior. But this patient begins meeting with a new therapist, who tells him, "I want to see you when things are going badly, not just when they are going well." The patient now begins to speak more freely of his failures and disappointments to the therapist. The therapist maintains these confidences, explaining the need for them to the curious case manager, who would like to know much more about the patient's vocational and social progress. However, the therapist does urge the patient to trust the case manager and reveal the "secrets" when he is ready.

The concentration of power in a therapist, who may become invested with transference-inspired fantasies, can also be detrimental to patients, including those with personality disorders and schizophrenia. For example, a patient who fails in job placement may assume that he has "disappointed" the case manager but can fall back on a "forgiving" therapist. Conversely, a patient heading into psychotic relapse may assume that she disappointed the therapist and may feel more comfortable in approaching the case manager for support.

Not surprisingly, then, when the therapist is given too much control over a patient's life, serious disturbances of the transference can result. Conflicts, for example, often arise over disability determinations. One patient avoided telling her therapist that a disability evaluation was in progress because she felt that the therapist could "see through her" and tell that she was too well for disability. In fact, the patient felt this was her very problem: she always came across better to others than she really felt. She sought to avoid the "inevitable" rejection by her therapist that would destroy their relationship.

We generally support the desirability of dividing some important functions between different members of the treatment team. The advantages and disadvantages in such arrangements have been widely discussed. Although we believe in distinctly different roles for therapist and case manager, we certainly agree with Harris and Bergman's (1987) supposition that case management may be a "mode of therapy" in which the patient is given a stable, rational, powerful, proactive, problem-solving model to internalize and identify with. Thus, it is no surprise that a study of the benefits and effects of case management highlighted the therapeutic effects of the case manager who develops a "supportive relationship" and teaches skills to the patient (Goering et al. 1988). However, some case management functions, such as money management and home visits, are too invested with power or fantasy to be regularly performed by therapists.

External Interfaces

Engagement With and Linkage to Outside Services

Although the task of coordinating services for a patient with outside services is in many instances assigned to a case manager, such coordination often serves a therapeutic purpose, such as giving the patient a real feeling of accomplishment when he feels he is ready for job training, independent living, or even "graduating" to fewer treatment sessions as his health improves. Indeed, the entire process of case management is to support the patient in achieving the goals of treatment and restore and enhance function in dealing with the illness and the recovery. Rapp (1998) describes what he calls the Strengths Model, which emphasizes that the desired outcome of case management is to aid clients in achieving the goals they set for themselves. This outcome is achievement and growth oriented, helping patients live healthy lives through identifying proper management of medication, identifying early warning signs of symptom exacerbations, and using strategies to reduce or eliminate their development, then helping the patients build a life that is satisfying and fulfilling. The goal of therapy is to help patients improve their quality of life through achievement, a sense of competency, life satisfaction, and empowerment.

Case Vignettes

A 26-year-old gay man at risk for AIDS went to a primary clinic to be tested for HIV status but was afraid to call for the results. He asked the therapist to make the call on his behalf. The therapist discussed the patient's fears, but the latter was still not inclined to call. At this point the therapist could have turned to other matters but concluded that it would be appropriately supportive to call the primary care clinic. As the therapist suspected, the clinic would not reveal the information over the phone. Nevertheless, the therapist's action showed his willingness to support the patient, who could not face the anticipated anxiety of the results. Two days later, the patient went to the primary care clinic, found out he was HIV negative, and called the therapist with the results. "I knew you would want to know," he explained.

A 36-year-old man with schizophrenia, who normally had a good working relationship with his therapist, became oppositional about accepting a new work assignment. He liked his current job and believed that he would lose his income by taking the new one. The therapist called the patient's vocational rehabilitation counselor and clarified the arrangements. The patient thanked his therapist several times in subsequent sessions for making the call, showing implicit recognition of the fact that the therapist had "stepped out of role" to help him out.

The therapist's decision in each of these cases was intuitive but not capricious. Probably, the patient was creating an interagency split (akin to the interpersonal splitting previously discussed) in which a "bad" external agency was seen as impeding the patient's progress in the "good" mental health clinic. The therapist's decision to intervene was based on the assumption that the intervention was necessary to mend the split. Such positive linkages must be balanced against the intervention that Kanter (1985a) calls "not linking," or allowing the patient to negotiate directly with the outside agency. Factors in the decision to assist a patient with a linkage include the urgency of the need and the patient's ability to meet it unassisted. For example, therapists who serve patients with severe illness should not shirk from helping them obtain Social Security or social benefits, even though they may be unaccustomed to such a facilitative role.

It should also be noted that interagency splits can arise independently of the patient as the result of ideological differences and the respective "orthodoxies" of the individual agencies.

Coordination and Continuity of Care

Many patients, particularly those who are more severely mentally ill, migrate through a variety of treatment modalities, from family care, to counseling at school, to formal psychotherapy in private practice or clinics and inpatient care. Providing continuity of such care requires an overall treatment plan that can help all the caregivers and the patient understand where in the process an individual might be. Assessing the activities and progress your patient is making to overcome weaknesses and understand the need for different levels of care is obviously an interactive process that may include setbacks and negotiating of level of care determinations. The key to successful treatment, then, is an awareness of the totality of the treatment process and your ability to coordinate with other professional, such as social workers, training personnel, other therapists, and attorneys, as well as inpatient units, family, and your patient, to ensure that each participant in the process is aware of what the others are doing and all are moving toward the planning goals (Mariush 2002).

Discharge Planning

Once a patient is assessed in the early stages of treatment and therapy begins, goals are set, milestones are reached, and progress is made toward the goals set. Discharge planning is the natural endpoint of the planning, therapy, revisions, and adaptations that you and your patient experience during the therapy. There comes a point when you, your patient, and the treatment team will determine that discharge from the program is appropriate. At that time, it is necessary to create a plan that helps the patient realize his goals and become more independent. The plan should include education about what to expect, job and social placement if necessary, resources the patient will need for coping with any remaining problems or relapses, and coordination with outside services that are available (Kennedy 2003).

Family Involvement in Assessment, Treatment, and Follow-Up

Families are the first caregivers for almost all of us—patients, therapists, bosses, workers, and the person on the street. As such, involvement of families is often a key step in treatment of a patient. Family members have unique insight into the symptoms, behaviors, and, in many cases, the techniques that will most help a patient. In addition, when coming up with a supportive therapy treatment plan, the family will often be the support system for encouraging progress and continuing care after formal therapy is reduced or no longer needed. Families for some patients may include the staff and cohabitants in settings such as group homes, rehabilitation centers, therapy groups, and school settings.

Heru and Drury (2007) discuss the importance of involving families in the treatment of psychiatric patients. Although their focus is on hospital settings, such involvement is often key to success in many treatment settings. The core competencies for general medical students established by the Accreditation Council for General Medical Education (ACGME) in 2004 include the ability to educate patients, families, and staff about medical, psychosocial, and behavioral issues and to establish a working alliance with patients and families. For psychiatric care, the patient's social system can yield valuable insights. The patient's position in the family, family attitudes toward the patient (and vice versa) and toward the patient's illness and behavior, and the ability of the family to support the treatment plan are variables that contribute to therapeutic process.

Family Matters

In psychotherapy as well as other health care specialties, the importance of the family in patient care cannot be denied. The ACGME, as discussed by Heru and Drury (2007), includes family matters in the core competencies. These include the following:

- Patient care, medical knowledge, interpersonal and communications skills, systems-based practice, professionalism, and practice-based learning and improvement
- Ability to educate patients, families, and staff about medical, psychosocial, and behavioral issues
- Ability to establish a working alliance with patients and families (For psychiatric patients, develop an understanding of the patient's position within the family and the social system, develop treatment plans within the psychosocial system, and support the system and educate the family.)

Although developed for medical residents, these principles are generally applicable to most health care professionals and are especially applicable to the supportive psychotherapeutic approach, which emphasizes the education of patients and caregivers.

Developing a Supportive Relationship With the Family

The decision to involve the family in a patient's treatment may itself be controversial. In order to keep the therapist's loyalties clear as well as to comply with privacy standards, the addition of the family should have the permission of, and promise some therapeutic benefit to, the patient. Thus, it may not be indicated for couples or for patients who do not live with their families and do not desire their assistance. In settings such as group homes, schools, and residential placements, the staff and fellow residents might be considered as the patient's family.

You may need to deal with both a reluctant, guilt-burdened patient and a family that does not want to exacerbate the acute stresses of the patient's illness by opening psychological wounds in acute confrontations. In many families, however, the members are important members of the treatment team. Engaging the patient and family requires interventions that support their self-esteem rather than more anxiety-provoking psychodynamic techniques. The occurrence of emotionally supportive interactions with the therapist has been found to be the strongest factor influencing family satisfaction with mental health professionals (Tessler et al. 1991). For a family to be successfully engaged in treatment, we also believe that there should be some perceived benefit *for them* other than the patient's welfare—that is, some alleviation of other family problems.

Interventions that offer such support have been termed *supportive family counseling* to distinguish them from family therapy per se (Bernheim 1982). In the former, didactic techniques are used and the family unit is treated as if it were basically healthy. In the latter, the approach is more indirect but evocative of underlying family conflicts and attempts to change the basic family structure.

Of the several types of supportive family programs, we shall highlight the family psychoeducational approach to schizophrenia developed by Anderson et al. (1986). This approach has been adopted by many hospitals and clinics for working with families of psychiatric patients generally (Compton and Broussard 2009). Patients with schizophrenia have been shown to relapse less frequently in families that are low in a characteristic called *expressed emotion*, the components of which are characterized as criticism, hostility, and intrusiveness. Family agendas for dealing with this issue will be discussed shortly. From the patient's perspective, the agenda usually involves reducing social contact with family members by providing alternative daytime and leisure activities (Leff 1989).

There is also evidence that in general, stress increases vulnerability and relapse in psychiatric illness, and that in particular, patients with schizophrenia suffer specific cognitive and information-processing deficits that make them vulnerable to novel and emotionally stressful situations.

The basic goals of a psychoeducational approach are outlined in Table 15–2. This model has also been applied to affective illness (Holder and Anderson 1990). A family psychoeducational program, like a social skills training program, involves considerable structure and detail, yet many of its elements can be incorporated into the therapist's ordinary contact with families.

Proper implementation of a psychoeducational approach requires much skill, for the process can be easily undermined if the following points are neglected:

- **Families have their own problems.** Exclusive focus on the patient as "the problem" is usually inaccurate. The psychoeducational approach has the "advantage" of providing the family with an explanation of its problem (e.g., scapegoating of the patient). This focus of attention may rally some families to a cause and preserve them from disintegration. It may, however, distract other families from the task of solving their own problems (which include the problems of the patient).

- **Other family problems result from the illness and require their own remedies.** These include the loss of income and the cost of the patient's support; the adoption of caregiving roles by other family members; and the family's isolation from neighbors and the community due to the stigma and burden of the illness.

- **Use of the psychoeducational model may exacerbate patterns of family dysfunction that will then need to be addressed.** Overinvolvement that has been found to raise levels of expressed emotion can itself be increased by implementation of the psychoeducational model.

- **Identification of the patient as the problem may be self-fulfilling.** As family counselors have long noticed, certain family members learn that by becoming "metaphors" of their family's problems, they serve to distract attention from other dysfunctional aspects. When the patient gets well, some

Table 15–2. Goals of the family psychoeducational approach

Form supportive treatment alliance with both patient and family.

Provide information and education about the illness.

Provide a low-key social environment (i.e., one that is low in expressed emotion).

Gradually integrate patient into family, social, and vocational roles

Oversee institutional transference and ensure continuity of care.

Source. Modified from Anderson et al. 1986, p. viii.

other family member may take on the role of dysfunctional family member in order to maintain this pattern.

- **Families may have a vested interest in sabotaging treatment.** The psychoeducational model, being community based, transfers the burden of care to the family, who may feel unable to handle it. It is sometimes in their perceived interest to hospitalize the patient and "prove" that the patient cannot be maintained in the community.

With these caveats in mind, the psychoeducational approach can be effective if attention on the patient is defocused. A corollary of this is that the therapist must regularly (even if infrequently) meet with the family alone, even if most meetings are conducted with the patient present. The therapist will never hear the family's full agenda if the patient is always there. On some occasions when the family members cannot physically be present, telephone or videoconferencing consultations may also be effective (Springer 1991).

The family structure, including its internal dynamic, is key to the success of family involvement. Therapists should assess the "power" structure within the family: who the leaders are, who the caregivers are, and who needs support and care. Some members of the family can be "difficult," domineering, likely to talk over the others, angry or controlling, or even silent and nonparticipatory, although willing and anxious to assist in the therapy (Heru and Drury 2007). Parents, siblings, and others in the family unit have their own functions within. In addition, families can be blended through remarriage, adoption, and fostering. Older children might be independent of the family in living arrangements but quite involved in caregiving, or more estranged or separate. Younger children might be in need of caregiving or temporary fostering. Work and school stressors might affect ability, time, and willingness to participate in therapy or caregiving.

Stages in Treatment

Goals for successful family involvement that lead to support of the psychotherapeutic process include the following[1]:

- Accepting the reality of the illness and understanding the current episode
- Identifying stresses of the current episode
- Identifying likely future stressors
- Identifying and describing the family interactions that may stress the patient
- Planning strategies for managing and minimizing stressors
- Accepting the need for continued treatment

Family responses to psychiatric illness parallel their responses to medical illness. We have divided such responses into three stages with appropriate interventions, as shown in Table 15–3.

Initially, some families react defensively to acute illness, with anger and denial. Their anger is often displaced onto mental health personnel, and their early expectations are of cure, with the family believing that the illness may be acute and a completely treatable disease, as are many physical medical problems. Sometimes their hopes are buoyed by the patient's rapid improvement under medication, but then their hopes are dashed and they experience anger and depression as the patient relapses. They may be angered further at insinuations that they are not being helpful with ensuring the patient's compliance. Such accusations may be factually correct, but verbalizing them will not help the situation. The rapidity with which antipsychotic or antidepressant medications are substituted for one another in some clinics and the multiple changes in dosages cause some families to think that the treating personnel are incompetent or do not appreciate the patient's history. Indeed, you should obtain the family's recollection of which medicines or strategies have worked. Because denial and resistance to diagnosis are strong, you should acknowledge the fallibility

---

[1]Adapted from Glick and Clarkin 1991.

Table 15–3. Stages in family management of psychiatric illness

Stage	Therapist interventions
Denial	Assess family.
	Build alliance.
	Establish partnership, not expert role.
	Use a tentative diagnosis.
Acceptance and adjustment to loss	Educate the family about the disease process.
	Reduce overinvolvement with and criticism of patient.
	Distinguish "salutary neglect" from limit setting.
Long-term coping and stabilized functioning	Develop the family's advocacy role for the patient.
	Return the family to maximized functioning.
	Enable family to identify warning signs and prodromal symptoms of relapse.
	Identify dysfunctional family roles and long-term psychodynamic issues.
	Support family caregiving role and prevent burnout.

of an initial diagnosis and present yourself as a partner in treatment rather than as an expert who knows the definitive solution.

Although the patient is your primary concern, you must establish a warm and supportive relationship with the family (and ideally with each family member) so that they are motivated to learn how to assist on the patient's behalf.

It is important to find out what the *family* (or the spokesperson for the family) sees as the problems to be addressed. This must be done by both insisting that family members speak for themselves and asking for the family spokesperson to state a consensus or summarize differences. For example, one patient's mother complained that her son did not take the garbage out of his room. His paranoid delusions were of little concern because they were not about her. Another family tolerated their son's reclusive behavior until he drilled a hole in the floor of his bedroom to observe the goings-on in the apartment downstairs. As

Vaughn and Leff (1976) discovered, the florid psychotic symptoms of disease were less important to families than were the disturbing character traits and socially inappropriate behaviors of the patient. Such inappropriate behaviors, which embarrass the family who may be trying to deny the need for treatment, can be made a focus of the individual therapy.

After acknowledgment of the seriousness of an illness, families react, as do individuals, with grief over lost function and guilt at its causation. Interventions of the second stage of treatment are most effective at this time. The therapist must address the sources of these feelings. The starting position should be that the illness is nobody's fault. The nature of many psychiatric diagnoses means that the condition is likely to be chronic and persist throughout the patient's life. Strategies for long-term care are of great importance to those who are going to be involved with the patient. Family factors, to be sure, contribute to the etiology of many illnesses, such as depression, but it is generally best to defer addressing these factors until the initial alliance with the family is secure.

Early interventions, therefore, need to stress the biological component, stating that family factors often exacerbate but usually do not cause the underlying disorder, and that it is natural to feel angry at the sick person for some of his behaviors and the disappointments that he generated in the family. For example, as disruptive as schizophrenic behaviors are, it is noteworthy that Holder and Anderson (1990) draw attention to the fact that depressive behaviors are most likely to be viewed by others as willful actions or personality traits. Thus, these behaviors are more likely to result in hostile or guilty responses instead of sympathetic family reactions. Educational materials and programs are especially relevant, because many families secretly hold their own theories or family myths about the origin of the patient's problem. It is therefore important to gauge the family's conception of the illness.

In both affective illness and thought disorder, other family members may react with criticism and overinvolvement in the patient's life. These criticisms may be reframed as positive attempts to improve the situation, but the psychoeducational strategy is for the family to reduce expectations for the patient, allow time for their activities as individuals, and, as any well-trained therapist does, avoid the assumption that they can cure the patient merely with an increased level of attention and care. A key task for many families is to practice "salutary neglect" of some psychotic behaviors to prevent these behaviors from provoking criticism and disrupting family life. The feasibility of such a task, however, is questioned by Kanter (1985b), because many patients are genuinely provocative. Perhaps the strategy should best be seen as the differentiation of tolerable and intolerable behaviors. Once the latter are the subject of limit setting, the former will be less provoking. Moreover, fairly high limits can be set if the family members can be helped to dissociate their self-esteem from the patient's illness behavior.

By the third stage of treatment, the family must be brought out of their isolation and shame by restoring their social connections. Strategies may include linking them up with a local self-help group or mental illness advocacy organizations such as NAMI (National Alliance on Mental Illness) that provide training or family therapy. Many hospitals and clinics do provide family education seminars to familiarize the families with what to expect, how to identify problems, and how to help (Heru and Drury 2007). Our society asks parents to be lifelong caregivers of their offspring. To do that, they must maintain their own psychological health, even if doing so requires solution of what has been called "the ethical and existential dilemma of how to balance their obligations to the ill family member with their own needs" (Grunebaum and Friedman 1988, p. 1187; see also Mechanic 1997).

Although some types of family therapy seek to "extrude" the patient from her family in order for her to achieve independence, this is often unrealistic with families in which a member is subject to recurrent psychiatric illness. We believe that such families have legitimate continuing roles. They may assist the patient in compliance with medications. A phone call between sessions may warn the therapist of a mood shift, of medication side effects, or of noncompliance. Thus, the family's role in crisis management may avert hospitalization. In addition, by the family's taking in of a family member who has made a (fairly benign) attempt at suicide, or by supplying food and housing to a usually independent offspring, a regressive crisis might be averted until the patient recovers enough strength to resume independent living.

Like clinicians, families are subject to burnout from prolonged caregiving. Long-term family support is frequently necessary and may end up as the major modality of treatment when the patient has a chronically worsening condition such as Alzheimer's disease. On the other hand, some families have the strength to tackle more systemic issues such as chronically dysfunctional family roles. Although mental illness does not result primarily from family miscommunication, it will often be appropriate to draw attention to patterns of nonverbal communication, metaphorical behaviors, the martyrdom role of caregivers, and scapegoating of the patient.

Therapists may wonder where they will find the time to perform all these functions with the family. It is clear that the clinician's commitment to the family is not merely a self-interested endeavor to help the patient. Rather, it is a social exchange; the therapist helps the family, and the family in turn helps the therapist. In Table 15–4, we have paired the related tasks in this process. For example, being responsive to crisis calls, even if it requires callback within the hour, is likely to prevent a minor crisis from escalating into hospitalization (Yee 1989). Also, by helping the family to become knowledgeable about the comprehensive services needed and to be available for the patient, the clinician can enable them as advocates for the improvement of mental health services. (For further discussion of this role, see Baker and Martens 2010; Compton and Broussard 2009; Intagliata et al. 1986.)

Peer Group Support

There are hundreds of national and local self-help organizations for patients with medical (including mental health) problems. Often it is desirable to refer a patient to one of them, such as Alcoholics Anonymous or Adult Children of Alcoholics, for adjunctive treatment. Within the mental health field, the therapist should be aware, however, that orientations toward psychiatric treatment vary. Emerick (1990) has proposed the following typology:

1. Groups that do not allow mental health workers membership
2. Groups that allow mental health workers in an auxiliary role
3. Partnership groups that accept mental health workers as leaders

As might be expected, separatist groups tend to interact very little with mental health professionals and tend to hold antiprofessional attitudes and espouse a social movement service model rather than one based on individual treatment. However, the point is not for therapists to steer their patients away from the more separatist groups (which would perhaps substantiate conceptions of therapeutic control). Rather, we believe that empowerment generally benefits the patient, and the therapist should be prepared to discuss the differences of opinion and establish better working relationship, with all outside groups.

Table 15–4. Benefits from therapist-family interaction

Therapist can	Family can
Address family's problems and agenda.	Provide therapist with a longitudinal picture of the illness.
Educate family about the disease; reduce self-blaming behaviors of family.	Learn appropriate behavioral strategies with patient that lower intrafamilial stress and relapse.
Help family to monitor compliance and prevent relapse.	Alert therapist to noncompliance and early symptoms of relapse.
Make services and support available in times of crisis.	Provide support to patient to avert crisis hospitalization.
Assist family and patient in developing social skills, thereby reducing the family's social dysfunction.	Assist patient with daily living tasks, including transportation of patient to clinic if necessary.
Link family to support groups and help them reestablish their own social networks.	Reduce overinvolvement with patient, fostering independence.
Give family an overall picture of the comprehensive needs and corresponding services for the patient.	Serve as an advocate for improved services, even in areas in which therapist cannot be effective.

Key Points

- Patients live and function in the community and with family (although sometimes estranged), as do the therapeutic professionals and staff.

- Communication among the community of providers, the patient, and family is key to successful implementation of therapy.

- Therapists can use the treatment planning process to bring together the multidisciplinary treatment team and to resolve differences between individual members.

- The process of splitting—separating mental contents into all-good and all-bad compartments—can be either detrimental to the therapy or used to the advantage of therapeutic progress.

- Linkages with outside agencies may be selective, but it is often vital for the therapist when doing supportive psychotherapy to understand the patient's family dynamics and involve some family in therapy.

- Peer group support and self-empowerment are important for persons with mental illness.

References

Anderson CM, Reiss DJ, Hogarty GE: Schizophrenia and the Family: A Practitioner's Guide to Psychoeducation and Management. New York, Guilford, 1986

Baker S, Martens L: Promoting Recovery From First Episode Psychosis: A Guide for Families. Toronto, ON, Canada, Centre for Addiction and Mental Health Services, 2010

Barton WE, Barton GM: Mental Health Administration: Principles and Practice, Vol 3. New York, Human Sciences Press, 1983, pp 695–744

Bernheim KF: Supportive family counseling. Schizophr Bull 8(4):634–641, 1982 7178851

Brenner AM: Teaching supportive psychotherapy in the twenty-first century. Harv Rev Psychiatry 20(5):259–267, 2012 23030214

Clinton H: It Takes a Village and Other Lessons Children Teach Us, 10th Anniversary Edition. New York, Simon & Schuster, 2006

Cole SA: Family treatment during brief hospitalization, in Less Time to Do More: Psychotherapy on the Short-Term Inpatient Unit. Edited by Leibenluft E, Tasman A, Green SA. Washington, DC, American Psychiatric Publishing, 1993, pp 59–88

Compton MT, Broussard B: The First Episode of Psychosis: A Guide for Patients and Their Families. New York, Oxford University Press, 2009

Dashoff J: JAMA study finds lower mortality rates at U.S. teaching hospitals. AAMC News, May 2017

Edenfield TM, Saeed SA: An update on mindfulness meditation as a self-help treatment for anxiety and depression. Psychol Res Behav Manag 5:131–141, 2012 23175619

Emerick RE: Self-help groups for former patients: relations with mental health professionals. Hosp Community Psychiatry 41(4):401–407, 1990 2332224

Gabbard GO: Splitting in hospital treatment. Am J Psychiatry 146(4):444–451, 1989 2648865

Glick ID, Clarkin JF: The family, in Inpatient Psychiatry: Diagnosis and Treatment, 3rd Edition. Edited by Sederer LI. Baltimore, MD, Williams & Wilkins, 1991, pp 255–276

Goering PN, Wasylenki DA, Farkas M, et al: What difference does case management make? Hosp Community Psychiatry 39(3):272–276, 1988 3356432

Grunebaum H, Friedman H: Building collaborative relationships with families of the mentally ill. Hosp Community Psychiatry 39(11):1183–1187, 1988 3224954

Harris M, Bergman HC: Case management with the chronically mentally ill: a clinical perspective. Am J Orthopsychiatry 57(2):296–302, 1987 3591914

Heru AM, Drury LM: Working With the Families of Psychiatric Inpatients. Baltimore, MD, Johns Hopkins University Press, 2007

Holder D, Anderson C: Psychoeducational family intervention for depressed patients and their families, in Depression and Families: Impact and Treatment. Edited by Keitner GI. Washington, DC, American Psychiatric Press, 1990, pp 157–184

Intagliata J, Willer B, Egri G: Role of the family in case management of the mentally ill. Schizophr Bull 12(4):699–708, 1986 3810069

Kanter JS: Case management of the young adult chronic patient: a clinical perspective. New Dir Ment Health Serv 27(27):77–92, 1985a 4058407

Kanter JS: Consulting with families of the chronic mentally ill. New Dir Ment Health Serv 27(27):21–32, 1985b 4058402

Kanter J: Clinical case management: definition, principles, components. Hosp Community Psychiatry 40(4):361–368, 1989 2714749

Keisling R, Peele R: Commitment to freedom. Paper presented at meeting of the American Academy of Psychiatry and the Law. Chicago, IL, October 17, 1980

Kennedy JA: Psychiatric Treatment Planning. Arlington, VA: American Psychiatric Publishing, 2003

Lamb HR: Treating the Long-Term Mentally Ill. San Francisco, CA, Jossey-Bass, 1982, pp 143–151

Leff J: Family factors in schizophrenia. Psychiatr Ann 19:542–547, 1989

Makover RB: Treatment Planning for Psychotherapists: A Practical Guide for Better Outcomes, 3rd Editon. Arlington, VA, American Psychiatric Association Publishing, 2016

Mariush ME: Essentials of Treatment Planning. New York, Wiley, 2002

Mechanic D: Improving Inpatient Psychiatric Treatment in an Era of Managed Care. San Francisco, CA, Jossey-Bass, 1997

Menninger WW: Dealing with staff reactions to perceived lack of progress by chronic mental patients. Hosp Community Psychiatry 35(8):805–808, 1984 6479915

Novalis PN: What supports supportive therapy? Jefferson Journal of Psychiatry 7(2):17–29, 1989

Rapp CA: The Strengths Model: Case Management With People Suffering From Severe and Persistent Mental Illness. New York, Oxford University Press, 1998

Schwartz SR, Goldman HH, Churgin S: Case management for the chronic mentally ill: models and dimensions. Hosp Community Psychiatry 33(12):1006–1009, 1982 7152491

Seeman MV, Pyke J, Denberg D, et al: Co-therapy in a clinic for schizophrenia. Can J Psychiatry 27(4):296–300, 1982 7104941

Springer AK: Telephone family therapy: an untapped resource. Family Therapy 18:123–128, 1991

Sun RC, Kulaylat AN, Grant SB: Improved communication techniques enable residents to provide better care now and in the future. Bull Am Coll Surg 98(8):26–32, 2013 24205572

Tessler RC, Gamache GM, Fisher GA: Patterns of contact of patients' families with mental health professionals and attitudes toward professionals. Hosp Community Psychiatry 42(9):929–935, 1991 1743664

Vaughn CE, Leff JP: The influence of family and social factors on the course of psychiatric illness: a comparison of schizophrenic and depressed neurotic patients. Br J Psychiatry 129:125–137, 1976 963348

Weiner MF: The Psychotherapeutic Impasse. New York, Free Press, 1982

Worden FG: Psychotherapeutic aspects of authority. Psychiatry 14(1):9–17, 1951 14816475

Yee WK: Psychiatric aspects of psychoeducational family therapy. Psychiatr Ann 19:27–34, 1989

16

Medication-Therapy Interactions and Medication Adherence

Both biological and psychosocial concerns must be addressed in behavioral health care. In this chapter, we first discuss some effects of medication on therapy and then turn to the effects of therapy on the patient's use of medication —particularly adherence with treatment. Treatment with the one-treater and two-treater models will also be examined. The side effects of medications will be discussed, because side effects will have an impact on adherence.

Medication-Therapy Interactions

The prescription or recommendation of medication has many possible meanings, messages, and effects, as outlined in Table 16–1. Actual effects vary with the medication, the individual patient, the illness, and the patient's response to it, and the therapist's implicit and explicit attitudes that are conveyed to the patient. These variables make it difficult to predict a patient's initial and subsequent reactions to medication, and the therapist must periodically reassess the patient's views. However, a few general guidelines are possible.

Table 16–1.   Meanings, messages, and effects of medication from the patient's perspective

Possible meanings (to the patient)

An earned gift

A gift of love

Transitional object or contact substitute

Substitute for the therapist's time

Sign of patient's dependence

Sign that patient is worsening

Therapist's attempt to poison

Danger of addiction

Indication of therapeutic failure

Harbinger of termination

Harbinger of successful therapy and final cure

Sign of therapist's competence/incompetence

Sign of therapist's nurturance, love, or interest

Evidence of therapist's power to cure (dominance, omnipotence) or power to control

Other possible messages (from the therapist)

"You have a serious illness." (legitimizing it or scaring patient)

"You're not responsible for your illness."

"I'm not sure what is wrong with you."

"At last I'm sure what is wrong with you."

"I'm not sure how to treat you."

"At last I'm sure how to treat you."

"Your treatment has been going poorly."

"Your treatment is going well."

Table 16–1.   Meanings, messages, and effects of medication from
the patient's perspective *(continued)*

Probable effects

When used initially, helps establish the supportive bond for verbal therapy

At any time, strengthens therapeutic alliance

Increases compliance with other aspects of treatment

Lessens anxiety, psychosis, or other symptoms, improving the verbal therapy

Note.   For additional discussion, see Waldinger and Frank 1989 and Cohen 1990.

First, knowledge of the patient's personality is helpful to the therapist in getting oriented to problems. For example, histrionic patients may overreact to side effects or experience unusual reactions, while obsessional patients may fear loss of control (Leibowitz et al. 1986). The reactions of patients with borderline personalities are particularly significant because of the potential dangers. According to one survey of therapists who work with such patients (Waldinger and Frank 1989), these patients are likely to overmedicate, overdose, or interpret the act of medication as a magical invocation of the therapist's powers. However, there was general agreement that medication strengthens the therapeutic alliance with borderline patients.

Second, the giving of medication with positive expectations usually creates a placebo effect that is a double-edged sword. A good therapist-patient relationship may enhance the placebo effect, but in just such an instance the patient may deny the effect because of fears it will end therapy.

Third, failure of the medication may hurt or help the therapeutic relationship, it being evidence not only of the therapist's fallibility but also of the primacy of the personal therapist-patient relationship as agent of change.

With patients for whom medication connotes an undesirable chronic dependence, the therapist may need to compare it to other chronic medical treatments such as insulin or a low-salt diet. With these treatments a normal life is possible; without them there is a serious risk of disability. You should also be mindful of several other guidelines when introducing medications (see Table 16–2).

Table 16–2.   Guidelines for discussing medication with the patient

Determine the meaning of the medication for the patient.

Discuss patient's expectations.

Explain why now (i.e., why medication is introduced at this stage).

Discuss effect on target symptoms before discussing side effects.

Document explanation of side effects and short-term and long-term benefits and costs.

Obtain consent for all medications, and in especial detail for those with long-term side effects such as tardive dyskinesia or for unusual usages not approved by the U.S. Food and Drug Administration or covered by general practice standards.

Reassess the patient's reaction to medication as the therapy proceeds.

Combined Therapy

Supportive psychotherapy is the most frequently employed form of psychotherapy and is often combined with pharmacotherapy. The research findings propose the benefit of combined therapy for patients with chronic, recurrent, severe, co-occurring, or treatment-resistant disorders. The benefits of combined treatment include better maintenance of diagnosed psychological disorders as well as enhanced psychosocial functioning (Hellerstein 2009).

The combination of pharmacotherapy and psychotherapy is the most commonly used approach, and most clinicians would acknowledge that the combination of these two is far more advantageous than each alone. However, combining the two therapies is not a simple task. In fact, it can be complicated with many variations and modifications. For example, pharmacotherapy could be combined with one of the multiple one-on-one or group therapies. Additionally, the pharmacotherapy and psychotherapy could be administered by one clinician (integrated treatment) or by two or more clinicians (collaborative or split treatment). The combination of these two could begin with either pharmacotherapy or psychotherapy. These many factors will need to be considered when pharmacotherapy and psychotherapy are being combined (Riba et al. 2018).

Most studies support the view that medication and therapy work additively. It is, however, not easy for most people to continue any task, such as maintaining an ideal weight, good grades, or top job performance. A crucial stage

Table 16–3. The therapist-prescriber split

Patients who usually benefit from a separate therapist and prescriber

Patients overwhelmed by authority

Patients with strong reservations against medication

Angry medical patients

Most borderline patients (because they get angry over medication issues and use nonadherence and medication abuse to express their feelings)

Patients who usually benefit from a single therapist/prescriber

Many patients with schizophrenia (see Chapter 6)

Manipulative patients (including some borderline patients)

Dependent patients

Depressed patients for whom the oral gratification of the medication improves the therapeutic alliance

Patients whose medication needs change frequently

Patients for whom the split is not relevant

Patients (if any!) for whom medication does not raise significant issues

in the treatment will be when your patient's condition has become stable while he is receiving medication and psychotherapy and both you and your patient may be satisfied with the advances. However, taking medications daily, regular visits with the therapist, and paying for medications and treatment when feeling well could generate a motive for your patient to make changes. This is an important time for you to understand that a concentrated effort must be made to safeguard that the patient's good progress continues (Riba et al. 2018).

The Therapist-Prescriber Split

Clinic policy or professional training often determines whether the therapist is the prescriber. When there is a choice, is there a reason to take the opportunity or turn it down? Table 16–3 lists factors that tend to favor or disfavor a therapist-prescriber split; however, the evidence is anecdotal, and the factors listed should be considered suggestions only and not as firm guidelines.

Certain patients (e.g., those with borderline personalities) tend to manipulate their prescribers, and this is often a reason for the therapist to be the prescriber or at least to work closely with the prescriber to suggest changes in the pharmacological regimen. In the treatment of schizophrenia, the therapist's role in monitoring symptoms and preventing psychological fragmentation also tends to favor a combined therapist-prescriber role.

The therapist, especially a supportive one, assumes a powerful role in the patient's mind, and the ability to give medication is an aspect of this role that concentrates the power of the clinic in the prescriber. The prescriber may also happen to have the power to hospitalize the patient. Combining all roles into one person can be a threat to a patient already overwhelmed by fears of losing control.

When patients have adherence problems, a split between therapist and prescriber is often beneficial, for it enables the patient to assume different roles with each professional. The patient may then find it easier to be honest about adherence problems with the nonprescriber, and if so, the therapist should make it clear that reported nonadherence will not result in a discontinuation of therapy. Therapist-prescriber splitting may foster primitive idealization or devaluation but may also reflect the assumption of a more genuine role with the therapist and a more constricted "formal" role with the prescriber, upon whom may be split the more negative elements of the patient's transference. Such a split enables the therapist and patient to talk about the negative transference in displacement (generally without revealing it to be what it is). Split transference between therapist and prescriber is one example of displaced transferences that occur when a patient is treated by multiple caregivers, and it is not limited to patients with primitive defenses.

When the therapist is the prescriber, the giving of oral medication is a form of feeding and can be gratifying to the patient. This has been found to improve adherence in most depressed patients (Schwartz 1988). However, the administration of injections is always painful, fraught with connotations of assault, and subject to transferential delusions; injections should be given by personnel who have less intense contact with the patient.

Advantages of Combining Treatment

According to Hollon and Fawcet (2007), there are four advantages of combining therapy over the single treatment approach. First, combined treatment may boost the quality of the response. Second, combined treatment increases the odds of a response. Third, combined treatment may improve the range of the response: the overall response may be superior to a response achieved with either treatment alone. Finally, combined treatment may reinforce the acceptance of and adherence to treatment. In summary, using combined therapy may contribute to improved adherence to medications and medications could increase the effectiveness of psychotherapy.

Adherence to Medications

Adherence is a major concern in all medical settings, including mental health. The development of the patient's maximum autonomy to make treatment decisions is a major goal of supportive therapy. Except in emergencies, or when courts or administrative bodies have ordered involuntary treatment, patients have the right to refuse treatment, and this right should never be misrepresented by the therapist. In most cases, however, adherence to the treatment plan is a goal of the treatment with which the patient struggles throughout the therapy.

Medication decisions involve complex balances of benefits and risks. It is clear, despite occasional claims to the contrary, that medication is a necessary adjunct at many stages in the treatment of many forms of mental illness. Low-dose, high-dose, targeted-symptom, and intermittent strategies have all been advocated in various circumstances. After an initial psychotic episode, some patients may not require further medications. Even a percentage of chronic patients (although it is difficult to predict which subset) can be taken off medication permanently. Therefore, you can only generalize when a patient asks if medication is really needed. Any uncertainties can be admitted to the patient and explored in more detail with the prescriber. In general, however, we believe that the therapist needs to act unambivalently in favor of adherence and not collude with the patient to outwit the prescriber, as sometimes happens.

With patients for whom medication connotes an undesirable deep-seated dependence, as mentioned earlier, you may need to compare medication to other chronic medical treatments such as insulin or a low-salt diet. With these treatments, a normal life is possible; without them, there is a serious risk of disability.

The effects of nonadherence to medications for your patients are complex but easy to identify and may range from a decreased quality of life to poorly managed symptoms, hospitalization, and death. However, the ramifications of nonadherence do extend into society, with far-reaching costs to society: $300 billion of avoidable health care costs as a result of nonadherence to medications have been identified (Zullig and Hayden 2017). A list of strategies to improve adherence is presented in Table 16–4.

A problematic task for many patients is adherence to a treatment plan, notably taking medication. Most people do not like to take medication (consider how many people will absolutely complete a full course of antibiotics). Generally, when they begin to feel better, patients will discontinue their medications. In primary care, most patients are not taking the full dose of antidepressant that was initially prescribed (Riba et al. 2018).

Nonadherence includes not filling prescriptions, not taking medication as prescribed (either taking too many or too few pills or not taking them at the correct times), taking medication with alcohol or other substances, or stopping the medication. Additionally, nonadherence may present in the form of missing appointments, arriving late, canceling appointments at the last minute, or not completing homework assignments. It is safe to assume that adherence will be difficult for most patients. Some of the causes of nonadherence could be related to the patients' psychopathology—for example, paranoia, suspiciousness, or psychosis; substance use disorder; cognitive deficits; severe depression that prompts psychomotor agitation and feelings of hopelessness or worthlessness; and pressure by family or friends to stop the medication (Riba et al. 2018).

In a survey of 205 psychiatric patients, Loria (2019) found that most patients had difficulty with medication adherence because of concerns about side effects. (Risk factors and side effects are discussed below.) Their second concern was the cost of the medication. Additionally, Loria found that as many as 80% of patients do not take their medications as prescribed.

Risk Factors and Causes of Nonadherence

The risk factors for nonadherence to medications are many, and there is no one single profile for a patient who may be at high risk for nonadherence. Theoretically, the risk factors can be divided into *patient-related, medication-related*, and *provider-related risk factors* (Lacro et al. 2002). Patient risk factors for nonadherence include substance use disorder, younger age, lower education level, and cognitive impairment (Depp et al. 2008). Medication risk factors include

Table 16–4. Ways to improve adherence

Psychosocial strategies

Discuss the patient's beliefs about the medication.

Reinforce the benefits of being well, but do not counteract necessary denial.

Entertain the patient's objections to medication.

Technical strategies

Personalize the treatment regimen to meet the patient's needs and health beliefs.

Simplify the regimen (e.g., fewer medications, fewer doses).

Maintain an effective regimen (e.g., do not change brands without a reason).

Monitor the regimen (unobtrusively if necessary; objectively by blood levels if needed).

Count the pills at clinic visits, or have the patient count and report by phone.

Counter concreteness and inflexibility by providing rules and answering questions regarding allowable variability in the regimen.

Provide the patient with instructions; write and repeat them as needed.

Attach specific instructions to each medication.

Arrange social supports to assist with adherence.

Do not assume the patient can read (or read small print).

Note. These guidelines are in addition to those general guidelines presented in Table 16–2.

side effects and frequent dosing (Sajatovic et al. 2006, 2007). Provider-related risk factors for poor adherence include a poor relationship with therapist or clinician, infrequent outpatient follow-up, and a deficient discharge plan (Lacro et al. 2002). Additionally, prescribers often do not devote an adequate amount of time to assess the risk factors for nonadherence. Limited psychoeducation to patients and family and a lack of shared decision making may also contribute to nonadherence (Kane et al. 2013).

A study of patients with schizophrenia found that one out of five patients was nonadherent with medications after discharge from an inpatient unit (Olfson et al. 2000). The contributing factors to the nonadherence were a history of nonadherence, a poor therapeutic relationship with inpatient staff, a poor family support system, substance use, and the patients' inability to recognize their own symptoms. Clinicians should be able to identify the risk factors and arrange proper preventive interventions for those patients during the transition from inpatient to outpatient care.

The failure to recognize symptoms or to accept the diagnosis of mental illness is often referred to as *denial*. However, individuals with an acute mental illness may not be thinking clearly enough to consciously choose denial. The medical term for this lack of awareness of the medical condition is *anosognosia*, from the Greek meaning "to not know a disease." The frontal lobe of the brain is responsible for updating and remembering self-image. In patients with schizophrenia, bipolar disorder, and dementia, the frontal lobe does not function at 100% and patients may lose the ability to update their self-image. For the person with anosognosia, the inaccurate insight of self-image feels real. This failure to recognize symptoms is a leading cause of nonadherence (National Alliance on Mental Illness 2015).

A common belief among providers is that persons with serious mental illnesses avoid treatment because of fears of involuntary hospitalization, stigma, or dissatisfaction with services. This belief is contradicted by a study by Kessler et al. (2001), who found that the main reason for nonadherence was by far anosognosia.

Managing Nonadherence and Suggestions to Improve Adherence

Educating your patients about their treatment is important. Written materials, information over the telephone and internet, and fact sheets will prove helpful. It is crucial for your patients to receive all information available, including on possible side effects, even though this may frighten them. To alleviate these fears, they must be given the opportunity to discuss their fears and questions with you. Encouraging participation in support groups may be of benefit for some patients. The involvement of family members may also be useful to help the patient adhere to treatment. It is important to ask about and monitor side effects of medications. You must continue to ask about any medical problems or new medications as some medications may interact with the psychotropic medications. If needed, you can make an adjustment to the psychotropics and perhaps prevent your patient from stopping the medication, which could lead to an increase in psychiatric symptoms. Finally, if you present as a competent and confident therapist, your patient will feel better about adhering to treatment (Riba et al. 2018). See Table 16–2 for guidelines for discussing medications with your patients.

In addition to the strategies listed in Tables 16–2 and 16–4, pharmacists can help in the following ways: arranging for 90-day supplies, educating patients about how their medications work, and instructing patients on how to administer doses and simplify drug regimens. Additionally, bubble packs, dosing alarms, and pill organizers will prove to be beneficial (Lamb 2006). And although you may have some control over your own time, investments in time and technology may be necessary to improve adherence within the multi-systemic setting that is typical of modern medical cases (Kini and Ho 2018).

According to Weiden and Rao (2005), there is minimal education in psychiatric residency programs on nonadherence because the topic does not fall into the area of psychopharmacology and it does not belong in any other formal role of psychiatric residency curriculum. Weiden and Rao suggest that discussion of medication adherence concerns should start with the patient's point of view, not the clinician's point of view. They also recommend that the clinician actively try to understand the patient's perspective and not correct the patient's beliefs.

Educating your patients about medications will prove to be a powerful intervention to increase adherence. According to Depp and Lebowitz (2007), the primary goal of medication education is to enhance knowledge about the properties of medications and understanding of the patient's role in managing medications. In addition, they suggest that the education on the medication include information about the basic properties of the medication, purpose, dosage and instructions, and factors that affect medication effectiveness. Jarboe (2002) identifies steps to improve patient education about medication and the beliefs of therapy and states that increasing the patient's control over medications could help enhance the therapeutic bond between the patient and clinicians.

Side Effects

Although side effects are not among the top reasons for nonadherence, as noted earlier in the text, they may be an obstacle to overcome for many of your patients. Again, education will be a key tool for clinicians to employ. Patients with schizophrenia suffer from higher rates of multiple medical problems and more difficulty in getting adequate health care (Meyer and Nasrallah 2003; Sartorius 2007). Side effects of antipsychotic medications may contribute to the poor health of these patients in general.

The first antipsychotic medications, including haloperidol, perphenazine, and chlorpromazine, now known as "typical" or "first generation" antipsychotics, were introduced in the 1950s. Chlorpromazine was developed in 1950 without any clinical trials and was the first effective treatment for schizophrenia. The first clinical trials of chlorpromazine and other antipsychotics were conducted in the United States in the early 1960s (Haddad et al. 2016). These early medications have troublesome side effects, including muscle rigidity, tremors, abnormal movements including tardive dyskinesia, photosensitivity, jaundice, seizures, and retinal pigmentation (Arana 2000; Psych Central Staff 2017).

The development of the "second generation" antipsychotics, also known as "atypical," occurred in the 1990s. Because of the perception then that they had fewer side effects or that they were more effective than the typical antipsychotics for schizophrenia, they are today often used as first-line treatment (Psych Central Staff 2017). However, the atypical antipsychotics are not without unpleasant and dangerous side effects either. Common side effects of the atypical antipsychotics include drowsiness, rapid heartbeat, hypotension, skin rashes, decreased libido, agranulocytosis, gynecomastia, diabetes, hyperlipidemia, myocarditis, and weight gain (Psych Central Staff 2017; Uçok and Gaebel 2008).

Weight Gain and Obesity as Side Effects of Antipsychotics

According to the World Health Organization (2018), obesity has nearly tripled worldwide since 1975, and in 2016 more than 1.9 billion adults were overweight; of these, 650 million were obese. The World Health Organization defines *overweight* as a body mass index (BMI) of 25 or greater and *obesity* as a BMI of 30 or greater.

According to Haupt (2006), 40%–62% of people with schizophrenia are overweight or obese. A study by Littrell et al. (2003) found that to prevent or decrease weight gain in patients, prevention programs need to be in place when patients begin antipsychotic medications. Seventy patients with a diagnosis of schizophrenia or schizoaffective disorder participated in the 6-month study. The patients were randomly assigned to an intervention group or a standard care group. The intervention group participated in classes regarding nutrition, exercise, and wellness. The intervention group was followed for 2 months to monitor any changes in weight. This study demonstrated positive outcomes of educational interventions to decrease or prevent the weight gain of patients with disorders for which antipsychotics were prescribed.

Side Effects of Antidepressants

The first-generation antidepressants—tricyclic antidepressants (TCAs) and monoamine oxidase inhibitors (MAOIs)—are effective because of enhanced serotonergic or noradrenergic mechanisms, or both. The unwanted side effects of the TCAs include weight gain, dry mouth, constipation, drowsiness, and dizziness. Although the TCAs are effective, they have a narrow therapeutic index and can cause seizures, heart block, arrhythmias, and death. The MAOIs interact with tyramine, causing possibly deadly hypertension and dangerous interactions with a plethora of medications (Feighner 1999).

The first selective serotonin reuptake inhibitor (SSRI), fluoxetine, was introduced in 1988, and the severity of the side effects was much lower (Ferguson 2001). The SSRIs do not cause cardiac conduction abnormalities with overdose and have a low tendency to trigger seizures (Feighner 1999). Although the efficacy of the SSRIs is superior to that of TCAs and MAOIs and the side effects are less severe, they do have troublesome, unwanted side effects.

The side effects of SSRIs are in most cases well tolerated and will decrease or vanish within the first few days to weeks of starting the medication. However, roughly 15% of patients will stop taking the medication because they cannot tolerate the side effects. The most common side effect of the SSRIs is sexual dysfunction. It is also important to note that psychiatric illness can affect sexual desire and performance. More than any of the other SSRIs, sertraline and fluvoxamine may cause more gastrointestinal side effects (Khawam et al. 2006).

Serotonin syndrome is a serious and possibly life-threatening side effect resulting from hyperstimulation of serotonin receptors. Patients with the syndrome present with mental status changes, nausea, diarrhea, restlessness, agitation, rigidity, delirium, seizure, and/or status epilepticus. The most severe case could result in cardiovascular collapse, coma, and death (Khawam et al. 2006; Volpi-Abadie et al. 2013). Serotonin syndrome can develop with the therapeutic use of an SSRI alone, after an intentional overdose, or as a result of the combination of two serotonergic drugs (Volpi-Abadie et al. 2013), This syndrome can also occur when an MAOI is combined with an SSRI, pentazocine, or L-tryptophan. Therefore, it is imperative, before the initiation of an MAOI, to wait at least 2 weeks after stopping an SSRI. Because of the long half-life of fluoxetine, the recommended wait time is 5 weeks (Khawam et al. 2006).

Supportive Psychotherapy Techniques When Addressing Side Effects of Medications

When using supportive psychotherapy, you should be building and maintaining a therapeutic alliance. Supporting the alliance includes expressing interest, empathy, and understanding. A priority topic for you and your patient, especially if the patient was recently hospitalized, will be medications. You should first ask if she is taking the medications as prescribed and whether she is experiencing any unpleasant side effects. Too often, when patients are not taking medications as prescribed, they are viewed as being nonadherent. A focus on the side effects will enable the transformation of the subject from adversarial to collaborative. Once you have addressed side effects, you can later discuss the psychological issues that may have an impact on taking medications (Winston et al. 2012). It is important to remember that patients may be too embarrassed to initiate a conversation about the sexual dysfunction side effects of medications and you should ask about these effects (Riba et al. 2018).

Key Points

- It is a challenge to determine the best method of coordinating medication and psychotherapy for patients. Complications of the split treatment include not just caring for the patient but also considering the other clinicians and obtaining the needed information from all involved.

- Medication adherence is essential for the treatment of your patients, and the combination of pharmacotherapy and psychosocial intervention may be your most powerful tool to assist patients with stabilization and recovery.

- Adherence to treatment is essential for the relief of symptoms in mental health patients.

- The methods to improve adherence are both pharmacological and psychosocial, and an important factor is to include patient education on psychotherapy and medications. This education must include discussion of potential side effects of the medication.

- Anosognosia, in addition to side effects, is an important factor to consider with the nonadherent patient, and the patient should not be labeled as "in denial."

- Obesity is a worldwide problem, and the side effect of weight gain with many of the antipsychotics can be a problem that must be addressed.

- The first-generation antipsychotics and antidepressants have the most troublesome, and sometimes life-threatening, side effects. It is important to remember that sexual dysfunction is a side effect of all the selective serotonin reuptake inhibitors and that the patient may be too embarrassed to bring up this topic. Again, education is important. Asking the patient about side effects could improve medication adherence.

References

Arana GW: An overview of side effects caused by typical antipsychotics. J Clin Psychiatry 61 (suppl 8):5–11, 2000 10811237

Cohen KD: Compliance with treatment transference and countertransference issues. Carrier Foundation Letter 148:1–2, 1990

Depp CA, Lebowitz BD: Enhancing medication adherence: in older adults with bipolar disorder. Psychiatry (Edgmont) 4(6):22–32, 2007 20711333

Depp CA, Moore DJ, Patterson TL, et al: Psychosocial interventions and medication adherence in bipolar disorder. Dialogues Clin Neurosci 10(2):239–250, 2008 18689293

Feighner JP: Mechanism of action of antidepressant medications. J Clin Psychiatry 60 (suppl 4):4–11, discussion 12–13, 1999 10086478

Ferguson JM: SSRI antidepressant medications: adverse effects and tolerability. Prim Care Companion J Clin Psychiatry 3(1):22–27, 2001 15014625

Haddad P, Kirk R, Green R: Chlorpromazine, the first antipsychotic medication: history, controversy and legacy. British Association for Psychopharmacology, October 31, 2016. Available at: https://www.bap.org.uk/articles/chlorpromazine-the-first-antipsychotic/. Accessed February 28, 2019.

Haupt DW: Differential metabolic effects of antipsychotic treatments. Eur Neuropsychopharmacol 16 (suppl 3):S149–S155, 2006 16872808

Hellerstein D: Combining supportive psychotherapy with medication, in Textbook of Psychotherapeutic Treatments. Edited by Gabbard GO. Washington, DC, American Psychiatric Publishing, 2009, pp 465–496

Hollon SB, Fawcet J: Combined medication and psychotherapy for mood disorders, in Gabbard's Treatments of Psychiatric Disorders, 4th Edition. Edited by Gabbard GO. Alexandria, VA, American Psychiatric Publishing, 2007, pp 439–447

Jarboe KS: Treatment nonadherence: causes and potential solutions. J Am Psychiatr Nurses Assoc 8:S18–S25, 2002

Kane JM, Kishimoto T, Correll CU: Non-adherence to medication in patients with psychotic disorders: epidemiology, contributing factors and management strategies. World Psychiatry 12(3):216–226, 2013 24096780

Kessler RC, Berglund PA, Bruce ML, et al: The prevalence and correlates of untreated serious mental illness. Health Serv Res 36(6 Pt 1):987–1007, 2001 11775672

Khawam EA, Laurencic G, Malone DA Jr: Side effects of antidepressants: an overview. Cleve Clin J Med 73(4):351–353, 356–361, 2006 16610395

Kini V, Ho PM: Interventions to improve medication adherence: a review. JAMA 320(23):2461–2473, 2018 30561486

Lacro JP, Dunn LB, Dolder CR, et al: Prevalence of and risk factors for medication nonadherence in patients with schizophrenia: a comprehensive review of recent literature. J Clin Psychiatry 63(10):892–909, 2002 12416599

Lamb E: Strategies and tools for promoting medication adherence. December 1, 2006. Available at: http://www.pharmacytimes.com/publications/issue/2006/2006-12/2006-12-6153. Accessed February 28, 2019.

Leibowitz MR, Stone MH, Turkat ID: Treatment of personality disorders, in Psychiatry Update: The American Psychiatric Association Annual Review, Vol 5. Edited by Frances AJ, Hales RE. Washington, DC, American Psychiatric Press, 1986, pp 356–393

Littrell KH, Hilligoss NM, Kirshner CD, et al: The effects of an educational intervention on antipsychotic-induced weight gain. J Nurs Scholarsh 35(3):237–241, 2003 14562491

Loria G: Guide to medication compliance in mental health patients. 2019. Available at: https://www.softwareadvice.com/resources/medication-compliance-mental-health/. Accessed February 28, 2019.

Meyer JM, Nasrallah HA: Medical Illness and Schizophrenia, 2nd Edition. Washington, DC, American Psychiatric Publishing, 2003

National Alliance on Mental Illness: Anosognosia. 2015. Available at: https://www.nami.org/Learn-More/Mental-Health-Conditions/Related-Conditions/Anosognosia. Accessed February 28, 2019.

Olfson M, Mechanic D, Hansell S, et al: Predicting medication noncompliance after hospital discharge among patients with schizophrenia. Psychiatr Serv 51(2):216–222, 2000 10655006

Psych Central Staff: Medications for schizophrenia and psychotic disorders. 2017. Available at: https://psychcentral.com/lib/antipsychotic-medications/. Accessed February 28, 2019.

Riba MR, Balon R, Roberts LW: Competency in Combining Pharmacotherapy and Psychotherapy: Integrated and Split Treatment, 2nd Edition. Arlington, VA, American Psychiatric Association Publishing, 2018

Sajatovic M, Bauer MS, Kilbourne AM, et al: Self-reported medication treatment adherence among veterans with bipolar disorder. Psychiatr Serv 57(1):56–62, 2006 16399963

Sajatovic M, Blow FC, Kales HC, et al: Age comparison of treatment adherence with antipsychotic medications among individuals with bipolar disorder. Int J Geriatr Psychiatry 22(10):992–998, 2007 17323327

Sartorius N: Physical illness in people with mental disorders. World Psychiatry 6(1):3–4, 2007 17342212

Schwartz LS: Psychosocial therapy for depression, in Psychiatry: Diagnosis and Therapy, '88/'89. Edited by Flahery JA, Channon RA, Davis JM. Norwalk, CT, Appleton & Lange, 1988, pp 35–41

Uçok A, Gaebel W: Side effects of atypical antipsychotics: a brief overview. World Psychiatry 7(1):58–62, 2008 18458771

Volpi-Abadie J, Kaye AM, Kaye AD: Serotonin syndrome. Ochsner J 13(4):533–540, 2013 24358002

Waldinger RJ, Frank AF: Clinicians' experiences in combining medication and psychotherapy in the treatment of borderline patients. Hosp Community Psychiatry 40(7):712–718, 1989 2777227

Weiden PJ, Rao N: Teaching medication compliance to psychiatric residents: placing an orphan topic into a training curriculum. Acad Psychiatry 29(2):203–210, 2005 15937268

Winston A, Rosenthal RN, Pinsker H: Techniques, in Learning Supportive Psychotherapy: An Illustrated Guide. Washington, DC, American Psychiatric Publishing, 2012, pp 53–89

World Health Organization: Obesity and overweight. February 16, 2018. Available at: http://www.who.int/mediacentre/factsheets/fs311/en/. Accessed February 28, 2019.

Zullig LL, Hayden B: Engaging patients to optimize medication adherence. May 14, 2017. Available at: https://catalyst.nejm.org/optimize-patients-medication-adherence/. Accessed February 28, 2019.

Ethical and Cultural Awareness in Supportive Psychotherapy

This chapter discusses a basic principle: Supportive psychotherapists should conduct therapy in an ethical and culturally sensitive manner.

Ethical Principles

Ethical issues in behavioral health relate to standards that go beyond the legal. The existence of such standards constitutes one basic difference between a *profession* and a *trade,* and psychotherapists doing supportive psychotherapy often face vexing ethical decisions because of their intense interactions with patients. Because ethical issues are often juxtaposed to legal ones, it is important at the outset for supportive psychotherapists to know the substantive legal issues that affect their work, not only for their own sake but as the core beneath which, as it were, one should not chip. Areas that we consider especially important include the following:

- Assessments of dangerousness and the concomitant duty to protect others from dangerous patients that leads to warnings and commitment actions
- The determination of competency to consent to treatment and to competently refuse it
- Related issues concerning the types of legal guardianship or conservatorship and the psychiatrist's role in contributing to legal and court proceedings
- The maintenance of confidentiality in treatment, often arising when obtaining information from patients' families
- The proper methods of terminating treatment
- Reporting of threats to others and past or future crimes
- Other reportable concerns, such as child, elder, or spousal abuse or abuse of vulnerable persons; spread of contagious diseases such as HIV infection; or ethical violations by other mental health professionals

Further information on these legal topics is available elsewhere (see, e.g., Bucky et al. 2005), and we shall assume the reader has a general familiarity with such issues when we introduce them below. We shall limit our discussion here to the ethical issues prominent in supportive psychotherapy that arise from its typically directive nature and the therapist's significant involvement in the patient's life.

The American Medical Association (AMA), in the preamble to the *Principles of Medical Ethics*, uses the term *ethical* to refer to "matters involving moral principles, values, and practices, as well as matters of social policy involving issues of morality in the practice of medicine" (American Medical Association 2001). As defined in that document, ethical standards of conduct may exceed legal requirements but do not oppose them. We shall let this definition stand without devising examples of ethical responsibilities that violate the law. For a discussion of the history and modernization of the AMA ethical code, see the article by Brotherton et al. (2016). The American Psychiatric Association has adopted the AMA's principles of medical ethics and provided annotations especially applicable to psychiatry (American Psychiatric Association 1989b). These principles and annotations, which have a long history (Musto 1981) and for which many changes could be suggested, are periodically revised by the AMA and the American Psychiatric Association. Supportive therapy, however, is practiced by therapists of many disciplines, so we have compiled a list of websites for ready access to the professional ethics of the organizations most relevant to the reader (Table 17–1). In Table 17–2 we provide a quick summary of some of the features found in various professional ethics codes.

Cultural Sensitivity

Culture, according to DSM-5, refers to

> systems of knowledge, concepts, rules, and practices that are learned and transmitted across generations. Culture includes language, religion and spirituality, family structures, life-cycle stages, ceremonial rituals, and customs, as well as moral and legal systems. Cultures are open, dynamic systems that undergo continuous change over time; in the contemporary world, most individuals and groups are exposed to multiple cultures, which they use to fashion their own identities and make sense of experience. (American Psychiatric Association 2013, p. 749)

To be culturally sensitive to his or her patient, the therapist should strive to have both general knowledge of the patient's culture (or cultures, plural) and knowledge of the patient's specific cultural beliefs. To aid in this, the American Psychiatric Association developed a Cultural Formulation Interview, which has evolved over 20 years into the present form (American Psychiatric Association 2013). This formulation is described and presented in DSM-5 and can be downloaded from the American Psychiatric Association's website (https://www.psychiatry.org/psychiatrists/practice/dsm/educational-resources/assessment-measures) for use with patients and in research. We recommend that all therapists have it readily available. It starts with 16 questions that arrange the patient's cultural information into four domains (DeSilva et al. 2015):

1. Cultural definition of the problem
2. Cultural perceptions of cause, context, and support (including cultural identity)
3. Cultural factors affecting self-coping and past help seeking
4. Cultural factors affecting current help seeking

Because the definition of culture includes religion, the culturally sensitive therapist is also urged to develop *religious competence*, which refers to "skills, practices, and orientations that recognize, explore, and harness patient religi-

Table 17–1.   Sources of professional ethics codes

American Psychiatric Association	www.psychiatry.org
American Medical Association	www.ama-assn.org
American Psychological Association	www.apa.org
American Academy of Psychiatry and the Law	www.aapl.org
American Association of Christian Counselors	www.aacc.net
American Association on Intellectual and Developmental Disabilities	www.aaidd.org
American Clinical Social Work Association	www.acswa.org
American Counseling Association	www.counseling.org
American Group Psychotherapy Association	www.agpa.org
American Mental Health Counselors Association	www.amhca.org
American Nurses Association	www.nursingworld.org
American Psychiatric Nurses Association	www.apna.org
American School Counselor Association	www.schoolcounselor.org
Madrid Declaration of Ethical Standards for Psychiatric Practice (World Psychiatric Association)	www.wpanet.org
NAADAC, the Association for Addiction Professionals (National Association for Alcoholism and Drug Abuse Counselors)	www.naadac.org
National Association of Addiction Treatment Providers	www.naatp.org
National Human Services Assembly	www.nationalassembly.org
National Organization for Human Services	www.nationalhumanservices.org
National Practice Standards for the Mental Health Workforce (Australian Government, Department of Health)	www.health.gov.au
Ontario College of Social Workers and Social Service Workers	www.ocswssw.org

Note.   This table lists many of the organizations of professionals in the various human services disciplines. This list is adapted and updated from one put together by the Illinois Institute of Technology (CSEP, http://ethics.iit.edu). There are, of course, other organizations, both in the United States and internationally. In addition, many national and state licensing and certification programs have their own codes of ethics. Most health care service organizations, such as the American Psychiatric Association, begin their codes with those of the American Medical Association, with modifications and annotations of particular relevance to their own mission. Since the codes are often updated, we have provided the link to the home page of each organization rather than specific links to the ethical standards themselves.

Table 17–2. Examples of important ethical rules derived from the many professional codes

Therapists should

Be competent in their disciplines and maintain their competency through continuing education.

Be honest in their relationships with patients.

Not exploit patients for financial or personal reasons.

Not exert undue influence upon their patients.

Treat patients according to a mutually developed treatment plan to the extent possible or to make patients aware of the differences between the therapist's goals and the patient's desired goals. (However, ethical rules covering involuntary treatment are also necessary.)

Treat patients to serve ethical goals so as to address patients' best interests in their personal and life development, to maintain or improve patients' physical and mental health, to maximize patients' ability to make life decisions after the therapy is completed, and to achieve similar goals as those of supportive psychotherapy.

Not engage in romantic or sexual relationships with present or former patients. (Codes may vary in time periods for relationships with former patients.)

Be culturally (including religiously) sensitive to their patients.

---

osity to facilitate diagnosis, recovery, and healing" (Whitley and Jarvis 2015, p. 14). This is certainly the impetus behind the admittedly brief intervention in treatment plans indicated by "Utilize faith-based coping skills."

Of particular interest to the field of psychiatry, it is important for international medical graduates who practice in the United States to become knowledgeable not only about the English language but also about American cultures and subcultures when treating Americans. This includes recognizing "regional patient dialects, colloquial speech, body language, and speech inflection" (Fiscella and Frankel 2000).

Supportive psychotherapists have a special role to play in utilizing culturally sensitive statements since they are in a position to reflect and elaborate upon their patients' own experiences. This includes the use of statements to "acknowledge differences and express a desire to understand the client's experience" (White et al. 2006, p. 310; in this article, White et al. offer many other recommendations).

Seven Permissive Guidelines

Consistent with the preceding principles, we shall offer two sets of guidelines to assist the supportive therapist who is concerned about the nature of his role. Each guideline is followed by a brief example or two and discussion. The first set of guidelines is permissive; it shall later be balanced by a set of limiting guidelines. The debate on such matters is voluminous; if readers disagree with our positions, we hope they will be motivated to develop their own reasoned viewpoints consistent with their relevant profession. (Some of these concepts were also discussed in Novalis 1989.)

Permissive Guideline 1: Therapeutic Influence Is Not in Itself Unethical

Example

A hypomanic patient is receiving supportive psychotherapy partially to increase adherence with medication orders as part of a mutually developed treatment plan. The prescriber discusses the benefits and risks of taking lithium. After the discussion, the patient is still unsure about taking it. The prescriber says firmly, "As your prescriber, I would say that you really ought to try it for a while."

This is a common scenario, in which the prescribing physician utilizes several kinds of power to influence a patient's medication decision. Raven (1986) elaborates a taxonomy of the options:

- *Informational power*, which requires the patient to have sufficient cognitive skills
- *Expert power* based on the psychiatrist's prestige or apparently superior knowledge
- *Legitimate power* that invokes social reciprocity or the inherent authority in the physician-patient relationship

- *Referent power* arising from the patient's identification with or modeling of the physician
- *Coercive and/or reward power*, which depends on the prescriber's ability to provide punishment or rewards contingent on the patient's use of the medication

In this case, the prescriber's role involves both informational (or educational) and expert power. These two functions of medical treatment express a venerable medical tradition, and it is generally assumed that in matters of fact, the patient's faculties of independent judgment are retained and, if anything, enabled to operate more effectively when the patient is given enough information to make an informed choice. The patient can, if desired, validate the factual information he receives at another source, and, perhaps more importantly, the information assumes an influence that is relatively independent of its source. The prescriber's taking an expert or advisory role and her use of *prestige suggestion* are fairly common and assume, reasonably, that the prescriber is an expert on medication matters and that the patient is not the primary decision-maker but gives informed consent to the prescriber's recommendation, as when a surgeon recommends that an exploratory laparotomy be made for a patient's abdominal pain.

Even this simple transaction is freighted with ethical questions. The patient's understanding and adherence to lithium treatment are affected by all three aspects of the therapist-patient relationship: supportive, transferential, and therapeutic alliance. Moreover, one wonders if a hypomanic patient is capable of giving truly informed consent to a medical treatment. When more personal decisions are called for, the patient may be unduly influenced by these relationship factors. In particular, the use of commands, prohibitions, or behavioral control methods, each of which shortcuts the route of therapist talk → patient insight → patient action, may deprive the patient of an opportunity to reflect upon courses of action and exercise independent judgment.

Note that in supportive psychotherapy, one typically assumes that 1) one is acting in the patient's best interests and 2) one's goal is eventually to achieve for the patient the maximum autonomy from the illness as is practical. However, it is certainly possible to encounter situations in which there is a conflict between those goals, and we discuss this later in the chapter. It helps to frame "best interests" to keep the goal in mind. Other motives that sometimes slip into supportive psychotherapy are discussed below.

Permissive Guideline 2: Specific Advice Is Not in Itself Unethical

Example

> The therapist tells a patient who has a history of poor financial planning, "You really can't afford a new car."

The possibilities of undue influence, not limited to sexual behavior, exist in all professional relationships, and therapists have been known to command their patients to stop using drugs, cease abuse of spouse or child, and obey the law. Therapists may suggest, advise, or comment on the patient's need to spend money more wisely or round up a new set of friends. At the other extreme, that of permission giving, a therapist's attempts to weaken an overly punitive conscience may influence the patient to engage in more aggressive, assertive, or sexual behavior.

When a therapist expresses opinions or offers direct guidance, there are many potential dangers. First, one may damage the therapeutic process, for the therapist's very expression of opinions can squelch the patient's participation; the therapist's words may hold the patient's thoughts hostage. Fearful of angering or offending—or even of pleasing and gratifying—the therapist, the patient may remain silent. This danger can be avoided, not by the therapist's silence or abstinence but by proper understanding of his role with respect to that particular patient.

Second, the advice may be mistaken; that is, if followed by the patient, the advice may be damaging in and of itself. But again, this danger cannot necessarily be avoided by the therapist's silence or inactivity, because failure to give advice may lead to a worse outcome. Rather, the danger can only be mitigated by the therapist's competence in offering but also limiting advice to appropriate matters for the particular patient. Taking a narrow view, Redlich (1986) argues that it is an abuse of power to exert influence on "activities about which patients ought to decide on their own" (p. 638). Yet the application of this admonition is uncertain in supportive therapy when a patient's decision-making capacity is impaired, for a patient's inability to give informed consent cuts both ways. As Redlich argues, it follows that the patient must be protected from a therapist's abuse of power; we argue that it also follows that she must be protected from damage caused by exercising her own powers, such as the power to destroy herself or damage her psychological health. Therapists should not respond to such calls for assistance with a deaf ear.

Third, the therapist's advice or opinions may be beneficial to the patient yet override some of the patient's values and change the patient's behavior. This effect is sometimes unavoidable but not necessarily bad. The advice may be valid and the behavioral change desirable *if it serves the interests of the patient*. We shall see this more clearly after discussing the next two guidelines.

Again, we would like to remind the reader that therapists, regardless of the type of therapy they practice, should always ask themselves, "Is this advice in the patient's interest or solely in mine?" We shall discuss this concern in greater detail later in this chapter.

Permissive Guideline 3: Treatment Goals Are Not Value-Free

Example

> After a month in community placement, a patient is criticized by her group home supervisor for failure to perform her chores. Angered and distraught, she approaches her therapist with the request that she be readmitted to the hospital. The therapist notes that living Independently has been a major goal of treatment. He urges that the patient make a stronger effort to work things out in the community and refuses admission.

As David Mechanic (1981) has pointed out, our current conceptions of mental health treatment are as much an ideology as previous conceptions. Even today's general goals of deinstitutionalization, maximum independence, and home treatment of chronic psychiatric patients create pressures to keep patients in the community and refuse them hospitalization. The therapist is influenced by these pressures in the very development of the treatment plan with the patient, even if it should seem that the patient has agreed to it.

Permissive Guideline 4: Treatment Goals May Override the Immediate Wishes of the Patient

Examples

> A patient asks for a 2-month supply of medication so he can go on an extended cross-country trip. The medicator feels that the patient will not reliably or safely

take medication for such an extended period of time and discusses this concern with the patient. The patient agrees to shorten his proposed trip and to call in periodically to the therapist.

Another patient in supportive psychotherapy, who receives depot medication every 2 weeks, has a habit of using his whole Social Security payment on hard liquor and other frivolous expenditures within a day or two of receiving his monthly check. The therapist and the patient's guardian agree to the checks coming to the clinic and the patient's being given a fourth of the funds at each weekly clinic appointment. The patient objects to this "totalitarian" approach, but the therapist insists on it to achieve better treatment adherence and ensure "better" expenditure of the patient's money.

For therapeutic reasons, therapists often oppose the immediate desires or plans of their patients. They cannot be indifferent to a patient's adherence to the treatment plan or to a patient's choice of destructive instead of constructive behaviors. These problems are particularly evident in supportive therapy involving patients with impaired judgment. At the extreme, when the patient is legally incompetent to make treatment decisions, the treatment team, or in some cases the courts, must do so.

In general, a therapist must allow the patient maximum autonomy to make treatment and life decisions. Nevertheless, benevolent direction may be in the patient's long-term interests. This may involve overriding the patient's immediate impulses and asking the patient to delay his current decisions. The comparison between models of autonomy and benevolence was elucidated by Beauchamp and McCullough (1984), who argued that neither principle is primary and that each may have an independent claim when ethical decisions are being made. In later elaborations from Beauchamp and Childress (2013), an ethical philosophy called *principlism* is developed that is also meant to reflect the belief that there actually is such a thing as a common morality of human beings. These principles are

> 1) *respect for autonomy* (a norm of respecting and supporting autonomous decisions), 2) *nonmaleficence* (a norm of avoiding the causation of harm), 3) *beneficence* (a group of norms pertaining to relieving, lessening, or preventing harm and providing benefits and balancing benefits against risks and costs), and 4) *justice* (a group of norms for fairly distributing benefits, risks and costs). (Beauchamp and Childress 2013, p. 18)

The origin of principlism actually dates back to a document called the Belmont Report produced by the National Commission for the Protection of Human Subjects of Biomedical and Behavioral Research (Bulger 2018). Although it might seem to outsiders that developments in ethics proceed at a glacial speed, there has been a substantial evolution in the concept of patient autonomy just within the past few decades (Kilbride and Joffe 2018). Additions to principlism have also been proposed, such as a mutuality principle: "Act to establish the mutual enhancement of all basic moral values" (DeMarco 2004).

Moreover, despite recent attempts to conceptualize the physician-patient relationship as a neutral provider interacting with an informed consumer, "psychiatrists know if philosophers do not that patients often are not reliable advocates of their own best interests" (Sider 1984, p. 393). Therefore, therapeutic influence retains its validity for patients who have complete autonomy if they have freely entered into a contractual agreement with the therapist to change their behavior. If so, in effect, they have given their consent to be influenced.

A paradoxical picture emerges of a therapist who is more powerful in some ways and less powerful in other ways than a friend. But the therapist must exercise some powers more than a friend ever could and others less so. This is because the therapist, on the one hand, has certain covert powers and sources of influence but, on the other hand, maintains a more limited relationship. For example, a friend of the patient may employ the relationship solely for self-gratification. But even the most friendly therapeutic relationship cannot be an actual friendship. The therapist must limit her use of influence to that which serves the interests of the patient and his treatment. Friendship follows a different set of rules: friends are able to impose their advice or opinions, and they are allowed to gratify their personal needs through the friendship.

The patient's right to be psychotic or different is not the issue here. The issue concerns the use of the therapist's influence to achieve the treatment plan, of which some of the goals may not be fully appreciated by the patient. As Webb (1988) observes, "[T]he psychiatric patient is seldom in a position to be an enlightened consumer who can really evaluate in a rational manner all aspects of a treatment contract" (p. 1089). For example, resolution of a manic state may involve the loss of satisfactions that, if asked about directly, a patient would not want to give up.

Permissive Guideline 5: Incidental Gratifications of the Therapist Are Not Always Unethical

Example

During the holiday season, the therapist's office manager does accept gifts of candies and treats from patients. A patient brings in a gift of candies on a serving tray. Once the candies are gone, the therapist is left with the serving tray, which she realizes is an expensive handmade item. She feels guilty and even tricked into having accepted this expensive item that, depending on its value, might violate the office's gift policy. She wonders if she should discuss this with the patient, offer it back to the patient, write a thank-you note for it, or give it to the office manager so as not to get a "gratification" out of the gift.

Therapists are paid for their work, and therapy is often an emotionally gratifying activity. The desire to help and change a patient is both altruistic and rewarding. When it fails to be the latter, professional burnout results. In supportive therapy, in which the helping role and real relationship to the patient may be significant, the therapist may become concerned that there is something wrong per se in having such a relationship. We have previously discussed gifts (see Chapter 5) and have ourselves recommended that therapists accept gifts from patients under certain circumstances. Looking back on those reasons, we see that they involve the acceptance of the gift as being of therapeutic benefit to the patient. More substantial gratifications, however, even if germane to a treatment plan, must be avoided on other principles, because they generate the appearance of corruption, which is inimical to the therapist's role as model for the patient. Sometimes one can meet ethical problems by directing substantial gifts to a neutral source, such as a patient fund or charity, but therapists in the public sector will first need to be sure that the laws allow such a transaction. Therapists in public or correctional settings may not be allowed to accept anything resembling a gift whatsoever. However, patients often offer items such as artwork or a drawing they made as a gift. We find that such items can be appreciated and returned, or, if the patient desires, placed in the appropriate section of the chart as with other external items and correspondence. Also see the posting by Newsome (2015) for a detailed account of a therapist who eventually (with advice from her professional ethics board) accepted an expensive gift from her patient.

Permissive Guideline 6: Supportive Psychotherapists May Ethically Be Advocates for Their Patients

Example

A patient tells his therapist, "I asked for a case manager, and they wouldn't give me one. Can you do something about that?" The therapist, who does believe that the patient's clinical situation meets the criteria for case management, picks up the phone to call the case management department.

This is not a "trick" example but a straightforward extension of what we have said about therapists linking to outside resources and serving as advocates for their patients. As discussed in Chapter 15, therapists may even be called upon to serve some case management functions themselves. This is not always desirable, but it is not wrong to make a phone call to obtain services for a patient. Or perhaps this may include calling the supported employment counselor to facilitate getting the patient a job. Later, under Limiting Guideline 6, we do discuss a counterpoint to this permissive guideline.

Permissive Guideline 7: The Therapist May Utilize the Patient's Own Beliefs In Treatment and Recovery From Mental Illness

Example

A patient from Nigeria is awaiting outcome of his asylum application. After several months of being a "model client" with no problems, he seems to have gone into an acutely manic state, with pressured speech, lack of sleep, and grandiose delusions. He thinks that the president of Nigeria is trying to contact him, and demands that the therapist call Nigeria to verify the contact and so forth. Reluctantly, the patient starts therapy including Western medication, but he requests that his family be allowed to send him traditional Nigerian medicines from home to supplement his treatment. The therapist is not a great "believer" in traditional medicines but decides to research the matter and discovers that traditional Nigerian medicines include a great number of treatments, several of which are alkaloid compounds that are undergoing research as antipsychotics. The therapist makes recommendations to the patient about which medicine might work best with Western treatments. The family is allowed to send the medicines to the patient, but the institution will not release the medicines until the patient leaves the institution. However, the patient agrees to continue the Western treatments until he is discharged.

We do not think many therapists would doubt that they have utilized and should utilize their patients' own beliefs to improve adherence to treatment, even when the therapist is not quite sure of the validity of the beliefs. However, the therapist in this vignette felt obliged to do some research and at least entertain the possibility that the traditional treatments would do his patient some good after he left the hospital. Of course, whoever "inherits" the outpatient therapy might still have to overcome the patient's objections to Western medicines. So the inpatient therapist might have saddled the outpatient therapist or clinic with a new problem. But we think this is just an example of the adage that "you do what you have to do when you have to do it." Inpatient care involves patients with impaired decision-making skills, and therapists need to invoke whatever powers they are comfortable with. So we say: Utilize your patients' beliefs when you need to. And argue to change them when you *have* to.

Seven Limiting Guidelines

While exercising a powerful and supportive role in shaping the patient's treatment, the therapist must constantly scrutinize the ongoing process and utilize or allow operation of additional checks and balances. We shall present the latter as a set of limiting guidelines that provide a counterpoint to the permissive ones.

Limiting Guideline 1:
The Patient's Autonomy Must Be Maximized

Example

Working with the hypomanic patient mentioned in the first permissive guideline, the physician provides the patient with information about the patient's illness and the uses and side effects of lithium carbonate and involves the patient in a support group. The physician shows willingness to openly discuss the patient's reactions to treatment, such as the feelings of chronic dependency that are created in treatment and the yearning to be "hyper" at times; the apparent effectiveness of the treatment so far; and the risks and benefits of alternative treatments.

The therapeutic use of authority can be likened to the orthopedist's use of a cast in treating a broken leg. The goal of casting is to restore the leg to proper function, and it is detrimental to that purpose to leave the cast on too long or to make it too tight (Mendel 1970). It is important to have clearly defined treatment goals that are periodically revised with the patient, but such revisions would be a sham unless the therapist made a concerted effort to help the patient become an active and involved partner in the treatment process. For this reason, we included in our definition of *supportive psychotherapy* in Chapter 1 the ongoing goal of maximizing the patient's treatment autonomy. A therapist who does that has gone a long way toward preventing undue dependency on therapeutic influence. Goldberg (1977) has also described a "therapeutic partnership," which is an explicit spelling out of what we would call the *working-alliance* aspects of the relationship.

It follows from this guideline that when it is difficult to specify the reason for an intervention, the therapist should generally refrain from the intervention. When the patient and therapist are opposed on an issue and a third party is needed, the therapist might seek consultation from another therapist or even a patient advocate office. In the community mental health setting, ethical consultations are most often obtained through clinical supervision, a process that may be less than ideal because neither supervisory time nor expertise may be sufficient; it may be more desirable to bring such problems before an ethics advisory and education committee (Handelsman 1989). If it is not possible to obtain consultation within the therapist's own agency, he can seek assistance from the ethics committee of his local professional organization. The Ethics Committee of the American Psychiatric Association also renders individual opinions to members regarding actual or hypothetical ethical violations; however, only a fraction of these are disseminated (American Psychiatric Association 1989a).

The availability of other mental health personnel as "auxiliary therapists" or of other negotiators such as patient advocates also helps to redress actual misuses of power and to provide the patient with the security that he can trust the therapist, because such mechanisms are available if needed. For example, patients who enter therapy often inquire if a therapist is a member of a relevant professional association so as to be reassured that the therapist is bound by the relevant code of ethics.

Limiting Guideline 2:
Some Treatment Goals Are Not Allowable

Example

A therapist tells a biologically male patient, who is thinking of becoming a transgender female, that "it is really not worth getting into that process. Let's work on maintaining your male gender identity."

Perhaps you assumed that we were suggesting the preceding as a recommended therapist behavior. But we were not. Our cultural values have changed (some would say, too rapidly) over the past few years. "Until the middle of the twentieth century, with rare exceptions, transgender presentations were usually classified as psychopathological" (Drescher 2015, p. 182). If this patient has distress about his gender identity, then there could be a therapeutic issue and a diagnosis of gender dysphoria. In the above example (although it is intentionally simplified and does not supply the details), it is likely that the therapist has made a value judgment on transgender identification for his patient and instead of treating a recognized mental disorder, the therapist has imposed his own values on the patient.

However, does it depend on the details? What is the age of the patient? Consider that "while most transgender children will outgrow their gender dysphoria (desisters) and grow up to be gay, lesbian, or bisexual, the minority do not (persisters) and develop into transgender adults" (Drescher 2015, p. 188). So on the assumption that the patient is an adult, should the therapist be "even-minded" about the possibility of changing genders? Would the negative advice ("It is really not worth getting into that process") be more appropriate if the patient were 13 years old? Or does that still impose the therapist's value system?

The existence of a mental disorder is one factor that can be used to justify therapeutic interventions, yet it is not the sine qua non of treatment, and many goals can be specified in treatment that are not related to the cure of a mental disorder. For example, almost any sort of dysfunctional behavior may be targeted for change, leaving the therapist to debate exactly what is "dysfunctional" and by whose standards it is dysfunctional. Indeed, there is no easy answer to such determinations. The determination of which goals are allowable involves an interplay of values ascribed to the patient and to society as a whole. For example, illegal activity *ought* not be counseled by an ethical therapist, and such activity also violates other principles of the ethical code. On the other hand, one can treat criminals (e.g., for depression) without demanding that they change their occupation, unless the occupation is clearly pertinent to their psychopathology.

In addition to being influenced by our concepts of disease and the considerations of legality, should advice-giving and behavioral-change strategies be addressed to the patient's stated needs? Not precisely, because as we found earlier, the patient's short-term stated needs may be greatly at variance with her long-term interests. For example, one would be loath to "help" a person who came into therapy to remain submissive to her abusive spouse, or to "teach" the child of an alcoholic parent how to "cover up" the family problem when friends visit.

To summarize, therefore, some treatment goals are not allowable because they impose inappropriate values on the patient. The therapist should be vigilant to avoid imposing her own values on the patient, or an idealized version of what the patient's values "ought" to be.

Limiting Guideline 3:
Patients Retain the Right to Refuse Treatment

Example

A patient who has been a street person is committed for treatment by psychiatrists who feel he has a chronic mental illness. After legal challenge it is decided that the patient is not a danger to others and should be released.

This common scenario in mental health systems varies with changes in social values as reflected in state commitment statutes. Even in cases in which it is clear that the therapist is acting in accordance with legal or medical standards, the patient retains the right to dispute those actions. This provides a balance to the undeniable fact that treatment goals are not value-free and involve elements of behavioral control that may infringe upon the constitutional rights of the patient. For example, giving medication that reduces disorganized or agitated behavior may represent a benevolent intervention to the therapist, but to the patient it may be an imposition and a violation of legal rights that are more important than the medical consequences.

Involuntary treatment standards are a reminder of our earlier point that ethical standards go beyond legal standards. In some places, one can involuntarily treat a homeless psychiatrically ill person who is unable to take care of his needs, and each jurisdiction has standards and procedures on giving treatment involuntarily. Thus, in some places, issues of the involuntariness of treatment are less ethical in nature than in other states because in the former, the law is closer to a typical therapist's values about the importance and usefulness of therapy. Nor should the therapist be shy about providing treatment because it is involuntary, because therapy under involuntary conditions is often successful.

Limiting Guideline 4:
The Need for Honesty in the Treatment Relationship May Override the Immediate Goals of Treatment

Example

A patient has been taking moderate quantities of an omega-3-rich fish oil supplement in the belief that it stabilizes his mood. He asks his prescriber for confirmation that fish oil is a potent drug. The prescriber is familiar with the slightly positive studies on fish oil as a mood stabilizer and says as strongly as he can muster: "It seems to be working for you, so I don't oppose your taking it."

If the therapist wields enough influence to override the patient's immediate wishes, as suggested in the fourth permissive guideline, such authority can be exercised legitimately only in a context of ongoing trust and honesty. This guideline also arises from the social and professional responsibilities of the therapist as a representative of the profession and as an individual model for his patients. It requires, we think, that a therapist usually not lie to a patient even if that would improve the patient's immediate functioning. At the same time, we recognize that support of a patient's denial may sometimes be allowable, such as when fostering adherence to a treatment plan (see Chapter 16). The dividing line may seem fuzzy, but as Eth (1990) observes, deceptions are now viewed as detrimental to the moral autonomy of the patient and to the doctor-patient relationship; despite justified temporizing delays or euphemisms, truthful explanations and options must eventually be forthcoming. Therefore, the "rightness" of the therapist's statement in the example above would seem to rest on what else is said in the session. Does the therapist review the (weak) evidence for use of fish oil as a mood stabilizer? Does the therapist explain how other medications have a stronger basis for recommendation? Or do the therapist and patient move on to other topics?

The therapist must be wary of proposing paradoxical courses of action that are confusing and thus detrimental to the therapist-patient relationship. Such interventions may work in certain situations but damage the patient's autonomy in the long term. Therapists skilled in such interventions, such as Milton Erickson, are perhaps less common than one would like to believe, and one should be cautious when trying to implement such techniques (see, e.g., Haley 1986).

Limiting Guideline 5: To Avoid Ethical Pitfalls, Therapists Must Understand Themselves as Well as Their Patients

Examples

A therapist who has been having a "difficult time" getting a patient to enter a vocational rehabilitation program notices a parallel in his personal life: He has been trying, without success, to get his daughter to go to a professional school. The therapist begins to realize that he has been imposing a program on the patient that may not be in the patient's best interests.

A lawyer with bipolar illness is located in a prominent legal office that sometimes is involved in actions that influence the work of the clinic. Moreover, the therapist enjoys hearing from the patient about the city leaders' conduct. The patient is considering retiring, as he would like to spend his time fully on singing, a life long wish. The therapist finds herself arguing with the patient not to retire.

An "escort" with histrionic personality disorder is thinking of getting married and returning to college. The therapist has enjoyed hearing from her about her sexual activities with prominent local businessmen and finds himself urging her not to change since she "needs" the $500 a night she has been earning.

Readers will probably object that the second two examples are rather blatant examples of therapy being contaminated by poor self-understanding of the therapist. But what about the first? Should the therapist's personal experience with his daughter change or reverse his recommendation to the patient?

We have already mentioned some of the pitfalls in making proper ethical decisions, but we shall discuss them in greater detail now.

Self-gratification is occasionally blatant and totally indefensible. Sometimes it is rationalized and unconscious to the therapist but obvious to everyone else.

We have observed that social values are often contained in or influence the development of psychiatric treatments. However, the therapist may have personal values that are different from the social values inherent in the patient's acceptance of the treatment plan. The danger faced by the patient with impaired autonomy, much greater than that of being brainwashed by social values (although some might call that process "acculturation" rather than brainwashing), is that of being overwhelmed by the imposition of (i.e., *contamination by*) the therapist's personal values or even voyeuristic or prurient interests.

Similarly, *contamination by personal needs* is a formidable danger in supportive work in which the desire to help may lead to projective identification and vicarious gratification from the patient's activities (whether socially desirable or not), paternalistic dominance, sadistic authoritarianism, or simply, as Marmor (1953) emphasizes, an unrealistic feeling of superiority. If one engages in supportive therapy, one ought to know the difference between altruism and moral masochism.

Dual agentry, in which the psychiatrist serves more than one role, is obvious in contexts where the psychiatrist serves a legal function for the court or an administrative role with respect to the patient. The prescriber in an HMO or managed care plan who "comes to believe" that most psychiatric disorders can be treated in brief psychotherapy or in monthly visits should examine both countertransference and cognitive dissonance and try to cleave his clinical judgment from his administrative and cost-containing role. Sometimes the role confusion is more insidious and less self-serving, as when the therapist treats both patient and family and it is no longer clear whose agenda is being furthered by specific interventions. The potential ethical conflicts in choosing between these modes of therapy are discussed by Sider (1984).

Certainly, interventions that serve different roles should be identified as such if the effects of dual agentry are to be minimized. Thus, the HMO prescriber above should present the treatment parameters honestly, without implying that the treatment will be curative. Similarly, therapists in most community mental health settings are saddled with the unshakable responsibility of allocating scarce time and resources to maximize benefits for the entire service population and not a particular patient. Many times, this involves dropping a patient from therapy or rehabilitation in lieu of another who stands to benefit. Such decisions are part of public mental health administration, but they should not be clouded with an illusory therapeutic rationale.

Technical errors do not necessarily represent ethical errors in treatment, but the therapist does have an ethical duty to be competent and avoid practicing types of therapy in which she does not have sufficient training. In the real world, of course, the sources of error are mixed. For example, through a combination of technical error, financial need, or paternalistic countertransference gratifications, the therapist may prolong therapy long after maximal benefits have been gained and even as the patient's dependency worsens (Karasu 1981).

Having previously provided guidelines for the therapist's actions, we now offer a similarly balanced set of guidelines for the therapist's attitudes that could warn of difficulties leading to either ethical abandonment of the patient (failure to make needed interventions; see Table 17–3) or ethical infringement on the patient's life (making interventions that are not needed; see Table 17–4).

Avoiding both abandonment and infringement, we think, requires a knowledge of the patient's values. A good example of this is the area of religion, which appears to be more important to patients than to their psychiatrists. One recent survey indicated that 90% of the general public and a similar percentage of psychiatric inpatients believe in God, but only 40%–70% of psychiatrists express the belief (Kroll and Sheehan 1989). Perhaps a nonreligious therapist may feel that a patient's religious statements are defensive, or the religious therapist may feel that the patient's religious beliefs should be unchallenged. In this regard, one prominent psychiatrist/minister points out the security as well as the danger of "mutual blind spots" when therapist and patient share the same religious views (Grosch 1985).

Unfortunately, psychiatrists often neglect to deal with religious issues when they should (Robinson 1986). Even more broadly, they fail to deal with their patients' questions about values. Such questions come up repeatedly. Moral scrupulosity is a factor in obsessive-compulsive disorder and obsessive-compulsive personality disorder. Religious preoccupation plays an especial role in schizophrenia, paranoia, and mood disorder. In the course of any therapy, the patient with even the most temporary problem will have questions about his or her goodness or badness, morality or immorality or amorality.

What is a therapist to do? The American Psychiatric Association, through its Committee on Religion and Psychiatry, considered this issue for some time and approved a set of guidelines urging psychiatrists to become knowledgeable about the religious or ideological orientations of their patients and to treat such beliefs with respect (American Psychiatric Association 1990). Various articles (see, e.g., Whitley and Jarvis 2015) provide more detail on taking spiritual assessments and interacting with patients on those topics.

Recent changes in conception of the doctor-patient relationship from an unequal authoritarian one to a negotiated egalitarian one reflect concomitant

Table 17–3. Attitudes that may lead to ethical abandonment

Experiencing a loss of empathy for the patient's position and needs

Trading one's role as therapist for the role of patient rights advocate

Assuming that all legally competent patients have equal decision-making capacities

Believing that suffering from one's mistakes is the only source of personal growth

Being fearful of exercising the awesome responsibility of giving medical or therapeutic advice that may be wrong or lead to a bad outcome

Equating the treatment negotiation process with one-sided behavioral control

changes in social attitudes toward physicians and medical practice itself. Despite this evolution, both overt and covert aspects of the therapist's influence, such as the powers in Raven's taxonomy (see the first permissive guideline discussed earlier) or the relationship elements discerned by Jerome Frank (see Chapter 2), must continue to operate if therapy is to be effective. It might even be argued that it is sometimes necessary to "mislead" the patient and promise more than one can deliver in order to deliver anything at all. For example, we know that placebo effects, nonspecific effects, and unconscious fantasies play a role in cure, as well as the more familiar transferential relationship. However, it should be clear by now that we believe that the sustenance provided by the real relationship in supportive therapy is more than a mirage from which the patient will never drink. Rather, it is a professional but genuine relationship providing understanding, support, hope, and benevolent direction in the patient's own interests.

Limiting Guideline 6:
Without Careful Scrutiny, the Advocacy Role Can Unethically Expand Into a Role That Exceeds the Therapist's Evidence-Based Standards of Treatment

Example

The therapist for an asylum-seeking person prepares an evaluation advocating that the patient be granted asylum based on the current legal standards for asylum (i.e., Refugee Act of 1980).

This example raises some obvious problems but also some more subtle ones; a spirited interchange of an article and letter brought this to our attention (Lustig

Table 17–4.   Attitudes that may lead to ethical infringement

Neglecting to find out the patient's values

Lacking respect for the patient as an individual locus of moral action whose autonomy must be maximized

Giving advice on matters when the outcome does not matter

Taking a "zero tolerance" approach to the patient's mistakes

Equating "successful patient" with "patient who agrees with the therapist"

Confusing the concepts of adherence and dependence in patients

Discovering a significant satisfaction when the patient is "disobedient" and gets hurt

2007; Morgan 2007). Asylum seekers often present stories of torture and abuse leading to a diagnosis of posttraumatic stress disorder (PTSD). However, there are no objective methods for validating a reported history of abuse, and in fact no good methods for validating the subjective symptoms of PTSD. While a therapist may feel comfortable treating the stress of a subjective psychological condition as reported by the patient, she may easily exceed her treatment role in becoming an advocate since the latter role may assume the truth of a history that is malingered, with the obviously high stakes of winning or losing legal proceedings. Expert witnesses may find themselves in such territory, but "ordinary" treating therapists should not. Most forensic standards therefore recommend separation of treatment and forensic roles for that reason.

Although this example is about asylum seekers, what about the example of a therapist advocating for case management (see example in Permissive Guideline 6)? What if the patient's situation is "at the borderline" between meeting the criteria for case management or not? Should the therapist still pick up the phone and advocate for the patient? What if the patient is an inmate seeking early release who, in the therapist's opinion, does "not really" meet the criteria? Should the therapist be a "good guy" and advocate for the early release? What if the inmate can and has made implicit threats to the therapist if he does not release him? If you have not already, you will have many instances of the "advocacy" problem in your life. Learning when to properly advocate and when not will depend on whether you can justify the advocacy based on your beliefs about the objective findings in your treatment.

Limiting Guideline 7: Cultural Sensitivity Must Be Balanced by the Relevance of Universal Principles of Equal Rights and Respect for the Dignity of Human Beings

Cultures are constantly evolving, as are individuals. And we believe that there are certain universal principles that cannot be overridden even by the most coherent and all-embracing culture. Some of the issues that have been in the forefront in the past 20 years are racism; sexism; genocide; murders of individuals who do not conform to their culture (e.g., homosexuals); genital mutilation; abuse of women, children, and the elderly; mistreatment of the poor, handicapped, or mentally ill; discrimination against immigrants; and segregation of the mentally ill in prisons. When therapists encounter such issues, we feel that they cannot agree completely with their patients and may want to tell their patients that they disagree with them. At least this can lead to a discussion of the differences between the patient's culture and the therapist's own. It may also lead to a disruption or termination of therapy. But as important as it is to be a successful therapist, we think it is also important to be a moral therapist.

Keying on that last concept, there can be found an argument that a therapist should cultivate qualities that are more than merely clinical skills and constitute moral virtues. The formulation of Radden and Sadler (Radden 2014; Radden and Sadler 2010) identifies 17 virtues for psychiatric practice: trustworthiness, empathy, self-knowledge, restraint, gender sensitivity, patience, imagination, fairness, integrity, propriety, *phronesis* (an ancient Greek word for a kind of practical wisdom or intelligence), groundedness, tact, compassion, caring, unselfing, and hopefulness. Perhaps we should rephrase our first sentence, as Radden notes, "A tenet of professional ethics is that clinical skills may be virtues as well"—that is, you are not going into a new moral realm when you practice your clinical skills, but rather your clinical skills comprise the virtues of your profession.

To conclude this chapter, we thought we would take just one of Radden's named virtues and elaborate on it. As we have said earlier about ethics, the literature on this subject is voluminous, so we just want to make a few points we think are particularly important for supportive psychotherapists to know.

Women's Issues

Despite the popular belief of laypersons and mental health professionals, women's issues were not attended to and resolved in the 1970s and 1980s. Numerous stressors remain today for women and girls that will need to be addressed by therapists, including violence, discrimination, limited economic resources, and unrealistic media images. Today, gender bias is still observed; however, it is usually covert (American Psychological Association 2007).

The collaboration with other health providers, family members, and outside agencies such as Child Protective Services and the court system with the care of female patients is compulsory and may be overwhelming. The therapist will be required to maintain confidentiality within legal and regulatory parameters, serve as an advocate to protect the patient's rights, and contribute to the resolving of ethical issues (American Nurses Association 2014; American Psychological Association 2017).

Generally, debates relating to the ethics of the care of the mentally ill center on a patient's rights and determining when the limiting of these rights is warranted. Such limitations of rights could occur to protect the patient or others from harm. As noted above, women's issues are numerous. So we will limit the present discussion to the ethical issues related to clinicians and their pregnant patients. Providers face ethical dilemmas when treating pregnant women with serious mental illnesses. Treatment and nontreatment will both pose risks, and if the mother cannot make decisions because of impaired capacity, the situation will be very challenging. The clinician will be required to adhere to privacy of the patient whose decision-making capacity is impaired and to protect the rights of the fetus (Desai and Chandra 2009).

Given deinstitutionalization, and with newer antipsychotic medications that do not reduce fertility, it is no longer a rare occurrence for women with serious mental illness to become pregnant (Oyserman et al. 2000). Many clinicians fear that women who did well during their pregnancies may become very psychotic after the baby is born. The murder of five children by their mother, Andrea Yates, is a classic example of the need for clinicians to understand culture, traditions, religious beliefs, and other information crucial to specific family interactions. A core value in the health care setting is respect for patient privacy. The functional approach to the ethics of balancing rights, benefits, and harms is that child safety will dominate all other values (Seeman 2004).

Conclusion

As we began this chapter, we end it (and this book) with advice to therapists to conduct therapy in an ethical and culturally sensitive manner. A response to this might very well be, "Of course, shouldn't all therapists, and all professionals for that matter, be advised to be ethical and culturally sensitive?" We agree, but in proposing this type of psychotherapy, namely supportive psychotherapy, we take on an added responsibility of being more directive than some of the older, so-called value-free modes of psychotherapy. And so it is that ethical and cultural sensitivity are even more important here.

There is no way we could teach this in one chapter, one book, or any number of books. Like most life skills, these sensitivities require experience in doing therapy, learning from patients and colleagues, and personal qualities that some therapists acquire more easily than others. Frankly, there are some therapists with a lifetime of experience who are (in our humble opinion) bad therapists both technically and ethically. And there are some therapists even at the beginning of their careers who seem to have an uncanny ability to be effective and sensitive with their patients, and to learn from each hour of their successes and failures in doing therapy. But having written this book, we do hope that we have helped some of our readers to become better therapists as well as more sensitive to the cultural issues and human values inherent in working with people's intimate wishes and needs.

References

American Medical Association: Current Opinions of the Council on Ethical and Judicial Affairs. Chicago, IL, American Medical Association, 1989; see subsequent editions at www.ama-assn.org

American Nurses Association: Psychiatric Mental Health Nursing: Scope and Standards of Practice, 2nd Edition. Silver Spring, MD, American Nurses Association, 2014

American Psychiatric Association: The Opinions of the Ethics Committee on the Principles of Medical Ethics. Washington, DC, American Psychiatric Press, 1989a; see subsequent editions at www.psych.org

American Psychiatric Association: The Principles of Medical Ethics With Annotations Especially Applicable to Psychiatry. Washington, DC, American Psychiatric Press, 1989b; see subsequent editions at www.psych.org

American Psychiatric Association: Guidelines regarding possible conflict between psychiatrists' religious commitments and psychiatric practice. Am J Psychiatry 147:542, 1990 11642759

American Psychiatric Association: Diagnostic and Statistical Manual of Mental Disorders, 5th Edition. Arlington, VA, American Psychiatric Association, 2013

American Psychological Association: Guidelines for psychological practice with girls and women. Am Psychol 62(9):949–979, 2007 18085843

American Psychological Association: Ethical principles of psychologists and code of conduct. January 1, 2017. Available at: https://www.apa.org/ethics/code/ethics-code-2017.pdf. Accessed February 28, 2019.

Beauchamp TL, Childress JE: Principles of Biomedical Ethics, 7th Edition. New York, Oxford University Press, 2013

Beauchamp TL, McCullough LB: Medical Ethics: The Moral Responsibilities of Physicians. Englewood Cliffs, NJ, Prentice Hall, 1984

Brotherton S, Kao A, Crigger BJ: Professing the values of medicine: the modernized AMA Code of Medical Ethics. JAMA 316(10):1041–1042, 2016 27415447

Bucky SF, Callan JE, Stricker G (eds): Ethical and Legal Issues for Mental Health Professionals: A Comprehensive Handbook of Principles and Standards. Binghamton, NY, The Haworth Maltreatment and Trauma Press, 2005

Bulger JW: Principlism. Available at: www.uvu.edu/ethics/seac/Bulger-Principlism.pdf. Accessed May 20, 2018.

DeMarco JP: Principlism and moral dilemmas: a new principle. J Med Ethics 31:101–105, 2004

Desai G, Chandra PS: Ethical issues in treating pregnant women with severe mental illness. Indian J Med Ethics 6(2):75–77, 2009 19517649

DeSilva R, Aggarwal NK, Lewis-Fernandez R: The DSM-5 cultural formulation interview and the evolution of cultural assessment in psychiatry. Psychiatr Times 32(6):9–13, 2015

Drescher J: Ethical issues in treating LGBT patients, in The Oxford Handbook of Psychiatric Ethics, Vol 1. Edited by Sadler JZ, Van Staden W, Fulford KWM. New York, Oxford University Press, 2015, pp 180–192

Eth S: Psychiatric ethics: entering the 1990s. Hosp Community Psychiatry 41(4):384–386, 1990 2185146

Fiscella K, Frankel R: Overcoming cultural barriers: international medical graduates in the United States. JAMA 283(13):1751, 2000 10755508

Goldberg C: Therapeutic Partnership: Ethical Concerns in Psychotherapy. New York, Springer, 1977

Grosch WN: The psychotherapist and religious commitment, in Psychotherapy and the Religiously Committed Patient. Edited by Stern EM. New York, Haworth, 1985, pp 123–127

Haley J: Uncommon Therapy: The Psychiatric Techniques of Milton H. Erickson, M.D. New York, WW Norton, 1986

Handelsman MM: Ethics training at mental health centers. Community Ment Health J 25(1):42–50, 1989 2721138

Karasu T: Ethical aspects of psychotherapy, in Psychiatric Ethics. Edited by Bloch S, Chodoff P. New York, Oxford University Press, 1981, pp 89–116

Kilbride MK, Joffe S: The new age of patient autonomy: implications for the patient-physician relationship. JAMA 320(19):1973–1974, 2018 30326026

Kroll J, Sheehan W: Religious beliefs and practices among 52 psychiatric inpatients in Minnesota. Am J Psychiatry 146(1):67–72, 1989 2912252

Lustig SL: Psychiatric evaluations of asylum seekers: it's both ethical practice and advocacy, and that's OK! (letter). Psychiatry (Edgmont Pa) 4(6):17–18, 2007 20711331

Marmor J: The feeling of superiority: an occupational hazard in the practice of psychotherapy. Am J Psychiatry 110(5):370–376, 1953 13104678

Mechanic D: The social dimension, in Psychiatric Ethics. Edited by Bloch S, Chodoff P. New York, Oxford University Press, 1981, pp 46–60

Mendel WM: Authority: its nature and use in the therapeutic relationship. Hosp Community Psychiatry 21(11):367–370, 1970 5475149

Morgan C: Psychiatric evaluations of asylum seekers: is it ethical practice or advocacy? Psychiatry (Edgmont) 4(4):26–33, 2007 20711325

Musto D: A historical perspective, in Psychiatric Ethics. Edited by Bloch S, Chodoff P. New York, Oxford University Press, 1981, pp 13–30

Newsome J: An ethical dilemma: when therapy clients accept gifts. Reconciling boundaries with the therapeutic alliance. Psychology Networker 2015. Available at: https://www.psychotherapynetworker.org/blog/details/517/an-ethical-dilemma-when-therapy-clients-give-gifts. Accessed May 4, 2019.

Novalis PN: What supports supportive therapy? Jefferson Journal of Psychiatry 7(2):17–29, 1989

Oyserman D, Mowbray CT, Meares PA, et al: Parenting among mothers with a serious mental illness. Am J Orthopsychiatry 70(3):296–315, 2000 10953777

Radden JH: Ethics and virtues in clinical psychiatry. Psychiatr Times 31(3):23–24, 2014

Radden JH, Sadler J: The Virtuous Psychiatrist: Character Ethics in Psychiatric Practice. Oxford, UK, Oxford University Press, 2010

Raven BH: A taxonomy of power in human relations. Psychiatr Ann 16:633–636, 1986

Redlich FC: The use and abuse of power in psychotherapy. Psychiatr Ann 16:637–639, 1986

Robinson LH: Therapist-clergy collaboration, in Psychiatry and Religion: Overlapping Concerns. Washington, DC, American Psychiatric Press, 1986, pp 21–31

Seeman MV: Relational ethics: when mothers suffer from psychosis. Arch Women Ment Health 7(3):201–210, 2004 15241666

Sider RC: The ethics of therapeutic modality choice. Am J Psychiatry 141(3):390–394, 1984 6703104

Webb WL Jr: Ethics and psychiatry, in The American Psychiatric Press Textbook of Psychiatry. Edited by Talbott JA, Hales RE, Yudofsky SC. Washington, DC, American Psychiatric Press, 1988, pp 1085–1096

White TM, Gibbons MBC, Schamberger M: Cultural sensitivity and supportive expressive psychotherapy: an integrative approach to treatment. Am J Psychother 60(3):299–316, 2006 17066760

Whitley R, Jarvis GE: Religious understanding as cultural competence: issues for clinicians. Psychiatr Times 32(6):13–16, 2015

Index

Page numbers printed in **boldface** type refer to tables.